# PHYTOCHEMICALS AND MEDICINAL PLANTS IN FOOD DESIGN

### Strategies and Technologies for Improved Healthcare

# PHYTOCHEMICALS AND MEDICINAL PLANTS IN FOOD DESIGN

## Strategies and Technologies for Improved Healthcare

*Edited by*

**Megh R. Goyal, PhD, P.E.**
**Preeti Birwal, PhD**
**Santosh K. Mishra, PhD**

**AAP** APPLE ACADEMIC PRESS

First edition published 2022

**Apple Academic Press Inc.**
1265 Goldenrod Circle, NE,
Palm Bay, FL 32905 USA
4164 Lakeshore Road, Burlington,
ON, L7L 1A4 Canada

**CRC Press**
6000 Broken Sound Parkway NW,
Suite 300, Boca Raton, FL 33487-2742 USA
2 Park Square, Milton Park,
Abingdon, Oxon, OX14 4RN UK

© 2022 Apple Academic Press, Inc.

*Apple Academic Press exclusively co-publishes with CRC Press, an imprint of Taylor & Francis Group, LLC*

**Library and Archives Canada Cataloguing in Publication**

Title: Phytochemicals and medicinal plants in food design : strategies and technologies for improved healthcare / edited by Megh R. Goyal, PhD, P.E., Preeti Birwal, PhD, Santosh K. Mishra, PhD.

Names: Goyal, Megh R., editor. | Birwal, Preeti, editor. | Mishra, Santosh K., editor.

Series: Innovations in Agricultural and Biological Engineering.

Description: First edition. | Series statement: Innovations in Agricultural and Biological Engineering | Includes bibliographical references and index.

Identifiers: Canadiana (print) 20210344245 | Canadiana (ebook) 20210344288 | ISBN 9781771889940 (hardcover) | ISBN 9781774639450 (softcover) | ISBN 9781003150336 (ebook)

Subjects: LCSH: Phytochemicals—Therapeutic use. | LCSH: Medicinal plants. | LCSH: Herbs—Therapeutic use.

Classification: LCC QK861 .P598 2022 | DDC 615.3/21—dc23

**Library of Congress Cataloging-in-Publication Data**

Names: Goyal, Megh R., editor. | Birwal, Preeti, editor. | Mishra, Santosh K., editor.

Title: Phytochemicals and medicinal plants in food design : strategies and technologies for improved healthcare / Megh R. Goyal, Preeti Birwal, Santosh K. Mishra.

Other titles: Innovations in Agricultural and Biological Engineering.

Description: 1st edition. | Palm Bay : Apple Academic Press, [2022] | Series: Innovations in Agricultural and Biological Engineering | Includes bibliographical references and index. | Summary: "Phytochemicals and Medicinal Plants in Food Design: Strategies and Technologies for Improved Healthcare explores the therapeutic potential of various natural and novel phytochemicals in the design of new foods. Divided into two parts, the first section discusses plant-based secondary metabolites for healthcare, focusing on the health aspects of herbs and medicinal plants and nutraceuticals for livestock production and for the treatment of diseases such as HIV and diabetes. The authors also address the benefits of preserving indigenous knowledge of medicinal plants and current consumer views of health issues from foods. The second part delves into the design and utilization of healthy foods. This section discusses the application of novel designs and herbal formulations in conjunction with other biomolecules for the development and utilization for food products with health benefits. Key features: Encourages the preservation of indigenous knowledge on herbs and medicinal plants Explains the health-promoting effects of some herbs and medicinal plants Discusses the therapeutics and their mechanisms of actions of the biological compounds for food safety This informative volume will be valuable for faculty, students, scientists, researchers, and industry professionals in the development of superfoods from phytochemicals and medicinal plants"-- Provided by publisher.

Identifiers: LCCN 2021050670 (print) | LCCN 2021050671 (ebook) | ISBN 9781771889940 (hardback) | ISBN 9781774639450 (paperback) | ISBN 9781003150336 (ebook)

Subjects: LCSH: Medicinal plants. | Phytochemicals. | Herbs--Therapeutic use.

Classification: LCC RS164 .P5339 2022 (print) | LCC RS164 (ebook) | DDC 615.3/21--dc23/eng/20211108

LC record available at https://lccn.loc.gov/2021050670

LC ebook record available at https://lccn.loc.gov/2021050671

ISBN: 978-1-77188-994-0 (hbk)
ISBN: 978-1-77463-945-0 (pbk)
ISBN: 978-1-00315-033-6 (ebk)

# ABOUT THE BOOK SERIES: INNOVATIONS IN AGRICULTURAL AND BIOLOGICAL ENGINEERING

Under this book series, Apple Academic Press Inc. is publishing book volumes over a span of 8–10 years in the specialty areas defined by the American Society of Agricultural and Biological Engineers (<asabe.org>). Apple Academic Press Inc. aims to be a principal source of books in agricultural and biological engineering. We welcome book proposals from readers in areas of their expertise.

The mission of this series is to provide knowledge and techniques for agricultural and biological engineers (ABEs). The book series offers high-quality reference and academic content on ABE that is accessible to academicians, researchers, scientists, university faculty and university-level students, and professionals around the world.

Agricultural and biological engineers ensure that the world has the necessities of life, including safe and plentiful food, clean air and water, renewable fuel and energy, safe working conditions, and a healthy environment by employing knowledge and expertise of the sciences, both pure and applied, and engineering principles. Biological engineering applies engineering practices to problems and opportunities presented by living things and the natural environment in agriculture.

ABE embraces a variety of the following specialty areas (<asabe.org>): aquaculture engineering, biological engineering, energy, farm machinery and power engineering, food and process engineering, forest engineering, information and electrical technologies, soil and water conservation engineering, natural resources engineering, nursery and greenhouse engineering, safety and health, and structures and environment.

For this book series, we welcome chapters on the following specialty areas (but not limited to):

1. Academia to industry to end-user loop in agricultural engineering
2. Agricultural mechanization
3. Aquaculture engineering
4. Biological engineering in agriculture
5. Biotechnology applications in agricultural engineering

6.  Energy source engineering
7.  Food and bioprocess engineering
8.  Forest engineering
9.  Hill land agriculture
10. Human factors in engineering
11. Information and electrical technologies
12. Irrigation and drainage engineering
13. Nanotechnology applications in agricultural engineering
14. Natural resources engineering
15. Nursery and greenhouse engineering
16. Potential of phytochemicals from agricultural and wild plants for human health
17. Power systems and machinery design
18. GPS and remote sensing potential in agricultural engineering
19. Robot engineering and drones in agriculture
20. Simulation and computer modeling
21. Smart engineering applications in agriculture
22. Soil and water engineering
23. Micro irrigation engineering
24. Structures and environment engineering
25. Waste management and recycling
26. Rural electrification.
27. Sanitary engineering
28. Farm to fork technologies in agriculture
29. Impact of global warming and climatic change on agriculture economy
30. Any other focus areas

For more information on this series, readers may contact:

Megh R. Goyal, PhD, PE
Book Series Senior Editor-in-Chief:
Innovations in Agricultural and Biological Engineering
E-mail: goyalmegh@gmail.com

# OTHER BOOKS ON AGRICULTURAL & BIOLOGICAL ENGINEERING BY APPLE ACADEMIC PRESS, INC.

Management of Drip/Trickle or Micro Irrigation
Megh R. Goyal, PhD, PE, Senior Editor-in-Chief

Evapotranspiration: Principles and Applications for Water Management
Megh R. Goyal, PhD, PE and Eric W. Harmsen, Editors

**Book Series: RESEARCH ADVANCES IN SUSTAINABLE MICRO IRRIGATION**
**Senior Editor-in-Chief: Megh R. Goyal, PhD, PE**
Volume 1: Sustainable Micro Irrigation: Principles and Practices
Volume 2: Sustainable Practices in Surface and Subsurface Micro Irrigation
Volume 3: Sustainable Micro Irrigation Management for Trees and Vines
Volume 4: Management, Performance, and Applications of Micro Irrigation Systems
Volume 5: Applications of Furrow and Micro Irrigation in Arid and Semi-Arid Regions
Volume 6: Best Management Practices for Drip Irrigated Crops
Volume 7: Closed Circuit Micro Irrigation Design: Theory and Applications
Volume 8: Wastewater Management for Irrigation: Principles and Practices
Volume 9: Water and Fertigation Management in Micro Irrigation
Volume 10: Innovation in Micro Irrigation Technology

**Book Series: INNOVATIONS AND CHALLENGES IN MICRO IRRIGATION**
**Senior Editor-in-Chief: Megh R. Goyal, PhD, PE**
- Engineering Interventions in Sustainable Trickle Irrigation: Water Requirements, Uniformity, Fertigation, and Crop Performance
- Fertigation Technologies for Micro Irrigated Crops: Performance, Requirements, and Efficiency
- Management of Drip/Trickle or Micro Irrigation
- Management Strategies for Water Use Efficiency and Micro Irrigated Crops: Principles, Practices, and Performance

- Micro Irrigation Engineering for Horticultural Crops: Policy Options, Scheduling and Design
- Micro Irrigation Management: Technological Advances and Their Applications
- Micro Irrigation Scheduling and Practices
- Performance Evaluation of Micro Irrigation Management: Principles and Practices
- Potential of Solar Energy and Emerging Technologies in Sustainable Micro Irrigation
- Principles and Management of Clogging in Micro Irrigation
- Sustainable Micro Irrigation Design Systems for Agricultural Crops: Methods and Practices

**Book Series: INNOVATIONS IN AGRICULTURAL & BIOLOGICAL ENGINEERING**
**Senior Editor-in-Chief: Megh R. Goyal, PhD, PE**

- Biological and Chemical Hazards in Food and Food Products: Prevention, Practices, and Management
- Bioremediation and Phytoremediation Technologies in Sustainable Soil Management
  - o   Volume 1: Fundamental Aspects and Contaminated Sites
  - o   Volume 2: Microbial Approaches and Recent Trends
- Dairy Engineering: Advanced Technologies and Their Applications
- Developing Technologies in Food Science: Status, Applications, and Challenges
- Emerging Technologies in Agricultural Engineering
- Engineering Interventions in Agricultural Processing
- Engineering Interventions in Foods and Plants
- Engineering Practices for Agricultural Production and Water Conservation: An Interdisciplinary Approach
- Engineering Practices for Management of Soil Salinity: Agricultural, Physiological, and Adaptive Approaches
- Engineering Practices for Milk Products: Dairyceuticals, Novel Technologies, and Quality
- Field Practices for Wastewater Use in Agriculture: Future Trends and Use of Biological Systems
- Flood Assessment: Modeling and Parameterization
- Food Engineering: Emerging Issues, Modeling, and Applications

- Food Process Engineering: Emerging Trends in Research and Their Applications
- Food Processing and Preservation Technology: Advances, Methods, and Applications
- Food Technology: Applied Research and Production Techniques
- Handbook of Research on Food Processing and Preservation Technologies:
  - o Volume 1: Nonthermal and Innovative Food Processing Methods
  - o Volume 2: Nonthermal Food Preservation and Novel Processing Strategies
  - o Volume 3: Computer-Aided Food Processing and Quality Evaluation Techniques
  - o Volume 4: Design and Development of Specific Foods, Packaging Systems, and Food Safety
  - o Volume 5: Emerging Techniques for Food Processing, Quality, and Safety Assurance
- Modeling Methods and Practices in Soil and Water Engineering
- Nanotechnology and Nanomaterial Applications in Food, Health, and Biomedical Sciences
- Nanotechnology Applications in Agricultural and Bioprocess Engineering: Farm to Table
- Nanotechnology Applications in Dairy Science: Packaging, Processing, and Preservation
- Novel Dairy Processing Technologies: Techniques, Management, and Energy Conservation
- Novel Strategies to Improve Shelf-Life and Quality of Foods: Quality, Safety, and Health Aspects
- Processing of Fruits and Vegetables: From Farm to Fork
- Processing Technologies for Milk and Milk Products: Methods, Applications, and Energy Usage
- Scientific and Technical Terms in Bioengineering and Biological Engineering
- Soil and Water Engineering: Principles and Applications of Modeling
- Soil Salinity Management in Agriculture: Technological Advances and Applications
- State-of-the-Art Technologies in Food Science: Human Health, Emerging Issues and Specialty Topics

- Sustainable Biological Systems for Agriculture: Emerging Issues in Nanotechnology, Biofertilizers, Wastewater, and Farm Machines
- Technological Interventions in Dairy Science: Innovative Approaches in Processing, Preservation, and Analysis of Milk Products
- Technological Interventions in Management of Irrigated Agriculture
- Technological Interventions in the Processing of Fruits and Vegetables
- Technological Processes for Marine Foods, from Water to Fork: Bioactive Compounds, Industrial Applications, and Genomics

# ABOUT SENIOR EDITOR-IN-CHIEF

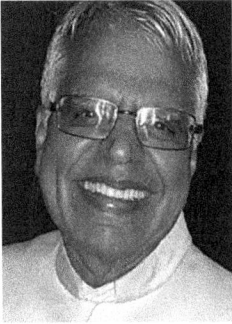

Megh R. Goyal, PhD, PE, is, currently a retired professor of agricultural and biomedical engineering from the General Engineering Department at the College of Engineering at the University of Puerto Rico–Mayaguez Campus (UPRM); and Senior Acquisitions Editor and Senior Technical Editor-in-Chief for Agricultural and Biomedical Engineering for Apple Academic Press Inc.

During his long career, he has worked as a Soil Conservation Inspector; Research Assistant at Haryana Agricultural University and Ohio State University; Research Agricultural Engineer/Professor at the Department of Agricultural Engineering of UPRM; and Professor of Agricultural and Biomedical Engineering in the General Engineering Department of UPRM. He spent a one-year sabbatical leave in 2002–2003 at the Biomedical Engineering Department of Florida International University, Miami, USA.

Dr. Goyal was the first agricultural engineer to receive the professional license in agricultural engineering from the College of Engineers and Surveyors of Puerto Rico. In 2005, he was proclaimed the "Father of Irrigation Engineering in Puerto Rico for the Twentieth Century" by the American Society of Agricultural and Biological Engineers, Puerto Rico Section, for his pioneering work on micro irrigation, evapotranspiration, agroclimatology, and soil and water engineering.

During his professional career of 51 years, he has received many awards, including Scientist of the Year, Membership Grand Prize for the American Society of Agricultural Engineers Campaign, Felix Castro Rodriguez Academic Excellence Award, Man of Drip Irrigation by the Mayor of Municipalities of Mayaguez/Caguas/Ponce and Senate/Secretary of Agriculture of ELA, Puerto Rico, and many others. He has been recognized as one of the experts "who rendered meritorious service for the development of [the] irrigation sector in India" by the Water Technology Centre of Tamil Nadu Agricultural University in Coimbatore, India, and Annual Meeting on August 01, 2018 in Detroit – MI, American Society of Agricultural & Biological Engineers (ASABE) bestowed on him Netafim Microirrigation

Award for his unselfish contribution. VDGOOD Professional Association of India awarded Lifetime Achievement Award at 12th Annual Meeting on Engineering, Science and Medicine that was held on 20-21 of November of 2020 in Visakhapatnam, India.

Dr. Goyal has authored more than 200 journal articles and edited more than 95 books.

Dr. Goyal received his BSc degree in Engineering from Punjab Agricultural University, Ludhiana, India, and his MSc and PhD degrees from the Ohio State University, Columbus, Ohio, USA. He also earned a Master of Divinity degree from the Puerto Rico Evangelical Seminary, Hato Rey, Puerto Rico, USA.

Readers may contact him at goyalmegh@gmail.com.

# ABOUT THE EDITORS

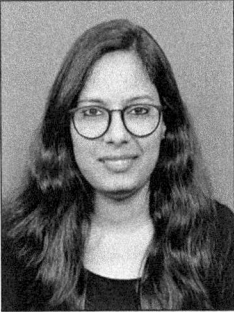

**Preeti Birwal, PhD**

Preeti Birwal, PhD, is a Scientist (Processing and Food Engineering) in the Department of Processing and Food Engineering, College of Agricultural Engineering and Technology, Punjab Agricultural Univer-sity, Ludhiana, Punjab, India.

She is currently working in the area of nonthermal food preservation, fermented beverages, food pack-aging, and technology of millet-based beer. She has served Jain Deemed to be University, Bangalore, as an assistant, where she has served as a member of the Board of Examiners and Placements. She has participated in many national and international conferences and seminars and won prizes for her oral and poster presentations. She has delivered lectures as a resource person on doubling farmers' income through dairy technology in training sponsored by the Directorate of Extension, Ministry of Agriculture and Farmers Welfare, Government of India. She is also serving as editor and reviewer of several journals and has been named "outstanding reviewer of the month" by the journal Current Research in Nutrition and Food Science. Recently she has organized a national conference. She has 18 research papers, an edited book, several book chapters, over 28 popular articles, several conference papers and abstracts, and several editorial opinions to her credit. She has successfully guided five postgraduate students for their dissertation work. She is also serving as external examiner for various Indian state agricultural universities.

Dr. Birwal earned her PhD (Dairy Engineering) on nonthermal pres-ervation of milk from ICAR-NDRI, Bangalore, and has received a merit certificate. She graduated with a degree in Dairy Technology from ICAR-National Dairy Research Institute (NDRI), Karnal, and master's degree in Food Process Engineering and Management from NIFTEM, Haryana, India. She is recipient of a university bronze medal under undergraduate program. She is the recipient of MHRD (2008), Nestle India (2009), GATE (2012–2014), UGC-RGN fellowships (2014–2018). She has successfully completed AUTOCAD 2D & 3D certification.

Readers may contact her at: preetibirwal@gmail.com

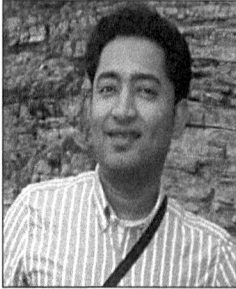

**Santosh Kumar Mishra, PhD**

Santosh Kumar Mishra, PhD, an Assistant Professor in the Department of Dairy Microbiology, College of Dairy Science and Technology, Guru Angad Dev Veterinary and Animal Sciences University, Ludhiana, Punjab, India. He is working presently on areas of functional foods and dairy products incorporating live probiotics and technology of functional lactic cultures for fermented and nonfermented dairy products. He served the dairy industry as Quality Assurance Executive at Mother Dairy, New Delh, India. He is also handling externally funded projects by DST, MoFPI, and UGC as PI or Co-PI. He has received several awards for best papers and posters/presentations. He is the recipient of junior and senior research fellowship during his master and doctoral programs at the National Dairy Research Institute, Karnal, Haryana, India. Recently, he received an award of honor at an international conference sponsored by Partap College of Education, Ludhiana, in association with the International Professionals Development Association, UK. He is the member of various scientific societies: life member of SASNET-Fermented Foods, Anand, and member of the Indian Dairy Associations, New Delhi. He has published several research, review, and popular articles in national and international journals as well several book chapters and teaching reviews in various training programs. He has recently completed the a young scientist project by DST, SEED Department, Government of India, New Delhi, on isolation and characterization of novel oxalate degrading lactic acid bacteria for potential probiotic management of kidney stone.

Dr Mishra received his BTech degree in Dairy Technology from Maharashtra Animal and Fisheries Sciences University, Nagpur, India, and his MSc and PhD degrees from the National Dairy Research Institute, Karnal, Haryana, India.

Readers may contact him at: skmishra84@gmail.com

# CONTENTS

# CONTRIBUTORS

**Luiz Domingues de Almeida Junior**
PhD, Laboratory of Phytomedicines, Pharmacology and Biotechnology (PhytoPharmaTech), Institute of Biosciences, São Paulo State University (UNESP), Rua Prof. Dr. Antonio C.W. Zanin, 250, Botucatu, 18618-689, São Paulo, Brazil; Mobile: +5514997289182; E-mail: domingues_luiz@hotmail.com

**Vedpriya Arya**
Scientist E, Patanjali Herbal Research Department, Patanjali Research Institute, University of Patanjali, Haridwar 249405, Uttarakhand, India; Mobile: +91-7060472471; E-mail: vedpriya.arya@prft.co.in

**Chellam Balasundaram**
Professor, Department of Environmental and Herbal Science, Tamil University, Thanjavur 613005, Tamil Nadu, India; Mobile: +91-9443821666; E-mail: bal333.chellam@gmail.com

**Acharaya Balkrishna**
Vice Chancellor, University of Patanjali, Haridwar 249405, Uttarakhand, India; Mobil: +91-7060830535; E-mail: achrayji@divyayoga.com

**Rachana Bhandari**
Research Associate, Patanjali Herbal Research Department, Patanjali Research Institute, University of Patanjali, Haridwar 249405, Uttarakhand, India; Mobile: +91-8650245110; E-mail: rachna.bhandari@prft.co.in

**Preeti Birwal**
Scientist, Department of Processing and Food Engineering, College of Agricultural Engineering and Technology, Punjab Agricultural University, Ludhiana-141004, Punjab, India; Mobile: +91-9896649633; E-mail: preetibirwal@gmail.com

**Rohit Bishist**
Assistant Professor (Veterinary Science), Department of Silviculture and Agroforestry, Dr Y S Parmar University of Horticulture and Forestry, Nauni, Solan 173212, Himachal Pradesh, India; E-mail: rohit.ndri@gmail.com

**Lekshmi V. Bose**
PhD Research Scholar, School of Environmental Sciences, Mahatma Gandhi University, Kottayam 686560, Kerala, India; Mobile: +91 9745366224; E-mail: lekshmivbose@gmail.com

**Vivek K. Chaturvedi**
PhD Research Scholar, Centre of Biotechnology, University of Allahabad, Prayagrag 211002, India; Mobile: +91-8737872479; E-mail: vivekchaturvedi2013@gmail.com

**Himani Chaurasia**
PhD Research Scholar, Bioorganic Research Laboratory, Department of Chemistry, University of Allahabad, Prayagrag 211002, India; Mobile: +91-9984098844; E-mail: himaniangel13@gmail.com

**Harita R. Desai**
Assistant Professor (Pharmacy), Department of Pharmaceutics, Bombay College of Pharmacy, Kalina (Santa Cruz East), Mumbai 400098, Maharashtra, India; E-mail: harita.desai@bcp.edu.in; hdesai27@gmail.com; harita.bcp@gmail.com

**Gunapathy Devi**
PhD Student, Department of Zoology, Nehru Memorial College, Puthanampatti 621007, Tamil Nadu, India; Mobile: +91-8489495193; E-mail: gunapathidevi40@gmail.com

**Bhupender Dutt**
Professor, Department of Forest Products, Dr Y S Parmar University of Horticulture and Forestry, Nauni, Solan 173212, Himachal Pradesh, India; E-mail: bdbfp@yahoo.co.in

**Krishan L. Gautam**
M.Sc. Student, Department of Silviculture and Agroforestry, Dr Y S Parmar University of Horticulture and Forestry, Nauni, Solan 173212, Himachal Pradesh, India; E-mail: krishanlalgautam99@gmail.com

**Kadakasseril V. George**
KSCSTE Emeritus Scientist, Department of Botany, St. Berchmans' College, Changanassery, Kottayam 686101, Kerala, India; Mobile: +91 9447409557; E-mail: kvgeorge58@yahoo.in

**Deepak K. Gond**
Scientist B, Patanjali Herbal Research Department, Patanjali Research Institute, University of Patanjali, Haridwar 249405, Uttarakhand, India; Mobile: +91-950608-8366; E-mail: Deepak.kumar@prft.co.in

**Nishant Gupta**
Research Associate, Patanjali Herbal Research Department, Patanjali Research Institute, University of Patanjali, Haridwar 249405, Uttarakhand, India; Mobile: +91-8077564732; E-mail: nishant.gupta@prft.co.in

**Solomon Habtemariam**
Director, Pharmacognosy Research Laboratories & Herbal Analysis Services, University of Greenwich, Chatham-Maritime, Kent ME4 4TB, UK; Tel: +44-208-3318302; E-mail: s.habtemariam@herbalanalysis.co.uk

**Ramasamy Harikrishnan**
Assistant Professor, Department of Zoology, Pachaiyappa's College for Men, Kanchipuram 631501, Tamil Nadu, India; Mobile: +91-8940283621; E-mail: rhari123@yahoo.com

**Megh R. Goyal**
Retired Faculty in Agricultural and Biomedical Engineering from College of Engineering at University of Puerto Rico—Mayaguez Campus; and Senior Technical Editor-in-Chief in Agricultural and Biomedical Engineering for Apple Academic Press Inc.; PO Box 86, Rincon, PR 006770086, USA; E-mail: goyalmegh@gmail.com

**Ankita Kataria**
PhD Scholar, Department of Food Science and Technology, Punjab Agricultural University, Ludhiana 141004, Punjab, India; Mobile: +91-8197247436; E-mail: ankitakataria92@gmail.com

**Lourthu Samy S. Mary**
PhD Student, Department of Biotechnology, Bharath College of Science and Management, Thanjavur 613005, Tamil Nadu, India; Mobile: +91-9094471422; E-mail: shanthimary1@gmail.com

**Jose Mathew**
Assistant Professor, Department of Botany, Sanatana Dharma College, Alappuzha 688003, Kerala, India; Mobile: +91 9744702847; E-mail: polachirayan@yahoo.co.in

**Murlidhar Meghwal**
Assistant Professor, Department of Food Science and Technology, National Institute of Food Technology Entrepreneurship & Management (NIFTEM), HSIIDC Industrial Estate, Kundli 131028, Sonepat, Haryana, India; Mobile: +91-9739204027; E-mail: murli.murthi@gmail.com; murli.mdm@niftem.ac.in

**Richa Mishra**
PhD Research Scholar, Bioorganic Research Laboratory, Department of Chemistry,
University of Allahabad, Prayagrag 211002, India; Mobile: +91-8765429587;
E-mail: richamay27@gmail.com

**Santosh K. Mishra**
Assistant Professor, Dept. of Dairy Microbiology, College of Dairy Science and Technology,
Guru Angad Dev Veterinary and Animal Sciences University (GADVASU), Ludhiana-141004,
Punjab, India; Mobile: +91-9464995049; E-mail: skmishra84@gmail.com

**Archana Sharma**
Assistant Professor, Department of Soil Science and Water Management, Dr Y S Parmar University of
Horticulture and Forestry, Nauni, Solan 173212 Himachal Pradesh;
E-mail: archanasharma201213@gmail.com

**Savita Sharma**
Senior Dough Rheologist, Department of Food Science and Technology, Punjab Agricultural University,
Ludhiana 141004, Punjab, India; Mobile: +91-9814769992; E-mail: savitasharmans@yahoo.co.in

**Ishwar P. Sharma**
Scientist B, Patanjali Herbal Research Department, Patanjali Research Institute, University of Patanjali,
Haridwar 249405, Uttarakhand, India; Mobile: +91-7579095587; E-mail: ip.sharma@prft.co.in

**Ramendra K. Singh**
Professor, Bioorganic Research Laboratory, Department of Chemistry, University of Allahabad,
Prayagrag 211002, India; Mobile: +91-9450304598; E-mail: rksinghsrk@gmail.com

**Vishal K. Singh**
PhD Research Scholar, Bioorganic Research Laboratory, Department of Chemistry,
University of Allahabad, Prayagrag 211002, India; Mobile: +91-7398146209;
E-mail: vishalkumarsingh922@gmail.com

**Luiz Claudio Di Stasi**
Full Professor in Pharmacology, Laboratory of Phytomedicines, Pharmacology and Biotechnology
(PhytoPharmaTech), Institute of Biosciences, São Paulo State University (UNESP),
Rua Prof. Dr. Antonio C.W. Zanin, 250, Botucatu, 18618-689, São Paulo, Brazil;
Mobile: +5514981333272; E-mail: luiz.stasi@unesp.br.

**Himanshi Solanki**
Assistant Manager—Research & Development, DFIL-CreamBell, Gurgaon 122002, India.
Mobile: +91-8901258573; E-mail: himanshisolanki42@gmail.com

**Ritika Srivastava**
PhD Research Scholar, Bioorganic Research Laboratory, Department of Chemistry,
University of Allahabad, Prayagrag 211002, India; Mobile: +91-8303191415;
E-mail: ritika.ritu.au@gmail.com

**Aparna Sudhakaran V.**
Assistant Professor, Department of Dairy Microbiology, College of Dairy Science and Technology,
Kerala Veterinary and Animal Sciences University, Thrissur Campus, Kerala 680651, India;
Mobile: +91-7558067959; E-mail: aparna@kvasu.ac.in

**Pragya Tiwari**
Assistant Professor, MG Institute of Management and Technology,
(Affiliated to Dr. APJ Abdul Kalam Technical University), Lucknow–Kanpur highway NH-24,
Lucknow-226401, Uttar Pradesh, India; Mobile: +91-9452165389;
E-mail: priyatiwari9452@gmail.com

**Ana Elisa V. Quaglio**
PhD, Laboratory of Phytomedicines, Pharmacology and Biotechnology (PhytoPharmaTech),
Institute of Biosciences, São Paulo State University (UNESP), Rua Prof. Dr. Antonio C.W. Zanin,
250, Botucatu, 18618-689, São Paulo, Brazil; Mobile: +5514998982403;
E-mail: anaequaglio@hotmail.com

# ABBREVIATIONS & SYMBOLS

| | |
|---|---|
| 2,4-D-2,4 | dichlorophenoxyacetic acid |
| A498 | human kidney carcinoma cell |
| ADC | AIDS associated dementia |
| ADI | acceptable daily intake |
| ADMET | absorption distribution metabolism excretion toxicity |
| AgNO3 | silver nitrate |
| AgNPs | silver nanoparticles |
| AIDS | acquired immuno deficiency syndrome |
| ALA | $\alpha$-linolenic acid |
| Apaf-1 | apoptotic protease-activating factor |
| ART | antiretroviral therapy |
| ATP | adenosine triphosphate |
| BAP | benzyl aminopurine |
| BBB | blood–brain barrier |
| BCAA | branched-chain amino acids |
| BHT | butylated hydroxytoluene |
| BIR | domains referred to as baculoviral iap repeats |
| BSA | bovine serum albumin |
| BSE | bovine spongiform encephalopathy |
| BSH | bile salt hydrolase |
| CAC | Codex Alimentarius Commission |
| CD | Crohn's disease |
| CNS | central nervous system |
| CRIs | co-receptor inhibitors |
| DAGA | deacylgymnemic acid |
| DC | dendritic cells |
| DCFH-DA | dichloro dihydro fluorescein diacetate |
| DHA | docosahexanoic acid |
| DLS | dynamiclight scattering |
| DMSO | dimethyl sulfoxide |
| DSS | dextran sodium sulfate |
| DTP | developmental therapeutics program |
| EC | emulsifying capacity |
| ECG | electrocardiogram |

| | |
|---|---|
| EDI | estimated daily intake |
| EDTA | ethylene diamine tetra acetic acid |
| EHEC | enterohemorrhagic *E. coli* o157: H7 |
| ELISA | enzyme-linked immunosorbent assay |
| EM8 | embryo maturation medium |
| EPA | eicosapentanoic acid |
| ES | emulsion stability |
| ESI-MS | electrospray ionisation mass spectrometry |
| EtBr | ethidium bromide |
| FACS | fluorescence activated cell sorting |
| FAO | Food and Agriculture Organization |
| FC | foaming capacity |
| FCC | face centered cubic |
| FIs | fusion inhibitors |
| FITC | fluorescein isothiocyanate |
| FMT | Facal microbiota transplantation |
| FOS | fructo-oligosaccharides |
| FS | foaming stability |
| FTIR | Fourier transform infrared spectroscopy |
| G3PDH | glyceraldehyde-3-phosphate dehydrogenase |
| GA | gymnemic acid |
| GALT | gut associated lymph tissue |
| GAP | good agricultural practices |
| GAPDH | glyceraldehyde-3-phosphate dehydrogenase |
| GC | gas chromatography |
| GC-MS | gas chromatography–mass spectrometry |
| GLP | glucagon-like peptide |
| GOS | galacto-oligosaccharides |
| GRAS | generally regarded as safe |
| GSH | glutathione |
| $H_2O_2$ | hydrogen peroxide |
| $H_3PO_4$ | phosphoric acid |
| HACCP | hazard analysis and critical control points |
| HAND | hiv-associated neurocognitive disorders |
| HBSS | Hank's Buffered Salt Solution |
| HCL | hydrochloric acid |
| HIV | human immunodeficiency virus |
| HMBC | heteronuclear multiple bond correlation |
| HPTLC | high performance thin layer chromatography |

| | |
|---|---|
| HSQC | heteronuclear single quantum coherence |
| IAA | indole acetic acid |
| IAP | inhibitor of apoptosis proteins |
| IBA | indole butyric acid |
| IBD | inflammatory bowel disease |
| IGN | intestinal gluconeogenesis |
| IMTECH | Institute of Microbial Technology |
| INIs | integrase inhibitors |
| IVPD | *in vitro* protein digestibility |
| $KH_2PO_4$ | potassium dihydrogen phosphate |
| KPL | Lumiglow Chemiluminescent Substrate System |
| LA | linoleic acid |
| LMPA | low melting point agarose |
| LP | lipid peroxides |
| MAC | microbiota accessible carbohydrates |
| MDA | lipid peroxidation |
| MHA | mueller-hinton agar |
| MNPs | metallic nanoparticles |
| MPs | metal particles |
| MRL | maximum level |
| MS medium | Murashige and Skoog medium |
| MSD | material safety data sheets |
| MSG | monosodium glutamate |
| mt | mitochondria |
| MTCC | microbial type culture collection |
| MTT | microbiota transfer therapy |
| MTT | thiazolyl blue tetrazolium bromide |
| NA | nutrient agar |
| NAA | napthalene acetic acid |
| NaOH | sodium hydroxide |
| NCI | National Cancer Institute |
| $NH_4NO_3$ | ammonium nitrate |
| NK | natural killer |
| NMR | nuclear magnetic resonance |
| NO | nitric oxide |
| NOAEL | no-observed adverse effect level |
| NPR | Natural Products Repository |
| NPs | nanoparticles |
| NRTIs | nucleoside reverse transcriptase inhibitors |

| | |
|---|---|
| NtRTIs | nucleotide reverse transcriptase inhibitors |
| O 96-w | opaque 96-well |
| O.D. | optical density |
| $O_2^-$ | superoxide radical |
| OAI | oil absorption index |
| PBMCs | peripheral blood mononuclear cells |
| Pd | platinum |
| PER | protein efficiency ratio |
| PG | prostaglandins |
| PI | propidium iodide |
| PI | propidium iodide |
| PPAR | peroxisome proliferator activated receptor |
| PSD | particle size distribution |
| PT | permeability transition |
| PUFA | polyunsaturated fatty acid |
| QSAR | quantitative structure activity relationship |
| RBI | relative band intensity |
| RCC | renal cell carcinoma |
| $R_f$ | retention factor |
| RLU | relative light units |
| ROS | reactive oxygen species |
| RT | reverse transcriptase |
| RT | room temperature |
| S.D. | standard deviation |
| SCFAs | short chain fatty acids |
| SDA | stearidonic acid |
| SEM | scanning electron microscopy |
| SHGM | standardized human gut microbiota |
| SPR | surface plasmon resonance |
| T2D | type-2 diabetes |
| T2D-Db | type-2 diabetes data-base |
| TBA | tert-butyl alcohol |
| TBARS | thiobarbituric acid reactive substances |
| TBP | tert-butyl hydroperoxide |
| TBS | tris buffer saline |
| TBST | tris buffered saline with tween 20 |
| TF | *Trigonella foenum-graecum* |
| TFAgNPs | AgNPs synthesis from root extract of *Trigonella foenum-graecum* |

| TIU | trypsin inhibitor units |
| TJ | tight junction |
| TL | telomere length |
| TMAO | trimethylamine oxide |
| TNBS | tri-nitrobenzene sulphonic acid |
| TNF-α | tumor necrosis factor alpha |
| UC | ulcerative colitis |
| UDP | uridine diphosphate |
| USDA | United States Department of Agriculture |
| UV | ultraviolet |
| WAI | water absorption index |
| WHO | World Health Organization |
| XIAP | X-linked inhibitor of apoptosis protein |
| XRD | X-ray diffraction |
| ZI | zone of inhibition |
| μg/ml | microgram per milliliter |
| μM | millionth of a meter |

# PREFACE

Phytochemicals, or secondary metabolites or bioactive compounds, are substances produced mainly by plants, and these substances have biological activities. In the pharmaceutical industry, plants represent the main source to obtain various bioactive ingredients, which exhibit pharmacological effects applicable to the treatment of bacterial and fungal infections and also chronic-degenerative diseases, such as diabetes and cancer. Thousands of phytochemicals have already been identified, and more are still being discovered year by year. Plants that are used for medicinal purposes are often less toxic and induce fewer side-effects than the synthetic medicines. In our world today, many commercially available drugs have plant-based origins with more than 30% of modern medicines directly or indirectly derived from medicinal plants. Indeed, plants can be a major source of pharmaceutical agents in the treatment of many life-threatening diseases.

The use of medicinal plants has largely increased because they are locally accessible, economical, and as well vital in promoting health. However, scientific data and information regarding the safety and efficacy of these medicinal plants are inadequate.

This book mainly covers the current scenario of the research and case studies and contains scientific evidence on the health benefits that can be derived from medicinal plants and how their efficacies can be improved. The findings reported in this book can be useful in health policy decisions. It will also motivate the development of healthcare products from plants. The book will further encourage the preservation of traditional medical knowledge of medicinal plants. Moreover, these plant products are drawing attention of researchers/policymakers because of their demonstrated beneficial effects against diseases with high global burdens such as diabetes, hypertension, cancer, and neurodegenerative diseases.

By searching the literature, one can find volumes of books and specialized publications on phytochemicals, herbs, and medicinal plants but only few of them have targeted health aspects of different foods using these biomolecules. Unfortunately, most of these publications have dealt with theoretical aspects of these strategies and technologies with little emphasis on real application in consumer and food products.

This book volume attempts to illustrate various aspects of herbs and medicinal plants and different health, safety, and preservation aspects of food by novel techniques and use of phytocompounds. This book has several potential users. It can be a reference book for those students who are taking a college- or university-level pharma, food safety, or quality assurance course for the first time. Our objectives were to compile information that pharma, dairy, and food-science students are expected to be familiar with as part of their college or university programs, before they seek career positions. This book will be further useful to pharma and food industry quality practitioners or employees, who need to become familiar with updated information pertaining to their routine work. This book is organized in such a way that each chapter treats one major application of an herb along with novel food designing techniques for health, food safety, and quality enhancement through various means.

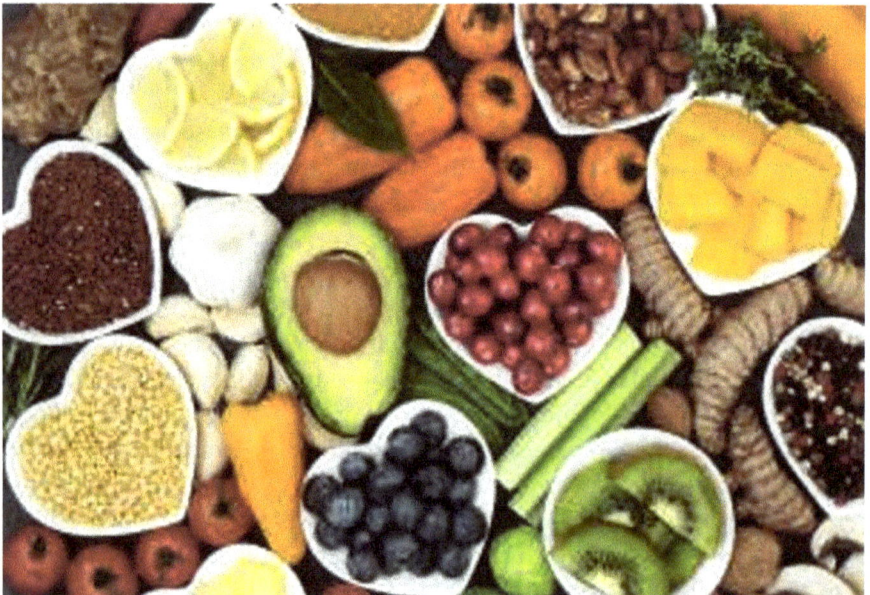

The book contains two main parts such as: (1) Plant-based secondary metabolites for healthcare: the concepts of health aspects of herbs and medicinal plants in livestock, nutraceutical, consumer survey of herbal foods, disease treatment like HIV, diabetes, etc., has been discussed. (2) Design and Utilization of Healthy Foods: the application of novel designs, herbal formulations with other biomolecules for healthcare food products development and utilization of these super foods for healthcare is elucidated.

We introduce this book volume under book series *Innovations in Agricultural & Biological Engineering.* This book volume is a treasure house of information and an excellent reference for researchers, scientists, students, growers, traders, processors, industries, and others for quality control and safety of food products during production, processing, and transportation in any food industry and boost their confidence in the area of safety and quality aspects of food products.

This book has surpassed our vision and expectations due to the contribution by all cooperating authors to this book volume, who have been most valuable in this compilation. Their names are mentioned in each chapter and in the list of contributors. We are grateful to all of them for their expertise, commitment, and dedication. We hope that this book will be a useful source for novel food developments using phytochemicals with a wide range of food and consumer product applications.

We would like to thank the staff at Apple Academic Press, Inc. for their valuable help and advice throughout this project.

We request readers to offer your constructive suggestions that may help to improve the next edition.

Also, we would like to thank our families, who have taught us the importance of working hard, having clear goals, and standing for what we believe is right. It is a lesson that guides us in everything we do. Last but not the least we wish to thank our better halves, for their understanding and patience throughout this project.

—*Megh R. Goyal, Editor*
*Preeti Birwal, Editor*
*Santosh K. Mishra, Editor*

PART I

# Plant-Based Secondary Metabolites for Healthcare

# CHAPTER 1

# ROLE OF HERBS IN LIVESTOCK PRODUCTION IN INDIA

KRISHAN L. GAUTAM*, ROHIT BISHIST, BHUPENDER DUTT, and ARCHANA SHARMA

## ABSTRACT

Animal rearing is a backbone of the rural livelihood of the Himalayan region and expansion of this sector is vital role for the improvement of life among the rural population. The indigenous knowledge and practice based on locally available bioresources are effective to cure diseases, and are easily administrable. Being natural supplements, these herbs are considered safe with no side effects, eco-friendly, and cost effective. This chapter introduces 14 effective and potential herbal medicines as feed additive and their effects on livestock performance.

## 1.1 INTRODUCTION

Animal husbandry is an important part of traditional agricultural systems in India. It plays an important role to increase the socioeconomic status of the farmer through the production of milk, milk products (butter, curd, butter-milk powder, and cheese), eggs, wool meat, skin, hides and manure, and so forth. India supports about 16% of the earth's human population and 10.71% of the world's livestock population. India is predominately an agricultural country, where about 70% of the Indian population lives in rural areas and their main profession is agriculture and animal husbandry. India's estimated milk production in 2016–2017 was 163.7 million tons. The share of gross value added of the livestock sector to total agriculture (crop and livestock) has increased from 23.8 in 2011–2012 to 26.7% in 2014–2015 at constant

*Corresponding author. E-mail: krishanlalgautam99@gmail.com.

prices. There are about 65.07 million sheep, 135.2 million goats, 300 million bovines, and 0.3 million pigs according to 19th Livestock Census in India [4].

Animal husbandry is a chief support of rural livelihood of the Himalayan region and the development of this sector is a vital role for the improvement of rural people [27]. The use of herbal feed additives in livestock production is an old tradition. There are number of medicinal herbs that have been used to improve feed palatability, utilization, and animal productivity [23, 30]. Whole plant or its parts (such as roots, rhizome. Latex, seeds, bark, leaves, and stem) are used as a raw material in different drugs and medicines.

It has been reported that over 35,000 medicinal herbs are used to treat various animal diseases [14, 32]. Apart from all modern medicines in today's world, the plants have gained prime importance in life of human beings as well as for animals due to their nutritional and medicinal value [15].

In India, ancient literature (such as Vedas and other written scriptures [i.e., Scand Puran (1000 BC), Devi Puran (2350 BC), Cherak and Shusruta (2500–600 BC)] have long documented the treatment of animal diseases by using medicinal plants [10, 20, 26, 31]. Modern research continues to contribute to knowledge on natural medicinal plants [7, 9, 13, 18]. Herbal preparations are helpful to enhance the digestion process and increase the milk yield.

Being natural supplements, the polyherbal preparations are safe, cost effective, and eco-friendly. Therefore, their incorporation in the livestock-diet encourages the animal's performance, better feed utilization, and attenuates unpromising consequences of environmental stress [6].

This chapter introduces 14 effective and potential herbal medicinal herbs (such as Giloe (*Tinospora cordifolia*), Shatavari (*Asparagus racemosus*), Chandrasur (*Lepidium sativum*), Jivanti (*Leptadenia reticulata*), Methi methi (*Trigonella foenum-graecum*), Erand (*Ricinus communis*), Kala jira (*Nigella sativa*), Saunf (*Foeniculum vulgare*), Bharingraj (*Eclipta alba*), Biskhapara (*Boerhavia diffusa*), Haldi (*Curcuma longa*), Bhumi Amla (*Phyllanthus niruri*), Manjishtha (*Rubia cordifolia*), and Karru (*Picrorhiza kurooa*)). The feed additives and their effects on livestock performance have also been discussed.

## 1.2  POTENTIAL HERBAL MEDICINES

### 1.2.1  T. CORDIFOLIA (GILOE)

It is commonly known as gulje, giloe, gurch, amrita, guduchi, amrita, gullawela, amrutvel, jiwantika, gulancha, ambarvel, giroli, shindilakodi, gulvel, gilo, amudam, and chittamritam. Giloe is a giant deciduous climber distributed throughout tropical India and Andamans. In Himachal Pradesh, it is found in Kangra, Hamirpur, Una, Paonta region of Sirmaur, Bilaspur, Mandi, Solan, and Chamba districts. Fresh or dried stems and leaves of giloe are used as a medicine.

The main biochemical ingredients of Giloe are essential oils, polysaccharides, glycosides, alkaloids, and mixtures of fatty acids. In giloe, the important phytoconstituents are clerodane furano diterpene, tinosporide, columbin, cordifolide, heptacosanol, cordifol, and b-sitosterol. Kavya et al. [16] reported that palmatine, magniflorine, tinosporin, berberine, tinosporin, and cholin are found in stem.

### 1.2.1.1   CULTIVATION

*T. cordifolia* is propagated either by seeds or vegetative cuttings. The stems having two nodes with 15–20 cm in length and small finger size thickness are used for vegetative propagation. It requires some support of trees for its better growth and development. Fast-growing species, such as neem (*Azadirachta indica*), jatropha (*Jatropha curcas*), moringa (*Moringa oleifera*), and so forth, can be grown to provide support for its growth and development.

*T. cordifolia* growing with neem (*A. indica*) is called as neem giloy that has chemical composition similar to neem as well as giloy and shows better therapeutic properties.

### 1.2.1.2   MEDICINAL USES OF GILOE

a.   Animals
    1.   Ground roots of *T. cordifolia* with water are useful to cure debility.
    2.   The medicinal plants are used as food or medicine in some tribal areas of India especially in Khedbrahma regions of North Gujrat.
    3.   In the treatment of cancer, powdered roots and stem of *T. cordifolia* are used with milk. It has been reported that dysentery and diarrhea can be cured by decoction of roots, while decoction of old stem is used in the treatment of periodic fever [28]. The extract of *T. cordifolia* and cyclophosphamide has a synergistic effect in reducing animal tumors.
    4.   Crushed stem is mixed with wheat flour and is fed to animal to cure mastitis.

          5.   Supplementation of *T. cordifolia* increases 10% milk yield, improves milk quality, and also enhances dry matter intake by 5% of lactating Murrah buffaloes [24].

  b.  Human Health

        1.   The quality of breast milk in lactating mothers is improved by decoction of stems of *T. cordifolia* [12].

        2.   Herbal drink is prepared by boiling branches of *T. cordifolia* and leaves of *Ocimum sanctum*, and this drink helps to increase the immunity of human body. It also increases platelet counts in case of dengue fever.

        3.   The people living in the sacred groves in Cuddalore district of Tamilnadu are accustomed to dry the leaves of *T. cordifolia* under shade. These dried leaves are ground into powder and mixed with hot water. The mixture is taken orally in the treatment of diabetes [16].

## 1.2.2   A. RACEMOSUS

*A. racemosus* is commonly known as Satavari, Sainsarmauli, Satawar, Satamuli, Shimai-shadavari, Ammaikodi, Kilwari, Challagadda, Pilligadalu, Kilwari, Majjige-gedde, Aheru balli Saatawari, Ekalakanto Satawarmul, Shatavali, Aswali, Shakakul, Abhiru, and Sainsarbuti. It is common throughout tropical and subtropical parts of India. In Himachal Pradesh, it is distributed in Una, Bilaspur, Chamba, Hamirpur, Kangra, Mandi, and Solan districts. Leaves and tuberous roots of *A. racemosus* are used as herbal drugs.

The main biochemical ingredients are isoflavones, asparagamine, racemosol, polysaccharides, saponins, vitamins A, $B_1$, $B_2$, P, Ca, Fe, C, E, Mg, and folic acid.

### 1.2.2.1   CULTIVATION

*A. racemosus* can be propagated from seeds or root suckers. Seedlings are ready for transplantation in 2 months. The field is irrigated once immediately after transplanting for establishment of seedlings. Being a climber, it requires proper support for its growth and development. A single plant may yield about 500–600 g of fresh roots.

## 1.2.2.2   MEDICINAL USES

**Animals:**
1.   The root extract of *A. racemosus* is used to increases milk secretion during lactation.
2.   Arthritis in cattle is cured by using 500 g of asparagus root powder with milk for 1 month.
3.   About 100 g/day of dried and powdered roots are useful for milching disorder.
4.   Prepartum supplementation of *A. Racemosus* root powder can significantly improve the postpartum animal productivity by enhancing milk production and total milk immunogloblulins [21]. Supplementation of milkplus (a Shatavari-based herbal preparation) has shown to increase milk yield from 8.26 to 10.11 l day$^{-1}$ in crossbred cattle [29].

**Humans:**
1.   It is regarded as a sacred plant and is considered auspicious in marriage ceremonies.
2.   Shatavari is also useful for hyperacidity, stomach ulcers, dysentery, and bronchial infections
3.   *It* helps in the healthy production of semen and can reduce other sexual problems in men, such as inflammation of sexual organs.
4.   It is also used for cough, dyspepsia, chronic fever, rheumatism, edema, cooling tonic antispasmodic, aphrodisiac, diarrhea, and dysentery.

## 1.2.3   L. SATIVUM

*L. sativum* is commonly known as Chandrasur, Candriki, Halim, Common cress, Aseriya, Aseliyo, Halon, Adityalu, taratej, and Aadalu. In India, it is distributed in Uttar Pradesh, Gujrat, Madhya Pradesh, Rajasthan, Gujarat, and Maharashtra. In Himachal Pradesh, it is distributed in Una, Kangra, Mandi Hamirpur, and Bilaspur. Whole plant, leaves, seeds, and roots of this plant are used to cure several diseases.

*L. sativum* contains protein, glutamic acid, leucine, methionine; and contains significant amounts of iron, calcium, nickel, cobalt, iodine, and folic acid in addition to vitamin A and C. Plant contains sinapine, sinapic acid, benzlycyanide, and glucotropoeoline.

## 1.2.3.1   CULTIVATION

*L. sativum* can be grown indoor or outdoor. It is propagated from seeds that may germinate approximately in 5–15 days depending on the ambient temperature. The leaves are ready for use after 2 or 3 weeks. There are ~350 seeds per gram.

## 1.2.3.2   MEDICINAL USES

**Animals:**
1.   *L. sativum* seeds are used to improve appetite and elimination of parasitic worms.
2.   *L. sativum* has a galactagogue effect in buffaloes; and supplementation with 100 g of seed powder daily to each buffalo was beneficial for improving the milk productivity [20]. The seeds of *N. sativa, L. sativum,* and Carum carvi are useful as galactagogue in lactating buffaloes [17].

**Humans:**
1.   The roots are used in the treatment tenesmus and secondary syphilis.
2.   *L. sativum* parts are used in the treatment of skin disorders, injuries, and eye diseases.
3.   The irritation of mucous membrane in diarrhea amoebic dysentery can be reduced by consumption of its seeds due to musilageous properties.
4.   Powder of dried seeds and leaves is used therapeutically for urine production, treating respiratory illness, bronchitis, inflammation, asthma, rheumatism bone fracture, and stimulation of urine production.
5.   It also has antiseptic, antibacterial, and therapeutic properties for the treatment of gastrointestinal complaints.
6.   To induce abortion, seeds boiled with milk are taken within 45 days of conception.

## 1.2.4   L. RETICULATA

*L. reticulata* is commonly known as Jeevanti, Dodi, Kharkhodi, Hiran vel, Palaikkodi, Kalasa, Palatheege balli, Nahanidodi, and Shinguti. It is distributed in Rajasthan, Punjab, Himachal Pradesh, Uttar Pradesh, Sikkim,

Karnataka, Kerala. Stems, leaves, and roots of *L. reticulate* are used for several health benefits.

This herb plant contains beta-sitosterol, cetyl alcohol, betaamyrin acetate, lupanol 3-*O*-diglucoside, and *n*-triacontane. Reticulin, Deniculatin, and Leptaculatin are three novel pregnane glycosides that are isolated from *L. reticulata*.

### 1.2.4.1   CULTIVATION

It can be propagated from stem cuttings that are planted in the nursery during February through March. About 5000 saplings are required for one ha at a spacing of $2 \times 1$ m. *L. reticulate* is shade-loving species; and being a twiner it requires a host or stalks. Gap filling is done 20 days after planting staking. Sandy loam to clay soil having pH 7.5–8.5 is good for cultivation of *L. reticulata*. Crop requires adequate amount of water for proper growth and development. The roots of *L. reticulate* can remain in the field for 10–15 years.

### 1.2.4.2   MEDICINAL USES

**Animals:**
1. Root and leaves of *L. reticulata* may significantly increase milk flow due to lactogenic, anabolic, and galactagogue effects.
2. *L. reticulata* produces significant galactopoietics response in goats, sheep, cows, and buffaloes [3].

**Humans:**
1. The fruits and tender stems are used as a vegetable for the improvement of vision.
2. It improves sperm count in males.
3. To treat fever, the decoction of root of *Leptadenia reticulate* is given with ghee @ of 40–50 mL.
4. *L. Reticulata* is used to improve the seminal quality, to enhance eyes, liver functions, and to treat fever, constipation, colitis, bleeding disorders, and bronchitis.
5. The 5 g each of dried powder of fruit pulp and turmeric powder is used with water to cure diabetes.
6. Daily intake of 10 g powder with water for long period is used to cure T.B., burning sensation in internal organs, leukoderma, skin

diseases, leucorrhoea, asthma, heart problems, blood impurities, and indigestion.

### 1.2.5   T. FOENUM-GRAECUM

*T. foenum-graecum* is commonly known as Methi, Venthayam, Vendhayam, Menthulu, Methika, and Greek hay. In India, it is grown in Rajasthan, Madhya Pradesh, Maharashtra Punjab, and Gujrat. More than 80% of this crop in the country is contributed by Rajasthan alone. Leaves and seeds of *T. foenum-graecum* are used for several health benefits.

Seeds contain protein, carbohydrate, minerals, vitamins, and amino acids. The bitterness in seeds is due to the presence of di-alkaloid. Leaves are rich source of sodium, calcium, phosphorus, protein, iron, vitamins A, B, C, and oxalic acid.

#### 1.2.5.1   CULTIVATION

Propagation of *T. foenum-graecum* is done by seeds. It can be grown throughout the year mostly during October 25 through November 25 and 30 kg of seed is required per ha. It requires lot of water and well-drained soils. Seeds yield is about 1000–1200 kg/ha.

#### 1.2.5.2   MEDICINAL USES

**Animals:**
1.  Leaves of *T. foenum-graecum*, rhizome of *C. longa* (Haldi), seeds of *Trachyspermum ammi* (Ajawaien), and powder of *Dendrocalamus strictus* (Bamboo) are mixed with *Piper nigrum* (black pepper) into water to increase the body temperature.
2.  Mixture of methi powder *(T. foenum-graecum)*, ajvain *(Trachyspermum ammi)*, saunth *(Zingiber officinale)*, and jiggery is fed to animals in case of food poisoning.
3.  It affects the lactation performance in ruminants. In goats, feeding 60 g of powder of fenugreek seeds per day may increase milk yield [2]. Supplementation of fenugreek seeds in buffalo's rations @ 200 g/buffalo/day leads to raise economic efficiency by about 7.89%. It improves feed efficiency and milk yield [22].

**Humans:**
1.  *T. foenum-graecum* is sometimes used as a poultice. It is wrapped in cloth, warmed, and applied directly to the skin to treat swelling, muscle pain, toe pain, leg ulcers, and swelling of lymph nodes.
2.  Leaves and shoots are used as vegetables.
3.  To cure constipation, fenugreek powder with jaggery is taken twice a day in morning and evening.
4.  *T. foenum-graecum* seeds have been used to promote lactation in lactating women due to presence of diosgenin.
5.  Boiled fenugreek seeds soaked overnight in coconut oil is applied on the head to prevent falling of hairs and to promote growth of hairs.

### 1.2.6  R. COMMUNIS

It is commonly known as Arandi, Palma christi, Arand, haralu, Eran, Castor bean, Erand, Krapata, castor oil plant, and Ricin. It is grown in Gujrat, Haryana, Karnatka, Kerala, Punjab, Sikkim, Tamilnadu Madhya Pradesh, Tripura, Manipur, Uttar Pradesh, Mizoram, West Bengal, Nagaland, and Rajasthan. Fruits, leaves, and seeds of this plant are used for several health benefits.

Leaves contain Ricinine, quercetin 3-O-β-rutinoside (rutin). Luoeol and 30-norupan-3B-OL-20-one in seed coats of castor beans. Castor oil contains stearic, hexadecenoic, palmitic, oleic, linoleic, linolenic, and dihydroxyste-aric acids as methyl esters.

#### 1.2.6.1  CULTIVATION

*R. communis* is cultivated from seeds that are planted just before the rainy season in the month of June. It requires 10–12 kg of seeds per ha. Depending on the soil type and weather conditions, irrigation may be given at 4–5 days interval. The crop is ready for harvesting in about 140–170 days. Seed yield is about 250–650 kg/ha.

#### 1.2.6.2  MEDICINAL USES

**Animals:**
1.  Juice composed of *R. communis* and leaves of *Ficus glomerata* has shown to enhance the milk production and is used as a dietary supplement for cattle and buffalo.

2.  To cure diarrhea, half cup of seed oil is administrated orally for 1 week.
3.  The seeds of *R. communis* are crushed and boiled to make the oil. The powder of dried leaves with oil can be used for covering the wounds to help in healing.
4.  The decoction of the fresh roots is taken orally to facilitate the expulsion of placenta or hasten parturition.

**Humans:**
1.  Fresh leaves or leaves warmed over a fire are applied to breasts of women to act as galactagogue.
2.  The powder of leaves is used for repelling mosquitoes, aphids, and white flies.
3.  The leaves in the form of a decoction or poultice are applied to increase the secretion of milk.
4.  Massage of warmed castor oil over the lower abdomen helps to relieve pain and cramping due to menstrual.
5.  It cures flatulence, dysentery, piles, cough, and leprosy.

### 1.2.7   N. SATIVA

It is commonly known as Jira, Kalo jire, Kalanijire, Karun-jiragam, Karun-shiragam, Fennel flower, kala jira, kalonji, Mugrela, Black seed, and Black Cumin. In India, it is grown in Punjab, Gujrat, Bihar, Uttar Pradesh, and Rajasthan. Seeds of this plant provide several health benefits

*N. sativa* seeds have saponin and alpha hederine and carvone, limonene, and citronellol in trace amounts.

### 1.2.7.1   CULTIVATION

*N. sativa* can be propagated by seeds. Proper time of sowing of *N. sativa* seed is during October. A seed rate of 8–10 kg is sufficient for 1 ha. The crop matures in 120–140 days after sowing depending on climatic conditions. Average yield of *N. sativa* is about 800–1000 kg per ha.

### 1.2.7.2   MEDICINAL USES

**Animals:**
1.  Supplementation of *N. sativa* seeds @ 100 mg per day per animal has shown to increase significantly milk fat percentage, protein

percentage and milk energy. Also, these milk components have been increased gradually with the advance of lactation until the end of the lactation period [1].

**Humans:**
1. A decoction of seeds is traditionally used to treat headache, asthma, cough, and fever.
2. Half table spoon of black seed oil mixed with water helps to treat the tooth pain.
3. Chewing two pieces of dry figs along with kalonji oil is used to treat backache, neck ache, and joint pain.
4. Drinking half tea spoon of kalonji oil twice a day is used to treat migraine headache.
5. Seeds of *N. sativa* are used to preserve the woolen clothes against attack of insects.

## 1.2.8  F. VULGARE

It is commonly known as Moti saunf, Saunf, Fennel, Indian sweet fennel, Mauri, Variari, BadiiSopu, Badi-shep, Sopn, Hop, Sompu, and Badian. It is distributed in Rajasthan and Gujrat. In Himachal Pradesh, it can be cultivated in lower and mid-hill slopes up to 2000 m. Branches, leaves, seeds, and roots of this plant provide several health benefits.

Main chemical ingredients are anethole, limonene, fenchone, estragole, safrole, α-pinene, camphene, β-pinene, β-myrcene, β-cymene, xanthotoxin, vanillin, and fenchone. Seeds are also rich in Vit. $B_1$, Vit. $B_2$, Vit. C, Vit. A, and niacin.

### 1.2.8.1  CULTIVATION

*F. vulgare* is cultivated by seeds. Proper time of sowing seed is from September to October. Sowing the seeds is done in rows at a spacing of 50 × 25 cm. A seed rate of 10–12 kg is sufficient for 1 ha. Small amount of water should be given immediately after sowing. The crop matures in 170–190 days after sowing. Yield is about 1200–1500 kg per ha.

### 1.2.8.2  MEDICINAL USES

**Animals:**
1. It is used to cure diarrhea.

2. Decoction from fresh leaves and fruits (150–200 g) of *F. vulgare* is mixed with jiggery. This mixture is given orally to animals for appetite and as a sedative for 5–6 days.

3. Polyherbal supplementation with *F. vulgare* seeds is given to lactating buffalo. It increases milk yield by 14.24% and improves general health [25].

**Humans:**

1. It increases lactation in nourishing mothers.
2. An infusion of roots is used to treat urinary disorders.
3. It is used as flavoring of foods, in toothpastes, soaps, perfumery, air fresheners, and so forth.
4. Fennel seeds have carminative, anticarcinogenic, antiinflammatory, antispasmodic, antimicrobial, and diuretic properties.
5. Chewing of fennel seeds after meals improves digestion and relieves symptoms of bloating and stomach ache.

### 1.2.9   E. ALBA

It is commonly known as Bharingraaj, False daisy, Maakaa, Keshore, Bhrun-garaja, Mochkand, Babri, Kaluganthi, Kesuti, Bhangra, Kadimulabit, and Bhangru. It is distributed throughout India up to an elevation of 2000 m in moist places. In Himachal Pradesh, it is mainly found along water channels, ditches, kuhls, and so forth, up to an elevation of 1500 m. Whole plant, leaves, and roots are used for several health benefits.

The major chemical constituents of *E. alba* are desmethyl-wedelolactone-7-glucoside, β-amyrin, luteolin-7-*O*-glucoside, hentriacontanol, heptacosanol, and stigmasterol.

### 1.2.9.1   CULTIVATION

*E. alba* can be propagated through seeds. Proper time of sowing is from February to March. Sowing the seeds is done manually in rows and small amount of water is given immediately after sowing. It is a common weed in rice fields, sugarcane fields, and coconut plantations. The plant is fast-growing and one can obtain about 17,000 seeds per plant.

### 1.2.9.2   MEDICINAL USES

**Animals:**
1. Fresh leaves are grinded and boiled with mustard oil. This paste is applied twice daily for 10–15 days on wounds for early healing [19].
2. Whole plant of *E. alba* is mixed with feed to improve body weight and milk production.

**Humans:**
1. The whole plant is used as an antiseptic, febrifuge, tonic, deobstruent in hepatic, and emetic.
2. The juice is given with honey to treat upper respiratory congestion in children.
3. Some local tribes of Mount Abu in Rajasthan, India use leaves and flowers of *E. alba* for the treatment of asthma, cough, and jaundice [11].

### 1.2.10   B. DIFFUSA

It is commonly known as Punarnava, Gadepurna, Dholisatudi, Ratka, Adakaputtana gida, Red hogweed, Tar vine, Red Spiderling, Wine flower, Saarai, khapara, Itsit, Shothagni, and Biskhapara. It is distributed in Bihar, Gujrat, Madhya Pradesh, Tamil Nadu, Punjab, Orrisa, Uttar Pradesh, and Assam. Seeds, leaves, roots, and aerial parts or the whole plant have several health benefits.

The chemical constituents of *B. diffusa* are flavonoid glycosides, alkaloids, lignin glycosides, and phenolic. The physicochemical properties of leaves have moisture content 84.5%, protein 6.1%, fat 0.9%, carbohydrates 7.2%, minerals 1.3 g/100 g, calcium 667, phosphorus 99, iron 18.4, vitamin C 27 mg/100 g, and energy 61 kcal/100 g.

### 1.2.10.1   CULTIVATION

*B. diffusa* can be propagated through seeds. Proper time of sowing seed is from November to December. During the rainy season, there is no need of irrigation; however, one or two during winter and two to three light irrigation during summer are needed. The extra plants are removed within 15–20 days after sowing in order to keep uniform plant spacing of 20 × 30 cm. The plant can produce fruits throughout the year, if sufficient water is available.

## 1.2.10.2   MEDICINAL USES

**Animals:**
1.   The aqueous extract significantly inhibits the increased serum amino-transferase activity in arthritic animals similar to hydrocortisone.
2.   Liver ATP phosphohydrolase activity also increases by aqueous extract and the alkaloid.
3.   The whole extract with raw sugar is used to cure stomach disorders, while leaves are boiled and used to bath cattle to cure skin diseases.

**Humans:**
1.   *B. diffusa* is used for abdominal pain, eye problems, fever, heart ailments, heart diseases, hemorrhages (at childbirth), urinary disorders, weakness, inflammation (internal), jaundice, kidney disorders, menstrual disorders, renal insufficiency, rheumatism, and snakebite. It is helpful as diuretic and expectorant [5].
2.   Decoction of roots is given orally to cure night blindness.
3.   Hot poultice of whole plant is used to expel guinea worms.

## 1.2.11   C. LONGA

It is also known as Haldi, Arisina, Manjal, Halad, Haladi, Haridra, and Halodhi, India is a leading producer and exporter of turmeric in the world. It is distributed in Andhra Pradesh, Tamil Nadu, Orissa, Karnataka, West Bengal, Gujarat, Meghalaya, Maharashtra, and Assam. Rhizomes have several health benefits.

   *C. longa* contains fat (5.1%), proteins (6.3%), minerals (3.5%), cineol, borneol, a-phellandrene, borneol, zingiberene, sabinene, and Sesquiterpenes.

## 1.2.11.1   CULTIVATION

*C. longa* can be propagated through rhizomes (roots). Proper time of sowing is from May to July. The small rhizomes with one or two buds are planted at 4–8 cm depth in soil. Subsequent irrigations are given at 7–10 days interval depending on soil. Harvesting consists of digging of underground clumps of rhizomes with pick-ax or digging fork. Yield is about 25,000–30,000 kg of fresh rhizomes per ha.

## 1.2.11.2  MEDICINAL USES

**Animals:**
1. The extract of fresh rhizome is applied externally on the affected eyes to cure eye diseases.
2. Rhizome of *C. longa* is crushed and warmed in oil to cure wounds.
3. *C. longa* is used as drench for retained placenta.
4. Rhizome of *C. longa* having size of 5–9 cm is grated and given as an infusion to bring down the brushed blood and to increase milk production.
5. The paste prepared from fresh rhizomes and mustard oil is used to treat naval infection of calf, foot, and mouth diseases of cow, and mastitis in lactating cows.
6. The powder of rhizomes is boiled in ghee. To relieve external and internal parasite, it is topically and orally used two times per day for 5–10 days.
7. Paste of *C. longa* is applied on broken horn to reduce the pain.

**Humans:**
1. Turmeric is helpful in the purification of breast milk and regulation of the female reproductive system.
2. *C. longa* is used as stomachic, tonic, and blood purifier [8].
3. *C. longa* possesses anticancerous property due to presence of curcumin that kills cancer cells but also prevents their formation and growth.

## 1.2.12  P. NIRURI

It is commonly known as Gale of the wind, Keezhar Nelli, Bhudhatri, Jar-amla, and Bhuin amla. It is distributed throughout the India mainly in Jharkhand, Bihar, and Chhattisgarh. Whole plant, shoot leaves, and roots are used for several phytochemical activities.

*P. niruri* contains flavonoids, lignans, alkaloids, triterpenes, phenols, terpenoids, polyphenols, tannins, coumarins, and saponins.

## 1.2.12.1  CULTIVATION

*P. niruri* can be propagated through seeds. Proper time of sowing seeds is from April to May. Due to small size of seeds, these are mixed with sand before sowing at a spacing of 10 × 15 cm. Irrigation is given two times daily for 15 days. The field should be free from weeds, for which regular hand weeding is required. Plants are harvested when the rainy season is over.

## 1.2.12.2 MEDICINAL USES

**Animals:**
1. Whole plant mixed with feed is used to improve the body weight and milk of cattle.
2. Decoction of roots given two times per day is used to cure cough and fever in sheep.
3. It is used as liver tonic to address conditions, such as jaundice and viral infections.

**Humans:**
1. *P. niruri* is used for the treatment of kidney stones and is also useful in chronic dysentery.
2. It is used for restricting the growth of hepatitis-B virus in the blood.
3. The extract of fresh roots is used in a case of jaundice.
4. Herbal tea prepared with fresh leaves of *P. niruri* is used to treat typhoid.
5. It helps in lowering high blood pressure.
6. Consumption of one spoon of fresh juice from the plant mixed with sugar and jeera helps to mitigate the pain in urination.

## 1.2.13  R. CORDIFOLIA

It is commonly known as Manjith, Bala-meshika, Manjit, Indian madder or Tushusho. It is distributed in temperate and sub-temperate parts of India up to an elevation of 3700 m. In Himachal Pradesh, it is found in Mandi, Kullu, Shimla and Chamba. Plant roots provide several health benefits.

*R. cordifolia* contains alizarin, anthraquinones, and their glycosides, terpenes, iridois, fructose, glucose,, sucrose, purpurin, carboxylic acids, and saccharides.

### 1.2.13.1  CULTIVATION

*R. cordifolia* can be propagated through seeds. Proper time of sowing seeds is in early summer. Propagation should be done through cuttings having two or three internodes. After seed germination, seedlings are transplanted in polythene bags for establishment. Optimum spacing between plants is $60 \times 75$ cm. Roots can be harvested in October through November. The crop yield is about 3000 kg of dry roots per ha.

### 1.2.13.2   MEDICINAL USES

**Animals:**
1.  Paste of whole plant of *Rubia manjith* or leaf paste of *Peoli Reinwardtia indica* is applied locally on the wounds.
2.  Juice of leaves is applied externally on the affected parts of foot.
3.  Extract of roots is effective to relieve discomfort.

**Humans:**
1.  The decoction of roots is used to treat irregular menstruation; and for eye and ear infections.
2.  Extract of *R. cordifolia* roots is antiinflammatory agent due to presence of rubimallin.
3.  The extract of roots reduces the blood sugar level.
4.  It is helpful to purify breast milk.
5.  It improves appetite and is useful in treating diarrhea, dysentery, bleeding ulcers, dyspepsia, parasitic worms, etc.
6.  Root powder mixed with honey is applied to brown spots of pityriasis versicolor.

### 1.2.14   PICRORHIZA KURROA

It is commonly known as Kaur, Kutki, Karru, Picrorhiza, Karvi, Tikta, Katuki, Kaud, Kadu, and Kali kutki. It is distributed in the Himalayan region from Jammu and Kashmir to Sikkim at an elevation of 2800–4500 m. In Himachal Pradesh, it is distributed in Kinnaur, Lauhal, Chamba, Kangra, Shimla, and Kullu districts. Rhizomes and stolons of this plant provide several phytochemical activities.

Biochemical constituents of *P. kurroa* are vanillic acid, apocyanin, picroside-I, picroside-II, kutkoside, Phenolic glycoside, Iridoid glycoside, alkanol, alkane, β-sitosterol Kutkin, and apocynin.

### 1.2.14.1　CULTIVATION

*P. kurroa* can be propagated through seeds or rhizomes in October to November. The small rhizomes with one or two buds are planted at 4–8 cm soil depth at 30 × 20 cm spacings. Irrigation is given on alternate days during the summer. The rotation period of *P. kurroa* is 3 years. For complete maturity of the seed, the plant needs about 1 year. The crop yield is about 1100 kg dry roots per ha.

### 1.2.14.2　MEDICINAL USES

**Animals:**
1. Paste of roots of *P. kurroa* is helpful to treat loss of appetite. It is also effective in dysentery.
2. Fresh root paste of *P. kurroa* is given to cattle during fever.
3. Aqueous extract of roots of *P. kurroa* is applied on the infected hooves.
4. It is helpful in to treat digestive disorders, alimentary disorders, intestinal worms, cough, tonsil, and diarrhea.

**Humans:**
1. It is used to treat cold, asthma, and cough; and also to cure liver complaints, anemia, and jaundice.
2. It is helpful in treating constipation.
3. It is a bitter tonic and is effective for nose bleeding.
4. It maintains blood sugar level in the body.
5. It helps to control the inflammatory conditions.

## 1.3　SUMMARY

This chapter introduces biochemical components and medicinal uses of

- Bharingraj (*E. alba*)
- Bhumi Amla (*P. niruri*)
- Biskhapara (*B. diffusa*)
- Chandrasur (*L. sativum*)
- Erand (*R. communis*)
- Giloe (*T. cordifolia*)
- Haldi (*C. longa*)

- Jivanti (*L. reticulata*)
- Kala jira (*N. sativa*)
- Karru (*P. kurooa*)
- Manjishtha (*R. cordifolia*)
- Methi (*T. foenum-graecum*)
- Saunf (*F. vulgare*)
- Shatavari (*A. racemosus*)

## KEYWORDS

- **animal husbandry**
- **Himalayan region**
- **livestock**
- **supplements**

## REFERENCES

1. Abd-El Moty, A.K.I.; Zanouny, A.I.; El-Barody, M.A.A.; Sallam, M.T. Effect of *Nigella Sativa* seeds supplementation on milk yield and milk composition in sheep. *Egypt. J. Sheep Goat Sci.,* **2015**, *10* (1), 19–26.
2. Alamer, M.A.; Basiouni, G.F. Feeding effects of fenugreek seeds (*Trigonella Foenum Graecum*) on lactation performance, some plasma constituents and growth hormone level in goats. *Pak. J. Biol. Sci.,* **2005**, *8* (11), 1553–1556.
3. Anjaria, J.V.; Gupta I. Studies on lactogenic property of *Leptadenia Reticulata* (Jivanti) and *Leptadenia* tablets in goat, sheep, cow and buffalo. *Indian Vet. J.,* **1967**, *44* (11), 967–974.
4. *Annual Report.* Department of Animal Husbandry and Dairying, PAU, Ludhiana India; **2016**; p. 81.
5. Bhalla, T.N.; Gupta, M.B.; Bhargava, K.P. Anti-inflammatory and biochemical study of *Boerhaavia Diffusa. J. Res. Ind. Med.,* **1971**, *6*, 11–15.
6. Bhatt, N. *Efficacy of Herbal Drugs in Rumen Metabolism, Growth and Milk Production in Crossbred Cattle.* M. Sc. Thesis. Pantnagar, India: G.B: Pant University of Agriculture and Technology; **2000**; p. 167.
7. Biswas, K. *Common Medicinal plants of Darjeeling and Sikkim Himalaya.* Alipore (WB), India: Government of West Bengal, Commerce and Industries Department, Superintendent, Government Printing, West Bengal Government Press; **1956**; p. 113.
8. Chopra, D.; Simon, D. *Herbal Handbook.* New York, NY: The Chopra Center, Three Rivers Press; **2000**; pp. 73–75.
9. Chopra, R.N.; Nayar, S.L.; Chopra, I.C. *Glossary of Indian Medicinal Plants.* New Delhi (India): Council of Scientific and Industrial Research, Government of India; **1956**; p. 273.

10. Dwivedi, S.K. Ethno-veterinary medicine in ancient India. In: *Veterinary Science and Animal Husbandry in Ancient India*; R. Somvanshi and M. P. Yadav, (Eds.); Izatnagar, India: Indian Veterinary Research Institute (IVRI); **2003**; pp. 103–106.

11. Frawley, D. *Ayurvedic Healing: A Comprehensive Guide*. Salt Lake City, UT: Passage Press; 1989; pp. 200–211.

12. Gaur, L.B.; Singh, S.P.; Gaur, S.C.; Bornare, S.S. basic information, cultivation and medicinal use of *Tinospora cordifolia*. *Popular Kheti* (Popular Farming), **2014**, *2*, 188–192.

13. Jain, S.K. *Glimpses of Indian Ethnobotany*. New Delhi, India: Oxford & IBH Publishing Co. Pvt. Ltd.; **1981**; pp. 75–82.

14. Jain, S.K. Plants in indian ethno-veterinary medicine: status and prospectus. *Indian J. Vet. Animal Sci. Res.*, *2000*, *2000*, 20–29.

15. Joshi, S.G. *Medicinal Plants*. New Delhi, India: Oxford and IBH Publishing Co. Pvt. Ltd.; **2000**; p. 491.

16. Kavya, B.; Kavya, N; Ramarao, V.; Vankateshwarlu, G. *Tinospora Cordifolia*: nutritional ethnomedical and therapeutic utility. *Int. J. Ayur. Res. Pharm.*, **2015**, *6* (2), 195–198.

17. Kholif, A.M.; Abd El-Gawad, M.A.M. Medicinal plant seeds supplementation of lactating goat's diets and its effect on milk and cheese quantity and quality. *Egypt. J. Dairy Sci.*, **2001**, *29* (1), 139–150.

18. Kirtikar, K.R.; Basu B.D. *Indian Medicinal Plants—with Illustrations*. 2nd edition; Volumes 1 to 4; Allahabad, India: Lalit Mohan Basu; **1935**; pp. 56–62.

19. Kumar, A.T. Veterinary Ayurveda in ancient Indian literature. In: *Veterinary Science and Animal Husbandry in Ancient India*; R. Somvanshi & M. P. Yadav (Eds.); Izatnagar, India: Indian Veterinary Research Institute (IVRI); **2003**; pp. 8–16.

20. Kumar, S.; Baghel, R.P.S.; Khare, A. Effect of chandrasoor (*Lepidium Sativum*) supplementation on dry matter intake, body weight and milk yield in lactating murrah buffaloes. *Buffalo Bull.*, **2011**, *30* (4), 262–266.

21. Kumar, S.; Mehla, R.K.; Singh, M. Effect of shatavari (*Asparagus Recemosus*) on milk production and immune modulation in karan fries crossbred cows. *Indian J. Trad. Knowl.*, **2014**, *13* (2), 404–408.

22. Mahgoub, A.A.S.; Sallam, M.T. Effect of extract crushed fenugreek seeds as feed additive on some blood parameters, milk yield and its composition of lactating egyptian buffaloes. *J. Animal Poultry Prod.*, **2016**, *7* (7), 269–273.

23. Maikhuri, R. K. Eco-energetic analysis of animal husbandry in traditional societies of India. *Energy* (Pergamon Press), **1992**, *17* (10), 959–967

24. Mir, N.A.; Kumar, P.; Rather, S.A.; Sheikh, F.A.; Wani, S.A. Effect of supplementation of *Tinospora Cordifolia* on lactation parameters in early lactating murrah buffaloes. *Buffalo Bull.*, **2015**, *34* (1), 17–20.

25. Patel, M.D.; Tyagi, K.K.; Sorathiya, L.M.; Fulsoundar, A.B. Effect of polyherbal galactagogue supplementation on milk yield and quality and general health of surti buffaloes of south gujarat. *Vet. World*, **2013**, *6* (4), 214–218.

26. Shirlaw, L.H. A short history of ayurvedic veterinary literature. *Ind. J. Vet. Sci.*, 1940, *10* (2), 1–39.

27. Singh, R. V. *Fodder Trees of India*. New Delhi, India: Oxford and IBH; **1982**; pp. 2–5.

28. Sinha, K.; Mishra, N. P.; Singh. J.; Khanuja, S. P. S. *Tinospora Cordifolia* (Guduchi): reservoir plant for therapeutic applications—review. *Ind. J. Trad. Knowl.*, **2004**, *3* (1), 257–270.

29. Sukanya, T.S.; Rudraswamy, M.S.; Bharat, K. T. P. Performance of Shatavari-based herbal galactagogue: milk plus supplementation to crossbred cattle of Malnad region. *Int. J. Sci. Nat.*, **2014**, *5* (2), 362–363.

30. Swarup, A.; Umadevi, K. Obs. & gynae. *India Today (III)*, **1998**, *6*, 369–672.

31. Swarup, A.; Pashu. Ayurveda during vedic period. In: *Veterinary Science and Animal Husbandry in Ancient India*; R. Somvanshi and M.P. Yadav (Eds.); Izatnagar, India: Indian Veterinary Research Institute (IVRI); **2003**; p. 107.

32. Yineger, H.; Kelbess, E.; Bekele, T.; Luleka, E. Ethno-veterinary medicinal plants at bale mountains national park, Ethiopia. *J. Pharmacol.*, **2007**, *112* (12), 55–70.

# CHAPTER 2

# ROLE OF PLANT-BASED ANTI-HIV AGENTS IN HIV-ASSOCIATED NEUROCOGNITIVE DISORDERS (HAND)

VISHAL K. SINGH, HIMANI CHAURASIA, RICHA MISHRA, RITIKA SRIVASTAVA, VIVEK K. CHATURVEDI, and RAMENDRA K. SINGH*

## ABSTRACT

The combination antiretroviral therapy (cART) is an effective tool to prevent human immunodeficiency virus (HIV) proliferation. Moreover, the emergence of drug resistance limits the cART, and hence novel drugs as well as newer objects are necessary. In this pursuance, the research for the drugs that attack HIV reservoirs (like brain, lymph nodes, blood, and digestive tract) has shifted the focus toward plant secondary metabolites (such as coumarins, terpenes, flavonoids, alkaloids, phenolics, lignans, quinones, saponins, etc.). These secondary metabolites have shown promising anti-HIV and neuroprotective activities. This chapter focuses on biodiversity of flora monarchy and presents an overview of the potential of plant extracts against HIV/AIDS along with their functional relationships of HIV-associated neurocognitive disorders.

## 2.1 INTRODUCTION

More than 36 million patients have died due to human immunodeficiency virus (HIV) infection on the global scenario along with 1.8 million new infections. Regrettably, still there is no treatment, which can completely clear the virus out of human body.

---

*Corresponding author. E-mail: rksinghsrk@gmail.com

It is a retrovirus, which has genetic material RNA. When this virus comes in contact with human cells, and then it makes new genetic material Ds-DNA, which is recognized by provirus. Then provirus gets entry into DNA of human and establishes several new infected sites. It is really tough to find a suitable cure, because the HIV life cycle is completed inside the host cell. Based on the literature survey, there are seven types of drugs (such as NRTIs, NtRTIs, NNRTIs, PIs, FIs, CRIs, and INIs) that may have preventive effects at various stages of HIV life expectancy.

However, HIV shows different behavior in different persons. It is caused due to occurrence of mutation in viral genetic material that leads to the development of several viral strains. Such mutated viral strains foster resistance against drugs on long-term exposure. In such a perilous phase, a combination therapy named by highly active antiretroviral therapy (HAART) has been employed [14, 16, 47, 52, 53].

Neurological disorders, which are accompanied with HIV/AIDS, are recognized as HIV-associated neurocognitive disorders (HAND) that possibly will have severe neurological disorders. A metabolic encephalopathy is persuaded through HIV infection and is driven via protected initiation of microglia is as a result of HAND [25, 30, 33, 48]. When the given cells get infected with HIV, they ooze out neurotoxins for host and viral origin.

The AIDS dementia complex (ADC) is featured by incapacitating cognitive mutilation accompanied with motor dysfunction, speech glitches, and behavioral transmutes. Cognitive mutilation is depicted by various deformities, such as deliberation of mental abilities, anxiety, loss of reminiscence, and impoverished attentiveness. Motor signs comprise of unwieldiness, deprived harmony besides trembles. Operational transformation can comprise of boredom, lassitude, and detracted emotional retorts and extemporaneity. Histopathologically, ADC is recognized through penetration of monocytes along with macrophages inside the central nervous system (CNS), hypertrophy of glial cells, paleness with whitish sheath around nerve fibers, anomalies related to branch like tree progressions, related to neuron forfeiture [3]. It is increased subsequently about HIV contagion, which is determined by the CD4 T-cell count and plasma viral load. Many times, these characteristics appear as the first symptoms of initiation of AIDS [20, 54].

In Western countries, the observed prevalence is about 10%–24% [65], out of which about 1%–2% are infections in India [65, 75]. As HAART is introduced, the prevalence of ADC has waned in the developed countries [21, 27]. HAART could preclude otherwise postponement of initiation based on ADC among the persons having HIV contagion. DTP belongs to NCI offered communications sustenance related to internal and extra-curricular (HIV) agents that act against HIV.

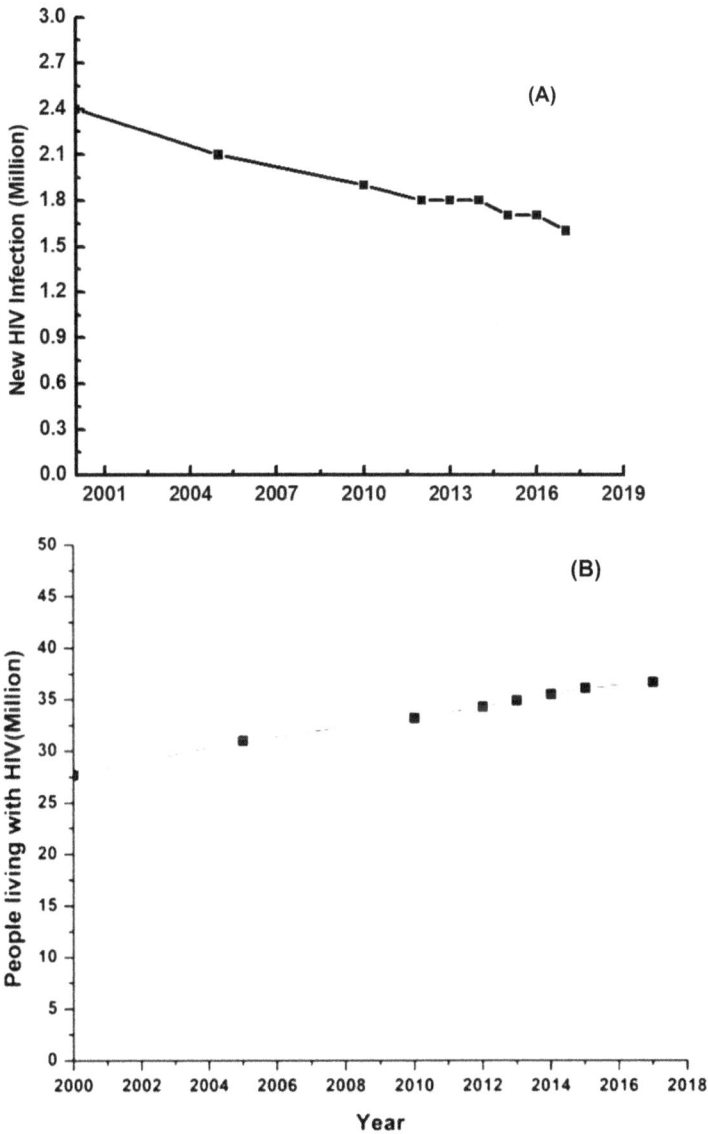

FIGURE 2.1  Global data on (A) new HIV infections; (B) patients with HIV infection.

It could be noteworthy to observe that there has been reduction in AIDS-related deaths in various parts of the world during the last 10 years (Figure 2.1), such as 39% reduction in Asia pacific, 45% reduction in central and west Europe and North America, 52% reduction in Caribbean, and 30% central and west Africa [14, 16, 41, 47].

This chapter highlights prominent anti-HIV findings and advancements, which were made possible through DTP sponsorship. The key instances are screening of plant-based biocompounds. Primary screening of anti-HIV agents has helped to recognize natural products that may stop the key phase in HIV lifecycle.

## 2.2 ANTI-HIV NATURAL PRODUCTS

Several medicinal plants have been identified with several anti-HIV charac-teristics. Assortment of plant-based secondary metabolites depicts promising anti-HIV activities (Table 2.1).

**TABLE 2.1**   Natural Plant Products: Sources and Anti-HIV Activities

| Natural Product | Source | Anti-HIV Activity |
|---|---|---|
| Carbohydrates | | |
| Galactansulphate | *Aghaedhella tenera* | 0.6–0.4 µg/mL[a,h] |
| Rhamnansulphate | *Monostroma latissimum* | * |
| Sulpahatedxylomannan | *Nothogenia fastigiata* | 13.7 µg/mL[a,d] |
| Coumarins | | |
| (−)-Calanolide B | *C. lanigerum* | 0.2 µM[b,h,k] |
| (+)-Calanolide A | *Callophuyllum lanigerum* | 0.2 µM[b,h,k] |
| Coriandrin | *Coriandrum sativum* | * |
| Imperatorin | *Ferula sumbul* | 1007 µg/mL[a] |
| Suksdorfin | *Lamatium suksdorfii* | 2.6 µM[b,d] |
| (−)7,8-Dihydrocalanolide B | *Callophyllum lanigerum* | 0.1 µM[b] |
| Phenolics | | |
| 8-C-Ascorbyl (−)-epigallocatechin | *Green and black tea* | 4 µg/mL[b] |
| Balanocarpol | *Hopea malibato* | * |
| Caffeic acid tetramer salts | *Arnebia eucbroma* | 1.5–4.0 µg/mL[b,d] |
| Calceolarioside B | *Fraxinus sieboldiana* | 0.1 µg/mL[a,l] |
| Camellia tannin H | *Camellia japonica* | 0.9 µM[a] |

**TABLE 2.1** *(Continued)*

| Natural Product | Source | Anti-HIV Activity |
|---|---|---|
| Corilagin | *Chamaesyce hyssopifolia* | 20 $\mu$M[a,e] |
| Diprenylatedbibenzyl | *Glycyrrhiza lepidota* | * |
| Guttiferone A | *Symphonia globulifera* | 8 $\mu$M[b,h] |
| Laxifloranone | *Marila laxiflora* | *[h] |
| Repandusinic acid | *Phyllanthus niruri* | *[e] |
| Theasinensin D | *Thea sinensis* | 8 $\mu$g/mL[b] |
| Vismiaphenone D | *Vismia cayennensis* | 11 $\mu$g/mL[b] |
| Alkaloids | | |
| 1-Methoxy canthinone | *Leitneria floridana* | 0.26 $\mu$g/mL |
| Buchapine | *Eudia roxburhiana* | 0.94 $\mu$M[b,h] |
| Casanmospermine | *Castenospermum austral* | >10 $\mu$g/mL[b,d,l,k] |
| Cepharanthine | *Stephania cepharantha* | *[d] |
| Crambescidin 826 | *Sponge monanchora* sp. | 1–3 $\mu$M[a,j] |
| Dehydocrambine | *Sponge monanchora* sp. | ~35 $\mu$M[a,j] |
| FK-3000 | *Stephania cepharantha* | 7.8 $\mu$g/mL[h] |
| Harmine | *Symplocos setchuensis* | *[d] |
| Hypoglaunine B | *Trypterigium hypoglaucum* | 0.1 $\mu$g/mL[b] |
| Michellamine | *Ancistrocladus korupensis* | 1 $\mu$M[b,e,j,k] |
| Nitidine | *Toddalia asiatica* | 14 $\mu$M[b,e] |
| O-Demethyl-buchenavianine | *Buchenavia capitata* | * |
| Trikendiol | *Trikentrion love* | 2 $\mu$g/mL[a,h] |
| Triptonine A | *Trypterigium hypoglaucum* | 2.54 $\mu$g/mL[b] |
| Triptonine B | *Trypterigium hypoglaucum* | <0.1 $\mu$g/mL[b] |
| Lignans | | |
| Anolignan A | *Anogeissus acuminata* | 60.4 $\mu$g/mL[b,g] |
| Retrojusticidin B | *P. myrtifolius* | *[e] |
| Flavonoids | | |
| 6,8-Diprenylaromadendrin | *Monotes africanus* | * |
| Xanthohumol | *Humulus lupulus* | *[h] |
| Saponins | | |
| Actein | *Cimicifuga racemosa* | 0.375 mg/mL[b] |
| Escins | *Aesculus chinensis* | * |
| Saponin B1 | *Soybean seeds* | 0.5 $\mu$g/mL[d,j] |
| Quinones | | |
| Conocurvone | *Conospermum incurvum* | 0.02 $\mu$M[b,h] |

**TABLE 2.1**  *(Continued)*

| Natural Product | Source | Anti-HIV Activity |
|---|---|---|
| Hypericin | *Hypericum perforatum* | * |
| Terpens | | |
| Cyanthiwigin B | *Myrmekiodermastyx* | 42.1 μM[b] |
| Celasdin B | *Celastrus hindsii* | 0.8 μM[b,d] |
| Cytosporic acid | *Fungus cytospora* sp. | 20 μM[a,g] |
| Clausenolide-1 ethyl ether | *Clausena excavate* | >20 μg/mL[k] |
| Clathsterol | *Clathria* sp. | 10 μM[a,e] |
| Dihydrobetulinic acid | *S. claviflorum* | 13 μM[a] |
| Garcisaterpene B | *G. speciose* | 37 μg/mL[b,e,k] |
| Garcisaterpene A | *Garcinia speciosa* | 5.8 μg/mL[b,e,k] |
| Halistanolsulphae G | *Pseudoxinissadigitata* | 3 μM[b,h] |
| Haplosamates B | *Xestospongia* sp. | 15 μg/mL[a,h] |
| Halistanolsulphae H | *Pseudoxinis sadigitata* | 6 μM[b,h] |
| Haplosamates A | *Xestospongia* sp. | 50 μg/mL[a,g] |
| Linearol | *Sideritis ekmanii* | 0.1–3.11 μg/mL[b,d] |
| Lancilactone | *Kadsuralancilimba* | 1.4 μg/mL[b,d] |
| Limonin | *Citrus* spp. | 60 μM[a,e] |
| Moronic acid | *Tripterygium wilfordii* | <0.1 μg/mL[b] |
| Maslinic acid | *Citrus* spp. | 17.9 μg/mL[a,f] |
| Nomilin | *Citrus* spp. | 52 μM[b,f] |
| Nigranoic acid | *Schisandra sphaerandra* | *e |
| Nortripterifordin | *Schisandra sphaerandra* | 25 μM[b,d] |
| Oxygenated triterpenes | *Myrceugenia euosma* | 0.17–0.23 μM[a,f,h] |
| Oleanolic acid | *Genum japonicum* | 21.8 μg/mL[a,d] |
| Prostratin | *S. claviflorum* | <0.132 μM[b] |
| Shinjulactone C | *Allanthus altissima* | 10.6 μM[b] |
| Suberosol | *Polyalthiasuberosa* | 3 μg/mL[a,d] |
| Uvaol | *C. pinnatifida* | 5.5 μM[a,f] |
| Ursolic acid | *Crataegus pinatifida* | 8 μM[a,e,f] |
| 16β,17-Dihydroxy-ent-kauran-19-oic acid | *Annona squamosa* | 0.8 μg/mL[b] |
| 12–0-Tetradecanoyl phorbol-13-acetate | *Croton tiglium* | 0.48 μg/mL[a,h] |
| 12-Deoxyphorbol-13-(3E,5E-decadienote) | *Excoecaria agallocha* | 6 nM[a,e] |

**TABLE 2.1**   *(Continued)*

| Natural Product | Source | Anti-HIV Activity |
|---|---|---|
| Proteins | | |
| Cyanovirin-N | *Nostoc ellipsosporum* | * |
| GAP31 | *Gelonum multiflorum* | 0.2–0.3 nM[b,g] |
| MAP30 | *Momordi cacharantia* | 0.2–0.3 nM[b,d,e,k] |
| MHL | *Myrianthus holstii* | 150 nM[b] |
| TAP29 | *Trichosanthes kirilowii* | 0.2–0.3 nM[b,d,e,k] |
| Trichosanthin | *Trichosanthes kerilowii* | *[d,k] |
| Peptides | | |
| [Leu7] surfactin | *B. s natto* | 14 μM[b,h] |
| Xanthones | | |
| Macluraxanthone | *Maclura tinctoria* | * |
| Swerti francheside (90) | *Swertia franchetiana* | 43 μM[a,e] |

[a]$IC_{50}$.

[b]$EC_{50}$.

[c]$ED_{50}$.

**Inhibitory action counter to:**

[d]HIV-1 copying.

[e]HIV-RTase.

[f]HIV protease.

[g]HIV integrase.

[h]HIV-induced cytopathic properties.

[i]Glycosylation.

[j]Cellular combination.

[k]Syncytium construction.

[l]Binding.

*$IC_{50}$, $EC_{50}$, $ED_{50}$ data are not available [5, 15, 70].

## 2.3   SELECTED PLANT-BASED SECONDARY METABOLITES AGAINST HIV

Several anti-HIV plant-based biocompounds (Figure 2.2) are calanolides that are also known as coumarins, betulinic acid (which is a triterpene), baicalin (a type of flavonoid), polycitone-A (a type of Alkaloid), lithospermic acid (with polyphenolic group). Withanolides (steroidal lactones: Figure 2.2) are therapeutic agents related to HAND [70].

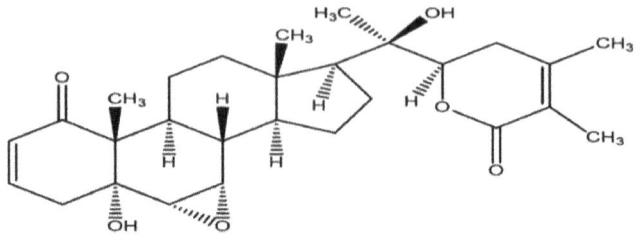

**FIGURE 2.2**   Chemical structure of Withanolide A.

## 2.3.1   COUMARINS

Calanolides, type of coumarin, exhibit its NNRTIs pursuit hostile to viruses. These are extracted from *Calophyllum lanigerum* species (Clusiaceae family) [42]. Calanolide-A (Figure 2.3: derivative of (7,8-dihydrocalanolide-B)) and Calanolide-B have capability to avert cytopathogenic response of HIV-1 in host cells. Cordatolide A and B from *Calophyllum cordato-oblongum* have some similarity in their structure with Calanolides and also have potential to impede HIV-1 replication [79]. The Suksdorfin (a pyro-coumarin derivative) is extracted from fruits of *Angelica morii* and *Lomatium suksdorfii* (both belong to apiaceae family) [51] and it also demonstrates some inhibitory effects on the viral replication in T-cell lines.

## 2.3.2   TERPENES

Few triterpenoids also exhibit antiretroviral activity by diverse mechanisms of action. Examples are betulinic acid (Figure 2.3), platanic acid along with oleanolic acid.

All these are extracted from leaves of *Syzigium claviflorum*; and have revealed activities against HIV and veteran upon H9 lymphocyte cells [77], where HIV-1 replication got inhibited with oleanolic acid that was extracted from *Xanthoceras sorbifolia* [36]. Maslinic acid from *Geum japonicum* has an operative inhibitory action counter to HIV-1 protease [64].

Celasdin B is extracted from *Celastru shindsii* and it has shown its bioactivity against HIV replication inside H9 cells [44]. Protostanes A and C (types of garcisa terpenes) can be extracted with ethyl acetate from stems and bark of *Garcinia speciose* and these can bottle up HIV-1 RTase activity [11].

Lanostane-type triterpene is a suberosol that can be obtained from leaves and stems of *Polyalthia suberosa*; and it has exhibited inhibitory activity on HIV replication in H9 cells. Triterpene lactone (lanci lactone C extracted from roots and stems of *Kadsuralancilimba*) may restrain HIV replication in veteran cells [50]. TPA (12-*O*-tetra-decanoylphorbol-13-acetate) is a phorboldi ester and is obtained with methanolic extract from *Croton tiglium*; and it shows inhibitory activity on cytopathogenic effects of HIV-1. Prostratin (phorbol ester, which is obtained from *Homalanthus nutans*) also exhibits anti-HIV properties.

### 2.3.3  FLAVONOIDS

Flavonoids also show anti-HIV activities besides other medicinal applications, such as antioxidant effects. Baicalin (Figure 2.3: it is extracted from *Scutellaria baicalensis*) is a flavonoid showing activity against HIV replication process and decelerating duplication of HIV in PBMC.

The 6,8-diprenylaromadendrin and 6,8-diprenylkaempferol (both prenylate flavonoids) are extracted from *Monotes Africanus* and both exhibit anti-HIV action during XTT-based, whole-cell assessment. The gallate ester is obtained from *Acer okamotoanum* and it retards the progression of integrase enzyme of HIV-1 [39]. Methanolic extracts obtained from leaves and twigs of *Rhus succedanea* comprise of some polymerase inhibitors of HIV-1 that are named as Hinokiflavone, robustaflavone, and bioflavonoids [44]. Biflavonoid (e.g., Wikstrol-B) is extracted from roots of *Wikstroemia indica* and it also reveals activity against HIV **[77]**. A prenylchalcone (named as *Xanthohumol*) is extracted from hops of *Humulus lupulus,* and it demonstrates inhibitory action against HIV-1 replication [45, 74].

### 2.3.4  ALKALOIDS

Numerous alkaloids are effective against HIV progression through several mechanisms. For example, Polycitone A is extracted from marine ascidians showing effects against reverse transcription process of HIV virus, RNA-, and DNA-guided DNA polymerases [45]. Papaverine decelerated the duplication process of HIV virion through *Papaver sominiferum*. Quinolone (is also called *Buchapine*) is obtained from *Eodia roxburghiana* and it demonstrates inhibitory effects against cytopathogenic parameters of HIV-1 [49]. Nitidine is obtained from roots of *Toddalia asiatica* and it is effective against HIV. A piperidine flavone (it is an associated alkaloid named as *O*-demethyl-buchenavianine) is extracted from *Buchenavia capitata* and it impedes normal activity of HIV [6]. Harmine is obtained from *Symplocos setchuensis* and it hinders the normal replication process of HIV inside H9 cells [34]. Some anti-HIV activities have also been shown by 1-methoxy canthionone that is attained from *Leitneria floridana* [76]. Sesquiterpene pyridine alkaloids (such as *Hypoglaumine B, Troponine B,* and *Troponine A*) can be extracted from *Tripterygium wilfordii* and *Tripterygium hypoglaucum*; and these demonstrate specific anti-HIV properties [19].

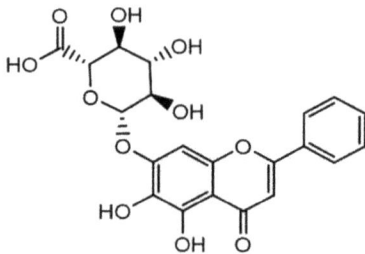

Baicalin

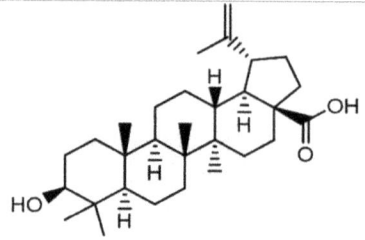

Betullinic acid

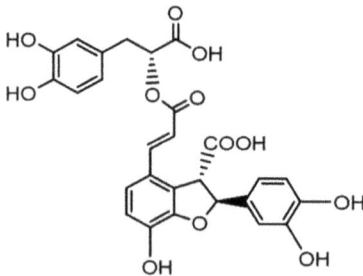

Polycitone A

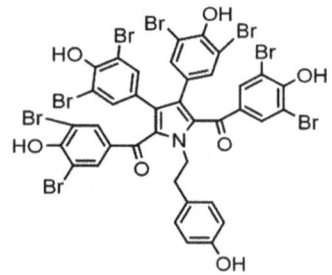

Lithospermic Acid

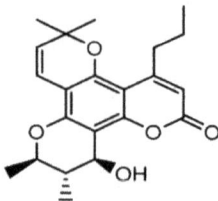

Calanolide A

**FIGURE 2.3**    Plant-based anti-HIV secondary metabolites.

### 2.3.5   PHENOLICS

Lymphocytic propagation is persuaded through phyto haemagglutinin-induction and prolonged supervision of polyphenol-rich fruit juices, which revealed bioactivities against HIV-positive patients. The annins and subsequent phenolic derivatives have also shown virucidal impression within numerous viral organizations, such as, Lithospermic acid (Figure 2.3), which is extracted *Salvia miltiorrhiza*; and this acid has been effective against HIV when subjected to H9 cells [1]. Punicalagin, chebulagic acid, and punicalin have shown hydrolyzing properties and all three compounds can be obtained by *Terminalia chebula* showing their anti-HIV activities [44]. Repandusinic acid is extracted from *Phyllanthus niruri* and it demonstrates inhibitory activity against HIV-1 RTase [59].

Monopotassium along with monosodium salts are isomeric caffeic acid tetramer that can be extracted with aqueous acetone from *Arnebia euchroma* demonstrating inhibitory action on replication process of HIV [35, 36, 75]. *Camellia*-tannin H extracts from *Camellia japonica* demonstrate inhibitory action against HIV-1 protease. Galloyl glucoses and gallic acid can be obtained from *Terminalia chebula* and these unveiled an impediment on HIV integrase [1]. Mallotojaponin is extracted from pericarps of *Mallotus japonicus* and it impedes HIV-1 RTase activity. Curcuminoids are obtained from rhizomes of *Curcuma longa* demonstrating inhibitory action against protease of HIV-1 and HIV-2. Peltatol A (prenylated catechol dimer) can be obtained from *Pothomorphe peltata* and has shown activity against HIV replication process [32].

### 2.3.6   LIGNANS

Antiviral activities have also been demonstrated by numerous lignans [10]. For example, Phyllamyricin B (along with its lactone such as retro justicidin B) can be isolated from *Phyllanthus myrtifolius*/and *P. urinaria* and these exhibit inhibitory action on HIV-RTase. Type A and B of Anolignan and dibenzylbutadiene lignans are extracted from *Anogeissus acuminata* and these display inhibitory activity on HIV-1 RTase [63]. Strongest inhibitor of HIV replication among lignans is Gomisin, which is obtained from *Kadsura interior* [11].

### 2.3.7   QUINONES

HIV inhibitory effects have also been manifested by naphthoquinones (such as Plumbagin, 1–4-naphthoquinone, juglone) and vitamin K3 [51]. Moreover, a trimeric naphthoquinone (named *Conocurvone*) has depicted impressive anti-HIV action and it can be extracted from *Conospermum incurvum*.

### 2.3.8 SAPONINS

Robust anti-HIV action has been illustrated by Actein, which is a tetracyclic triterpenoid saponin that is obtained from rhizomes of *Cimicifuga racemosa* (black cohosh).

## 2.4 PHYTOCOMPOUNDS THAT PROMOTE HAND

HIV/AIDS can often enter the nervous system, where contaminated white-blood cells drift a semipermeable membrane separating the blood from the cere-brospinal fluid via "Trojan horse" mechanism for prospective viral ingression. Subsequently, contaminated monocytes emigrate and traverse the endothe-lium, where all reconcile as contaminated perivascular macrophages. Finally, the viral escalation leads through cell-to-cell interplay between microglia cells and macrophages [38]. Multinucleated prodigious cells (fused microglia cells) and macrophages are responsible for the sustenance of viral replication in the brain [37]. A protean spurt is fortified inside the brain along with intermittent subjection that leads to fervid viral replication within microglia. The building blocks of brain tissues, where viral proteins are free-spirited, are the locus of production of cytokines, chemokines, along with various inflammation stimulating factors that in turn are result of stimulation of astrocytes and microglia [2, 58]. Viral proteins are exonerating and additionally galvanized through specific cell-encoded markers, which encourage the escalation of HIV replication within microglia cells resulting in neuronal dysfunction as well as neuronal damage. Although factors are collectively approachable besides HIV infection, yet an idiosyncratic neuropathological moniker has been noticed. Observed pathological amendments are customarily minor along with incon-sistency, lastly resulting in HAND [68]. Several investigations have proposed that accompanying risk factors of this disarray in patients of HIV and spot this disorder in a fewer cases. Prominent HIV plasma viral load [8, 17, 71] is associated with neurocognitive impairment count [28, 69]. HIV-positive individuals also express shorting of telomeric length [46, 60], which acts as a biomarker for aging. This telomeric shorting induces neurocognitive impair-ment along with the recurrence of dementia. This situation is worse as serious cognitive decline is related to the age factor [72].

## 2.5  HAND: INFLAMMATION AND HIV NEUROTOXICITY

Although dynamic inflammation has not been observed constantly in HAND, yet it is predominant near the initial phase of disease progression. Extensive spectrum neuropathological studies about HAND by Navia *et al.* [56] are summarized as "There was extended paleness with in white matter, which then extends to lymphocytes along with coffee-colored histiocyte and ultimately sophisticate distances via clumps formed by foamy macrophages and multinucleated cells allied in the midst of multifocal rarefaction belonging to white matter. The CNS system in the brain is also severely affected by HIV infection. Nevertheless, in about 33% of cases of dementia, the histopathological investigation remains devoid of clinical dysfunction of brain."

In the patient on combination antiretroviral therapy (cART) treatment, pathological studies do not always support the recurrence of paleness in brain tissues. However, very minute changes toward neuro-dyenation can be noticed, which augments severity in older population having long history of infection [9, 43, 67]. Stimulated circulating monocytes play a vital role, mutually intended for insertion of HIV inside head through means of drifting beyond blood–brain barrier as a result of chemo approach indication shuttered as long as the parenchyma and successive setting up of inflammation inside CNS perivascular macrophages [24, 26, 43], microglia [66] and astrocytes [13]. Despite the fact astrocytes do not appear killed by yielding integral virions beneath ordinary circumstances; however, they are able to generate along with nonstructural proteins carrying tat *Rev*, including *Nef* due to these infections and spoilage of nerve cells [12, 62].

A question still remains unanswered: why does CNS infection remain constant even after the maiden induction of viral reconstructions is obscured by CART [61, 73]. It is hypothesized that the inflammatory responses originated by HIV lead the proteasome to turn out to be an immune proteasome, which blocks conveyance of bend proteins inside the nerve cells that changes cellular stability and retorts toward strain [57] thus aiding to HAND. Another argument regarding constant CNS infection is glial cells that are derived from moving microorganism translocation production resulting due to gut bacilli and a troubled microbiome [23]. It is recommended that the CNS infection in CART-medicated folks can diminish the configuration toward immune re-formation infection disorder [22]. The work of genetic control in response to inflammations, predominantly, gene encoding with CCL3L1 and CCR5 (named polymorphisms) has been documented to elucidate the distinct eroticism during progression of HAND, in addition to incidence connected with HAND in HIV+ folks [27].

## 2.6   HAND AND ART

HAND deals for the neurological disorders associated with HIV infections, which are found in HIV patients [56]. Brain perivascular macrophages show vital character for incursion and reconstruction of HIV in innate neurological tissues; and infected neurological cells can start progress of disease based on nervous system like HAND [67].

Activation of cellular component of immune system of residentglia and swelling in neuronal cells are linked through this disease. The ART helps to completely diminish the effect of serious stage of HAND [9, 14], yet associated infections persist at high level. The main reason behind the severe infection of HAND is the HIV reconstruction and increase of swelling in CNS [4, 7, 18, 26].

Auxiliary effect of aging can enhance the nerve cell damage that is related with HAND. The relocation of triggered monocytes, complete stimulation of immune responses along with misapplication of drugs are subsidiary impacts of growing older that can be enhanced due to damages occurring in neuronal tissues continuously under conditions of HAND and may endure in spite of proper application of effective ART [24].

Active regeneration of damaged nervous system is known as neuroprotection. It can reverse the fundamental activation of cellular components of immune system and combined swelling within brain [6, 12, 13, 62]. The neuroprotection against HAND can be facilitated by the use of medicine that interferes with cellular pathways involved CNS. Hence the effect of ART neurotoxicity can be minimized by using effective CNS penetrating HIV drugs.

## 2.7   SUMMARY

Natural products have been used for the treatment of several syndromes together with HIV and other neurological disorders. Many plant-based phytocompounds are highly effective to treat HIV patients. There is an urgent need to come up with new anti-HIV medicines with minimum side effects, minimum toxicity, and minimum conflict, and with innovative way of action. This chapter serves as a repository of information on plant products.

Before the formation of any new anti-HIV drug candidate, we must carefully evaluate its side effects, toxicity and conflict. However, reasonable survey of natural products against HIV/AIDS and well-designed scrutiny process must be adopted before entering into clinical trials and subsequent steps of drug formulation.

## KEYWORDS

- **acquired immunodeficiency syndrome**
- **AIDS-associated dementia**
- **antiretroviral therapy**
- **fusion inhibitors**
- **HIV-associated neurocognitive disorders**
- **nucleoside reverse transcriptase inhibitors**
- **reverse transcriptase**
- **telomere length**

## REFERENCES

1. Abd-Elazem, I.S.; Chen, H.S.; Bates, R.B.; Huang, R.C.C. Isolation of two highly potent and non-toxic inhibitors of HIV-1 integrase from *Salvia miltiorrhiza*. *Antiviral Res.*, 2002, *55*(1), 91–106.
2. Achim, C.L.; Wiley, C.A. Inflammation in AIDS and role of macrophage in brain pathology. *Curr. Opin. Neurol.*, 1996, *9* (3), 221–225.
3. Adle-Biassette, H.; Levy, Y.; Colornbel, M.; Poron, F.;Natchev, S.; Keohane, C.; Gray, F. Neuronal apoptosis in HIV infection in adults. *Neuropathol. Appl. Neurobiol.*, 1995, *21* (3), 218–227.
4. Ancuta, P.;Kamat, A.; Kunstman, K.J.; Kim, E.Y.; Autissier, P.; Wurcel, A., Singer, E. J. Microbial translocation is associated with increased monocyte activation and dementia in AIDS patients. *PLOS One*, 2008, *3* (6), e2516.
5. Antinori, A.; Arendt, G.; Becker, J.T.; Brew, B.J.; Byrd, D.A.; Cherner, M.; Gisslen, M. Updated research nosology for HIV-associated neurocognitive disorders (HAND). *Neurology*, 2007, *69* (18), 1789–1799.
6. Beutler, J.A.; Cardellina, J.H.; McMahon, J.B.; Boyd, M.R.; Cragg, G.M. Anti-HIV and cytotoxic alkaloids from *Buchenavia capitata*. *J. Nat. Prod.*, 1992, *55* (2), 207–213.
7. Brown, A. Understanding the MIND phenotype: macrophage/microglia inflammation in neurocognitive disorders related to HIV infection. *Clin. Transl. Med.*, 2015, *4* (1), 7–11.

8. Chang, L.; Ernst, T.; Witt, M.D.; Ames, N.; Gaiefsky, M.; Miller, E. Relationships among brain metabolites, cognitive function and viral loads in anti-retroviral-naıve HIV patients. *Neuroimage*, 2002, *17* (3), 1638–1648.

9. Chang, L.; Wong, V.; Nakama, H.; Watters, M.; Ramones, D.; Miller, E.N.; Ernst, T. Greater than age-related changes in brain diffusion of HIV patients after one year. *J. Neuroimmune Pharmacol*, 2008, *3* (4), 265–274.

10. Charlton, J.L. Antiviral activity of lignans. *J. Nat. Prod.*, 1998, *61* (11), 1447–1451.

11. Chen, D.F.; Zhang, S.X.; Wang, H.K.; Zhang, S.Y.; Sun, Q.Z.; Cosentino, L.M.; Lee, K.H. Novel anti-HIV lancilactone C and related triterpenes from *Kadsura lancilimba*. *J. Nat. Prod.*, 1999, *62* (1), 94–97.

12. Chompre, G.; Cruz, E.; Maldonado, L.; Rivera-Amill, V.; Porter, J.T.; Noel Jr, R.J. Astrocytic expression of HIV-1 Nef impairs spatial and recognition memory. *Neurobiol. Dis.*, 2013, *49*, 128–136.

13. Churchill, M.J.; Wesselingh, S.L.; Cowley, D.; Pardo, C.A.; McArthur, J.C.; Brew, B.J.; Gorry, P.R. Extensive astrocyte infection is prominent in HIV-associated dementia. *Annals Neurol.*, 2009, *66* (2), 253–258.

14. Coffin, J.M. HIV population dynamics *in vivo*: implications for genetic variation, pathogenesis and therapy. *Science*, 1995, *267* (5197), 483–489.

15. Cos, P.; Maes, L.; VandenBerghe, D.; Hermans, N.; Pieters, L.; Vlietinck, A. Plant Substances as anti-HIV agents selected according to their putative mechanism of action. *J. Nat. Prod.*, 2004, *67* (2), 284–293.

16. De-Clercq, E.R.I.K. Antiviral therapy for HIV infections. *Clin. Microbiol. Rev.*, 1995, *8* (2), 200–239.

17. Devlin, K.N.; Gongvatana, A.; Clark, U.S.; Chasman, J.D.; Westbrook, M.L.; Tashima, K.T.; Cohen, R.A. Neurocognitive effects of HIV, hepatitis C, and substance use history. *J. Int. Neuropsychol. Soc.*, 2012, *18* (1), 68–78.

18. Dharmaratne, H.R.W.; Tan, G.T.; Marasinghe, G.P.K.; Pezzuto, J.M. Inhibition of HIV-1 reverse transcriptase and HIV-1 replication by calophyllum coumarins and xanthones. *Planta Medica*, 2010, *68* (1), 86–87.

19. Duan, H.; Takaishi, Y.; Imakura, Y.;Jia, Y.; Li, D.; Cosentino, L.M.; Lee, K.H. Sesquiterpene alkaloids from *Tripterygium Hypoglaucum* and *Tripterygium Wilfordii*: new class of potent anti-HIV agents. *J. Nat. Prod.*, 2000, *63* (3), 357–361.

20. Ellis, R.J.; Badiee, J.; Vaida, F.; Letendre, S.; Heaton, R.K.; Clifford, D; McCutchan, J.A. CD4 nadir is a predictor of HIV neurocognitive impairment in the era of combination antiretroviral therapy. *AIDS (London, England)*, 2011, *25* (14), 112–118.

21. Ellis, R. Langford, D.; Masliah, E. HIV and antiretroviral therapy in brain: neuronal injury and repair. *Nat. Rev. Neurosci.*, 2007, *8* (1), 33–36.

22. Fauci, A.S.; Marston, H.D. Ending HIV-AIDS pandemic: follow the science. *New Engl. J. Med.*, 2015, *373* (23), 2197–2199.

23. Ferrington, D.A.; Gregerson, D.S. Immunoproteasomes: structure, function, and antigen presentation. In: *Progress in Molecular Biology and Translational Science*; New York: Academic Press; 2012; Vol. 109; pp. 75–112.

24. Fischer-Smith, T.; Bell, C.; Croul, S.; Lewis, M.; Rappaport, J. Monocyte/macrophage trafficking in acquired immunodeficiency syndrome encephalitis: lessons from human and nonhuman primate studies. *J. Neurovirol.*, 2008, *14* (4), 318–326.

25. Gannon, P.; Khan, M.Z.; Kolson, D.L. Current understanding of HIV-associated neurocognitive disorders (HAND) pathogenesis. *Curr. Opin. Neurol.*, 2011, *24* (3), 275–280.

26. Gelman, I.H.; Zhang, J.; Hailman, E.; Hanafusa, H.; Morse, S.S. Identification and evaluation of new primer sets for detection of lenti-virus-proviral DNA. *AIDS Res. Hum. Retrovir.*, 1992, *8* (12), 1981–1989.

27. Gonzalez, E.; Kulkarni, H.; Bolivar, H.; Mangano, A.; Sanchez, R.; Catano, G.; Murthy, K. K. The influence of CCL3L1 gene-containing segmental duplications on HIV-1/AIDS susceptibility. *Science*, 2005, *307* (5714), 1434–1440.

28. Gonzalez, R.; Heaton, R.K.; Moore, D.J.; Letendre, S.; Ellis, R.J.; Wolfson, T. Computerized reaction time battery versus traditional neuropsychological battery: detecting HIV-related Impairments. *J. Int. Neuropsychol. Soc.*, 2003, *9* (1), 64–71.

29. González-Scarano, F.; Martín-García, J. The neuro pathogenesis of AIDS. *Nat. Rev. Immunol.*, 2005, *5* (1), 69–72.

30. Gray, F.; Adle-Biassette, H.; Chretien, F.; de la GrandmaisonLorin, G.; Force, G.; Keohane, C. Neuropathology and neurodegeneration in HIV infection: pathogenesis of HIV-induced lesions of the brain, correlations with HIV-associated disorders and modifications according to treatments. *Clin. Neuropathol.*, 2001, *20* (4), 146–155.

31. Grovit-Ferbas, K.; Harris-White, M.E. Thinking about HIV: the intersection of virus, neuro inflammation and cognitive dysfunction. *Immunol. Res.*, 2010, *48* (1–3), 40–58.

32. Gustafson, K.R.; Cardellina, J.H.; McMahon, J.B.; Pannell, L.K.; Cragg, G.M.; Boyd, M.R. HIV inhibitory natural products: peltatols. *J. Org. Chem.*, 1992, *57* (10), 2809–2811.

33. Heaton, R.K.; Franklin, D.R.; Ellis, R.J.; McCutchan, J.A.; Letendre, S.L.; LeBlanc, S.; Collier, A.C. HIV-associated neurocognitive disorders before and during the era of combination antiretroviral therapy: differences in rates, nature, and predictors. *J. Neurovirol.*, 2011, *17* (1), 3–16.

34. Ishida, J.; Wang, H.K.; Oyama, M.; Cosentino, M.L.; Hu, C.Q.; Lee, K.H. Anti-HIV Principle from *Symplocos Setchuensis* and its derivatives. *J. Nat. Prod.*, 2001, *64* (7), 958–960.

35. Jung, M.; Lee, S.; Kim, H. Recent studies on natural products as anti-HIV agents. *Curr. Med. Chem.*, 2000, *7* (6), 649–661.

36. Kashiwada, Y.; Wang, H.K.; Nagao, T.; Kitanaka, S.; Yasuda, I.; Fujioka, T.; Ikeshiro, Y. Anti-HIV activity of oleanolic acid, pomolic acid, and structurally related triterpenoids. *J. Nat. Prod.*, 1998, *61* (9), 1090–1095.

37. Kaul, M. HIV-1 associated dementia: update on pathological mechanisms and therapeutic approaches. *Curr. Opin. Neurol.*, 2009, *22* (3), 315–318.

38. Kaul, M.; Garden, G.A.; Lipton, S.A. Pathways to neuronal injury and apoptosis in HIV-associated dementia. *Nature*, 2001, *410* (6831), 988–992.

39. Kim, H.J.; Yu, Y.G.; Park, H.; Lee, Y.S. HIV gp41 binding phenolic components from *Fraxinus Sieboldiana* var. Angustata. *Planta Medica*, 2002, *68* (11), 1034–1036.

40. Kraft-Terry, S.D.; Buch, S.J.; Fox, H.S.; Gendelman, H.E. Neuroimmune crosstalk in HIV infection. *Neuron*, 2009, *64* (1), 133–145.

41. Kurapati, K.R.V.; Atluri, V.S.; Samikkannu, T.; Garcia, G.; Nair, M.P. Natural products as anti-HIV agents and role in HAND). *Front. Microbiol.*, 2016, *6*, 1444.

42. Lee-Huang, S.; Huang, P.L.; Chen, H.C.; Huang, P.L.;Bourinbaiar, A.; Huang, H.I.; Kung, H.F. Anti-HIV and anti-tumor activities of recombinant MAP30 from bitter melon. *Gene*, 1995, *161* (2), 151–156.

43. Lentz, M.R.; Peterson, K.L.; Ibrahim, W.G.; Lee, D.E.; Sarlls, J.; Lizak, M.J.; Hammoud, D. A. Diffusion tensor and volumetric magnetic resonance measures as biomarkers of brain damage in small animal model of HIV. *PLOS One*, 2014, *9* (8), e105752.

44. Lim, Y.A.; Mei, M.C.; Kusumoto, I.T.; Miyashiro, H.; Hattori, M.; Gupta, M.P.; Correa, M. HIV-1 reverse transcriptase inhibitory principles from *Chamaesyce hyssop Ifolia. Phytoth. Res.*, 1997, *11* (1), 22–27.
45. Loya, S.; Rudi, A.; Kashman, Y.;Hizi, A. Polycitone: novel and potent general inhibitor of retroviral reverse transcriptases and cellular DNA polymerases. *Biochem. J.*, 1999, *344* (Part-1), 85–90.
46. Malan-Müller, S.; Hemmings, S.M.J.; Spies, G. Correction: shorter telomere length-a potential susceptibility factor for HIV-associated neurocognitive impairments in South African women. *PLOS One*, 2013, *8* (4), 101371; https://doi.org/10.1371/annotation/53ec3c1c-3247–452d-85c7–576fb35bdbe3;
47. Matthée, G.; Wright, A.D.; König, G.M. HIV reverse transcriptase inhibitors of natural origin. *Planta Medica*, 1999, *65* (6), 493–506.
48. McArthur, J.C.; Steiner, J.; Sack tor, N.; Nath, A. HIV-associated neurocognitive disorders: mind the gap. *Annals Neurol.*, 2010, *67* (6), 699–714.
49. McCormick, J.L.; McKee, T.C.; Cardellina, J.H.; Boyd, M.R. HIV inhibitory natural products: quinoline alkaloids from *Euodia Roxburghiana. J. Nat. Prod.*, 1996, *59* (5), 469–471.
50. Meragelman, K.M.; McKee, T.C.; Boyd, M.R. Anti-HIV prenylated flavonoids from *Monotes Africanus. J. Nat. Prod.*, 2001, *64* (4), 546–548.
51. Min, B.S.; Miyashiro, H.; Hattori, M. Inhibitory effects of quinones on RNase H-activity associated with HIV-1 reverse transcriptase. *Phytoth. Res.*, 2002, *16* (S1), 57–62.
52. Mocroft, A.; Lundgren, J.D. Starting highly active antiretroviral therapy: why, when and response to HAART. *J. Antimicrob. Chemoth.*, 2004, *54* (1), 10–13.
53. Montessori, V.; Press, N.; Harris, M.; Akagi, L.; Montaner, J.S. Adverse effects of antiretroviral therapy for HIV infection. *Can. Med. Assoc. J.*, 2004, *170* (2), 229–238.
54. Muñoz-Moreno, J.A.; Fumaz, C.R.; Ferrer, M.J. Nadir CD4 cell count predicts neurocognitive impairment in HIV-infected patients. *AIDS Res. Human Retrovir.*, 2008, *24* (10), 1301–1307.
55. Nath, A.; Schiess, N.; Venkatesan, A.; Rumbaugh, J. Evolution of HIV dementia with HIV infection. *Int. Rev. Psych.*, 2008, *20* (1), 25–31.
56. Navia, B.A.; Cho, E.S.; Petito, C.K.; Price, R.W. AIDS dementia complex, II: neuropathology. *Annals Neurol.*, 1986, *19* (6), 525–535.
57. Nguyen, T.P.; Soukup, V.M.; Gelman, B.B. Persistent hijacking of brain proteasomes in HIV-associated Dementia. *Am. J. Pathol.*, 2010, *176* (2), 893–902.
58. Nottet, H.S.; Gendelman, H.E. Unraveling the neuroimmune mechanisms for the HIV-1-associated cognitive/motor complex. *Immunol. Today*, 1995, *16* (9), 441–448.
59. Ogata, T.; Higuchi, H.; Mochida, S.; Matsumoto, H.; Kato, A.; Endo, T.; Kaji, H. HIV-1 reverse transcriptase inhibitor from *Phyllanthus niruri. AIDS Res. Human Retrovir.*, 1992, *8* (11), 1937–1944.
60. Paul, R.; Flanigan, T.P.; Tashima, K.; Cohen, R.; Lawrence, J.; Alt, E.; Hinkin, C. Apathy correlates with cognitive function but not CD4 status in patients with HIV. *J. Neuropsych. Clin. Neurosci.*, 2005, *17* (1), 114–118.
61. Peluso, M.J.; Meyerhoff, D.J.; Price, R.W.; Peterson, J.; Lee, E.; Young, A.C.; Robertson, K. Cerebrospinal fluid and neuroimaging biomarker abnormalities suggest early neurological injury in subset of individuals during primary HIV Infection. *J. Infect. Dis.*, 2013, *207* (11), 1703–1712.

62. Pu, H.; Tian, J.; Flora, G.; Lee, Y.W.; Nath, A.; Hennig, B.;Toborek, M. HIV-1 Tat protein upregulates inflammatory mediators and induces monocyte invasion into the brain. *Mol. Cell. Neurosci.*, 2003, *24* (1), 224–237.

63. Rimando, A.M.; Pezzuto, J.M.; Farnsworth, N.R.; Santisuk, T.; Reutrakul, V.; Kawanishi, K. New lignans from *Anogeissusacuminata* with HIV-1 reverse transcriptase inhibitory activity. *J. Nat. Prod.*, 1994, *57* (7), 896–904.

64. Rukachaisirikul, V.; Pailee, P.; Hiranrat, A. Anti-HIV-1 protostanetri terpenes and di-geranyl-benzophenone from trunk bark and stems of *Garcinia speciosa*. *Planta Medica*, 2003, *69* (12), 1141–1146.

65. Satishchandra, P.; Nalini, A.; Gourie-Devi, M.; Khanna, N. Profile of neurologic disorder associated with HIV/AIDS from Bangalore, India (1989–96). *Ind. J. Med. Res.*, 2000, *111*, 14–20.

66. Schuenke, K.; Gelman, B.B. Human microglial cell isolation from adult autopsy brain: brain pH, regional variation, and infection with HIV-1. *J. Neurovirol.*, 2003, *9* (3), 346–357.

67. Seider, T.R.; Gongvatana, A.; Woods, A.J. Age exacerbates HIV-associated white matter abnormalities. *J. Neurovirol.*, 2016, *22* (2), 201–212.

68. Sharer, L.R. Pathology of HIV-1 infection of the central nervous system. *J. Neuropathol. Exper. Neurol.*, 1992, *51* (1), 3–11.

69. Simioni, S.; Cavassini, M.; Annoni, J.M.; Abraham, A.R.; Bourquin, I.; Schiffer, V.; Du Pasquier, R.A. Cognitive dysfunction in HIV patients despite long-standing suppression of viremia. *AIDS*, 2010, *24* (9), 1243–1250.

70. Singh, I.P.; Bharate, S.B.; Bhutani, K.K. Anti-HIV natural products. *Curr. Sci.*, 2005, *2005*, 269–290.

71. Tozzi, V.; Balestra, P.; Galgani, S.;Narciso, P.; Ferri, F.; Sebastiani, G.; De Felici, A. Positive and sustained effects of highly active antiretroviral therapy on HIV-1 associated neurocognitive impairment. *AIDS*, 1999, *13* (14), 1889–1897.

72. Valdes, A.M.; Deary, I.J.; Gardner, J.; Kimura, M. Leukocyte telomere length is associated with cognitive performance in healthy women. *Neurobiol. Aging*, 2010, *31* (6), 986–992.

73. Van Marle, G.; Henry, S.; Todoruk, T.; Sullivan, A.; Silva, C.; Rourke, S.B.; Power, C. HIV-1 Nef protein mediates neural cell death: neurotoxic role. *Virology*, 2004, *329* (2), 302–318.

74. Vitiello, B.; Goodkin, K.; Ashtana, D.;Shapshak, P.; Atkinson, J.H.; Heseltine, P.N.; Lyman, W.D. HIV-1 RNA concentration and cognitive performance in cohort of HIV-positive people. *AIDS*, 2007, *21* (11), 1415–1422.

75. Wadia, R.S.; Pujari, S.N.; Kothari, S. Neurological manifestations of HIV disease. *J. Assoc. Phys. India*, 2001, *49*, 343–348.

76. Xu, H.X.; Wan, M.; Dong, H.; BuT, P.P.H.; Foo, L.Y. Inhibitory activity of flavonoids and tannins against HIV-1 protease. *Biol. Pharm. Bull.*, 2000, *23* (9), 1072–1076.

77. Xu, Z.; Chang, F.R.; Wang, H.K.; Kashiwada, Y.;McPhail, A.T.; Bastow, K.F.; Lee, K.H. Anti-HIV and antitumor agents; two new sesquiterpenes, leitneridanins A and B, and cytotoxic and anti-HIV principles from *Leitneria floridana*. *J. Nat. Prod.*, 2000, *63* (12), 1712–1715.

78. Yang, S.S.; Cragg, G.M.; Newman, D.J.; Bader, J.P. Natural product-based anti-HIV drug discovery and development facilitated by NCI developmental therapeutics program. *J. Nat. Prod.*, 2001, *64* (2), 265–277.

79. Zhou, P.; Takaishi, Y.; Duan, H.; Chen, B.; Honda, G.; Itoh, M.; Lee, K.H. Coumarins and bicoumarin from *Ferula sumbul*: anti-HIV activity and inhibition of cytokine release. *Phytochemistry*, 2000, *53* (6), 689–697.

# CHAPTER 3

# TRITERPENOIDS FROM *GYMNEMA SYLVESTRE* R.BR. (PERIPLOCA OF THE WOODS): BIOLOGICAL SIGNIFICANCE IN THE TREATMENT OF DIABETES

PRAGYA TIWARI*

## ABSTRACT

Diabetes is a devastating metabolic disorder causing socioeconomic concerns. Extensive research studies on bioactive molecules for their pharmacological significance have been attempted. *Gymnema sylvestre* R. Br. (Hindi: gurmar) has been studied for its triterpenoids (known as Gymnemic acids analogs) and polypeptide Gurmarin, which is gaining immense popularity as herbal medication for treatment of Type-II diabetes. The herb exhibits physiological properties ranging from regulation of blood sugar levels, control sugar cravings, and regeneration of pancreas. This chapter provides a comprehensive insight on the significance of triterpenoids from *G. sylvestre* R. Br., their potential mechanism of action in the treatment of diabetes, and its prospects and challenges in diabetes therapy.

## 3.1 INTRODUCTION

The rising frequency of diabetes is imposing a major threat and alarming concerns worldwide. The present era has witnessed the prevalence of diabetes in low- and middle-income population, and has been attributed as a major cause of heart attacks, blindness, kidney failure, and so forth [73]. The National Diabetes Statistics Report of 2017 suggested that 84.1 million American adults showed prediabetic conditions [www.cdc.gov/features/

---

*Corresponding author. E-mail: priyatiwari9452@gmail.com.

diabetes-statistic-report], while 30.3 million Americans are affected from the disease. Type-II form of the disease constitutes 90% of the cases [20].

With the alarming rise in the prevalence of diseases, naturopathic medication is being explored extensively by the researchers all over the world. The era of "herbal medicine" has been a revolution in the field of medicine, owing to safety and effectiveness as compared to commercially available drugs [22, 65].

Secondary metabolites in plant parts exhibiting antidiabetic properties demonstrate antihyperglycemic and hypoglycemic activities. Studies have suggested that pharmacological functions of a phytomolecule can be attributed to its structural organization and several bioactive constituents from plants, such as flavonoids, terpenoids, and saponins, which have been effective in reducing blood glucose levels [23]. Metformin (from *Galega officinalis*) is a naturopathic medication showing significant efficacy in the regulation of sugar levels in the blood of diabetic patients.

This chapter discusses the significance of triterpenoids from *Gymnema sylvestre* R. Br., its mechanism of action and prospects of development as "herbal medicine" in diabetes management.


## 3.2   AN OVERVIEW OF *G. SYLVESTRE* R.BR.

*G. sylvestre* R. Br. or Gurmar has been used as a naturopathic treatment for diabetes [43]. The plant belongs to the "milkweed family" and is a source of several bioactive substances [17, 51]. The plant's habitat suggests a warm tropical climate in southern parts of India, Malaysia, China, and so forth [19, 52, 57]. It is cultivated worldwide for its multiple therapeutic importance, ranging from diabetes, arthritis to cancer, and dental caries [60, 61]. The triterpenoids (such as Gymnemic acids, Gymnemasaponins, Deacylgymnemic acid, and Gymnemasins A to D) are key phytomolecules imparting sweet-suppression activity to the plant. *G. sylvestre* R. Br. in Indian subcontinent was traditionally used to treat "Honey urine".

Several techniques from commercial breeding to plant tissue culture have been employed for plant propagation due to poor germination [44]. In vitro techniques include in vitro regeneration through nodal explants [44], production of Gymnemic acids employing bioelicitors [11], mass multiplication [58], etc. (Table 3.1).

**TABLE 3.1** Summary of Methods for Growth and Multiplication of *G. sylvestre* R. Br. and In Vitro Production of Gymnemic Acids

| Explant | Method | Media Composition | Significance | Ref. |
|---|---|---|---|---|
| Callus culture | Callus induction and flavonoid detection | MS medium | Flavonoid detection | [69] |
| Callus culture | In vitro shoot morphogenesis | MS medium | Shoot bud sprouting and indirect plant regeneration | [21] |
| Callus cultures (leaf) | GA production through cell culture | MS medium | Production of GA | [24] |
| Cell suspension cultures | Suspension culture were employed for production of GA | MS medium | GA secretion | [42] |
| *G. sylvestre* suspension culture, *A. niger* extract | *A. niger* cell extract with suspension culture (elicited culture) | MS medium | GA production (high conc.) | [11] |
| Globular/heart-shaped embryos | Somatic embryogenesis | EM8 medium | Whole plant regeneration | [29] |
| Young leaf, stem and petiole | Callus induction and GA estimation | MS medium | Production of GA | [4] |
| Leaf explant | Callus induction and culture | MS medium | Production of GA | [12] |
| Leaf discs | Agrobacterium mediated Transformation | MS medium | Plant propagation through callus induction | [45] |
| Leaf explant | Somatic embryogenesis and plant regeneration | MS medium | Development of somatic embryogenesis system | [3] |
| Leaf explant | Induction and GA production in callus cultures | MS medium | GA production | [32] |

**TABLE 3.1**    *(Continued)*

| Explant | Method | Media Composition | Significance | Ref. |
|---------|--------|-------------------|--------------|------|
| Leaves | Production of Gymnemagenin from suspension culture | MS medium | Production of biomass and Gymnemagenin | [66] |
| Nodal cultures | Multiple shoot production | Half strength MS medium | Multiple shoot and GA production | [84] |
| Nodal explant | Micropropagation for shoot regeneration | MS medium | Plant propagation | [44] |
| Nodal explants (leaf discs) | Callus initiation and Micropropagation | MS medium | Initiation of callus, phytochemical screening | [37] |
| Plant twigs | Micropropagation | MS medium | Micropropagation of *G. sylvestre* R. Br. | [49] |
| Seedlings | In vitro propagation | MS medium | In vitro propagation | [10] |
| Nodal explant and leaf | The induction of multiple shoots from nodal segments | MS medium | Mass multiplication and callus induction | [58] |

## 3.3  PRESENCE OF PHYTOCONSTITUENTS

The plant family includes 40 species, namely *Gymnema yunnanense, Gymnema inodorum, Gymnema montanum*, etc., and has demonstrated medicinal properties [41, 50, 74]. Phytochemical studies suggested that the oleanane-type triterpenoids are Gymnemasaponins and Gymnemic acids, while Gymnemasides represents example of dammarane type structure [15, 26]. In addition, some other phytoconstituents (such as flavones, anthraquinones, phytin, resins, β-amyrin glycosides, stigmasterol, etc.) have also been found in the plant. Among the plant parts, shoot tips comprise of highest percentage of Gymnemic acids (54.29 mg $g^{-1}$ of dry weight) and least percentage is present in seed of the plant (1.31 mg $g^{-1}$ of dry weight). The triterpenoid structure of Gymnemic acids plays a significant, functional role in its activity showing that ester group in genin portion of the molecule is important for its antisweet activity.

The Gymnemic acid molecules confer antisweet property to the plant, thereby exhibit prospects as "lead molecules" in the drug designing for

Type-II diabetes. The secondary metabolites show variation in their chemical structure and are designated as Gymnemosides, Gymnemic acids, Gymnemasins A to D, Gymnemagenin, Deacylgymnemic acid, and various analogs, etc. Gurmarin (35 amino acid peptide) was isolated from the plant and its antisweet activity was shown electrophysiologically in rats [16]. Gymnemasins A to D are derivatives of Gymnemic acids and an important class of triterpenoids that were isolated from the leaves [56]. In addition, the plant also consists of different kinds of phytomolecules, such as gymnemanol, stigmasterol, anthraquinones, coumarols, lupeol, and hydroxycinnamic acids. A lupane-type triterpenoid was isolated from aerial tissues and the compound was named as (3β, 16β)-lupane-3,16,20,23,28-pentol [82].

Furthermore, four new pregnane glycosides (namely, Gymsylvestrosides A–D) were also identified from the stem [75]. The availability of plethora of bioactive compounds from plants, their identification, and experimental validation is enriching our knowledge and opening new avenues of the plant for diabetes treatment. Table 3.2 indicates Triterpenoids from *G. sylvestre* R. Br., chemical structure, and bioactive concentration of antidiabetic activity [61].

**TABLE 3.2** Triterpenoids from *G. sylvestre* R. Br. their Chemical Structure and Active Concentration of Antidiabetic Activity

| Phytomolecule with molecular structure | Active (antidiabetic) concentration | Ref. |
|---|---|---|
| Gymnemic acid I | 0.5 mM solution, active | [78] |

**TABLE 3.2** *(Continued)*

| Phytomolecule with molecular structure | Active (antidiabetic) concentration | Ref. |
|---|---|---|
| Gymnemic acid II | 0.5 mM solution, active | [78] |
| Gymnemic acid III | 1 mM solution, active | [78] |
| Gymnemic acid IV | 1 mM solution, active | [78] |

**TABLE 3.2** *(Continued)*

| Phytomolecule with molecular structure | Active (antidiabetic) concentration | Ref. |
|---|---|---|
| Gymnemic acid V | 1 mM solution, active | [77] |
| Gymnemic acid VI | 1 mM solution, active | [77] |
| Gymnemic acid VII | 1 mM solution, inactive | [77] |

**TABLE 3.2**   *(Continued)*

| Phytomolecule with molecular structure | Active (antidiabetic) concentration | Ref. |
|---|---|---|
| Gymnemic acid VIII | 0.5 mM solution, active | [80] |
| Gymnemic acid IX | 0.5 mM solution, active | [80] |
| Gymnemic acid X | 0.5 mM solution, active | [80] |

**TABLE 3.2**   *(Continued)*

| Phytomolecule with molecular structure | Active (antidiabetic) concentration | Ref. |
|---|---|---|
| Gymnemic acid XI | 0.5 mM solution, active | [80] |
| Gymnemic acid XII | 0.5 mM solution, active | [80] |
| Gymnemic acid XV | 0.5 mM solution, active | [81] |

**TABLE 3.2** *(Continued)*

| Phytomolecule with molecular structure | Active (antidiabetic) concentration | Ref. |
|---|---|---|
| Gymnemic acid XVI | 0.5 mM solution, active | [81] |
| | | |
| Gymnemic acid XVII | 0.5 mM solution, active | [81] |
| | | |
| Gymnemic acid XVIII | 0.5 mM solution, active | [81] |
| | | |

**TABLE 3.2** *(Continued)*

| Phytomolecule with molecular structure | Active (antidiabetic) concentration | Ref. |
|---|---|---|
| Gymnemasaponin I | 1 mM solution, inactive | [79] |
| Gymnemasaponin II | 1 mM solution, inactive | [79] |
| Gymnemasaponin III | 1 mM solution, active | [79] |

**TABLE 3.2**  *(Continued)*

| Phytomolecule with molecular structure | Active (antidiabetic) concentration | Ref. |
|---|---|---|
| Gymnemasaponin IV<br> | 1 mM solution, active | [79] |
| Gymnemasaponin V<br> | 1 mM solution, active | [79] |
| Gymnemagenin<br> | – | [54] |

**TABLE 3.2** *(Continued)*

| Phytomolecule with molecular structure | Active (antidiabetic) concentration | Ref. |
|---|---|---|
| 23-hydroxylongispinogenin | – | [2] |
| Gymnemoside I | – | [36] |
| Gymnemoside II | | [36] |

**TABLE 3.2**  *(Continued)*

| Phytomolecule with molecular structure | Active (antidiabetic) concentration | Ref. |
|---|---|---|
| Deacylgymnemic acid | | [6] |

| Dihydroxy gymnemic triacetate | 20 mg/kg | [8] |

| Gymnemoside-W1 | – | [83] |

**TABLE 3.2**  *(Continued)*

| Phytomolecule with molecular structure | Active (antidiabetic) concentration | Ref. |
|---|---|---|
| Gymnemoside-W2 | – | [83] |

## 3.4  BIOSYNTHESIS OF TRITERPENOIDS

Significant work has been attempted to investigate therapeutic significance of this plant. The phytomolecules demonstrating sweet-suppression activity were isolated and characterized via metabolic profiling and phytochemical analysis, but the biosynthetic mechanism of Gymnemic acid analogs in the plant was not reported (Figure 3.1). The structural elucidation of the phyto-molecules highlights that sugar chain is linked to sapogenin (aglycone part). Glycosylation of a sapogenin is critical in biological function, suggesting that glycosylation mechanism imparts antidiabetic activity to Gymnemic acid analogs [61]. These phytomolecules possess special significance in the naturopathic treatment of Type-II diabetes, therefore studies to delineate the biosynthetic mechanism of Gymnemic acid analogs highlight an important area of study. Gymnemic acid analogs were identified employing different plant metabolomic techniques (Figure 3.1).

Saponins comprise of steroidal aglycone or triterpenoids that are present in these plants [72] and demonstrate pharmacological properties, namely, Ginsenosides and Saikosaponins, and so forth [35, 38]. Studies have suggested that the biosynthesis of triterpene saponins occurs through the mevalonate pathway, resulting in β-amyrin and similar glycosides. The meta-bolic pathway steps defining β-amyrin biosynthesis is well characterized.

However, the final transformation of triterpenoids by P450's and uridine diphosphate (UDP)-dependent glycosyltransferases, is not known. Significant interest and investigation on the identification of the metabolic pathway leading to Gymnemic acid biosynthesis have been hypothesized [61]. It was suggested that glycosylation of aglycone sapogenin by UDP-dependent glycosyltransferases leads to biosynthesis of Gymnemic acid analogs. The suggested hypothetical pathway provided better insights into the biosynthesis and physiological mechanism of the molecules, pertaining to antidiabetic property (Figure 3.2). Research on similar platforms also suggested the glycosylation of secondary metabolites of triterpenoid origin [61, 62].

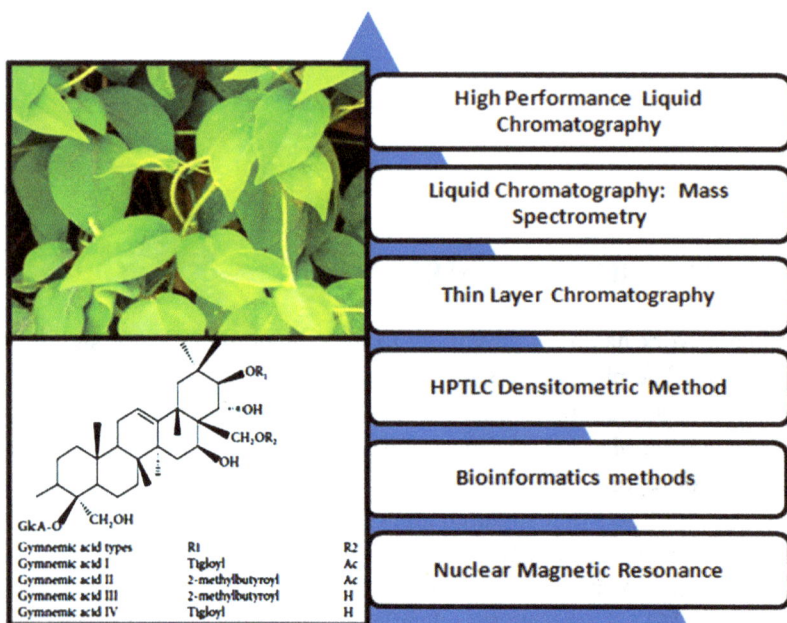

**FIGURE 3.1** Use of various plant metabolomics techniques for the identification of Gymnemic acids.

## 3.5 TRADITIONAL AND PRESENT USE OF *G. SYLVESTRE* R.BR.

*G. sylvestre* R. Br. is an indigenous plant and is designated as "miracle herb" [33]. The herb is gaining popularity as natural medication owing to its immense benefits ranging from Diabetes to use in arthritis, anemia, heart diseases, asthma, microbial infections, and so forth [60, 61]. Literature reviews have highlighted the importance of the plant in the treatment of various disorders [33, 34, 71]. Besides key therapeutic application for Type-II diabetes, the herb exhibits promising effects in the treatment of inflammation, indigestion, hypercholesterolemia, osteoporosis, etc. Traditionally, the plant was used for malaria and snakebite treatment, obesity, dental caries, as antibiotic in rheumatism, and as blood purifier. The leaves, roots, and stems include bioactive constituents and were used in Ayurvedic system of medicine as "herbal medication." A comprehensive review providing key insights on multiple pharmacological properties of the plant has been discussed extensively [60, 61].

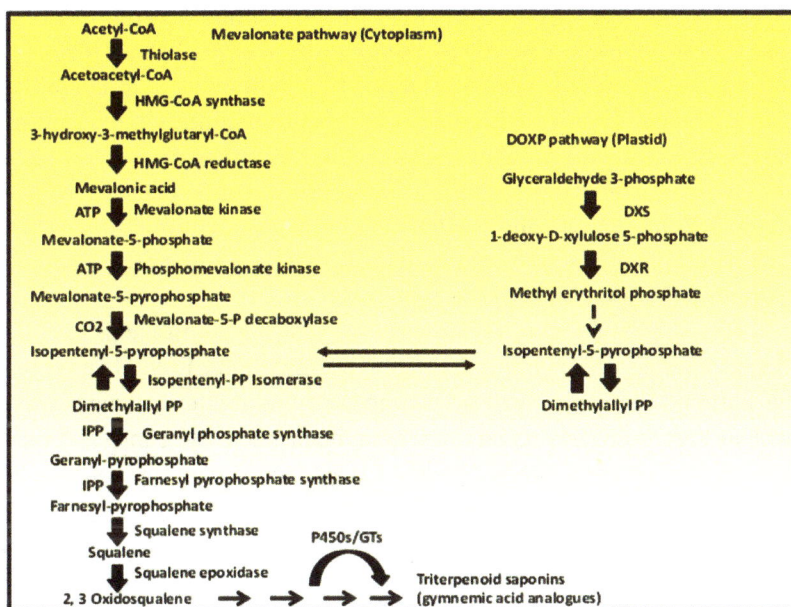

**FIGURE 3.2**   Biosynthetic pathway of Gymnemic acid.

Studies have shown the isolation of bioactive compounds as pure molecules or plant extracts and their experimental validation, showing effectiveness in the treatment of multiple health ailments. The plant has proved extremely beneficial in the treatment of Type-II diabetes on animal models [13, 30, 31, 39], antimicrobial activity [9, 59], neuroprotective [14], anticancer and cytotoxic [67], hepatoprotective [70], wound healing [27], immunomodulatory [46, 53], and ethnobotanical uses [5, 28]. The leaves were used for the treatment of diabetes; and bark and flowers were used for throat problems

[28]. The book, *Sushruta*, described sugar suppression activity of the plant during the ancient period. The multiple medicinal properties of the plant include use in jaundice, cardiopathy, asthma, stimulant, laxative, antipyretic, and so forth [5, 61]. Also, the plant was used for leucoderma, dyspepsia, astringent, jaundice, cardiotonic, uterine tonic, diuretic, cough dyspepsia, hemorrhoids, hepatosplenomegaly, and so forth [47].

### 3.5.1 ANTIDIABETIC ACTIVITY OF GYMNEMIC ACIDS

Several studies highlighted the antidiabetic property of Gymnemic acid analogs from the plant. Gymnemic acid I to XVIII and several derivatives/ analogs (Table 3.2) comprise of key bioactive molecules that are responsible for antidiabetic property. The structure of the Gymnemic acid is similar to a sugar molecule. Therefore it exhibits competitive inhibition by binding to the taste receptors; and regulates sugar intake. Another research suggested role of Gymnemic acid derivatives in decreasing sugar levels in blood due to interaction with GAPDH and G3PDH enzymes [55]. Gurmarin, a polypeptide, with antidiabetic activity exerts its action through interfering with taste sensation (sweet and bitter) of the taste buds.

Research studies on Gymnemic acids and its antisaccharine effects provided valuable insights into their role in regulation of blood sugar levels in the patient. Phytochemical screening and metabolic profiling coupled with plant metabolomics techniques have been significant in isolation and validation of pure compounds/extracts for antidiabetic activity, which were further validated scientifically on animal models. An interesting study highlighted the efficacy of the plant in decreasing blood sugar levels in berrylium nitrate and streptozotocin treated rats, respectively [68]. Other significant work includes the characterization of functional role of Gymnemic acid in diabetes [1], leaf extract administration in streptozotocin diabetic rats [7], hypoglycemic activity of a polyherbal formulation in Wister Albino rats [40, 48], etc. Similarly, Kumar et al. [33] showed the sugar suppression activity of the extract on Albino rats [33]. The administration of aqueous leaf extract in rats improved the metabolic profile [33]. Recently, Hazare [18] investigated the sugar decreasing effect of the plant extract on normal and diabetic mice (diabetes induced with alloxan). Such studies are crucial in determination and validation of antidiabetic activity of the plant and its bioactive phytoconstituents.

## 3.6    GYMNEMIC ACID AND DRUG DESIGNING FOR DIABETES

With unprecedented advancement in technologies and scientific break-throughs, the development and screening of "natural product-based thera-peutics" is gaining momentum in the present era. Computational biology together with in silico prediction methods have contributed immensely in science of natural products and drug designing for diabetes. The emergence and popularity of natural products (low costs, efficacy, and minimum side effects) has opened new avenues for pharmacological applications. Several bioinformatics methods including databases and repositories constitute a collection of related information on a particular disease and its treatment strategies. Some popular databases for diabetes include T2D-Db (Type-II diabetes Database), Attie Lab Diabetes Database [25], Pima Indians Diabetes Database, and Type-II diabetes database [76]. The comprehen-sive information for online databases and resources has been extensively studied to provide key information on diabetes and potential drug targets [60, 64].

The research studies on Gymnemic acid analogs [63] and on different antidiabetic plants, and their phytomolecules have highlighted the impor-tance of natural products as therapeutics agents. The automated sequencing of whole genomes of biological organisms has put forth enormous informa-tion "Big data" and its decoding for identification of key drug targets, thereby development of target-based therapeutics. Gymnemic acid analogs were in silico investigated and analyzed for their prospects as "lead molecules" in drug discovery studies, employing quantitative structure–activity relation-ship (QSAR) studies [63].

The use of bioinformatics resources namely databases information on diabetes, molecular modeling approaches, QSAR and softwares, have contributed in identification of novel "drug-like" molecules and the analysis of their pharmacokinetic properties (absorption, distribution, metabolism, excretion, and toxicity) [63, 64]. The study discussed the prediction of anti-diabetic activity of phytomolecules by QSAR model, a statistical approach in prediction of "drug-like" molecules. Molecular docking and ADMET analysis showed active Gymnemic acid analogs. However, poor bioavail-ability of molecules requires further optimization. The in silico screening methods provide an important tool to gain insights on the potential of natural "lead molecules" for drug designing in diabetes.

## 3.7 SUMMARY

Several research studies have highlighted the significance of *G. sylvestre* R. Br. in diabetes management, as "herbal model" for research programs. Metformin, the first antidiabetic drug of plant origin (from *G. officinalis*), is an effective medication for diabetes, since then several plants have been explored for their pharmacological properties. Research work on *G. sylvestre* has extensively discussed the chromatographic isolation and metabolite analysis of Gymnemic acid analogs; however, scarce information is available on the biosynthetic pathways and functional mechanism of the phytomolecules. Considering the growing popularity of the plant and respective molecules, as an effective medication for diabetes, both in silico prediction strategies as well as their experimental validation, forms a prime area of research. The pharmacokinetic properties of Gymnemic acid molecules suggested oral bioavailability concerns in ADMET studies. A prospective solution includes designing and chemical synthesis of new Gymnemic acid analogs and their pharmacokinetic analysis employing in silico methods. Moreover, another key area of research should focus on delineating the biosynthetic pathway of Gymnemic acid, which would provide key information about their antidiabetic mechanism in planta.

## KEYWORDS

- **computational biology**
- **diabetes**
- **drug designing**
- ***Gymnema sylvestre* R. Br.**
- **gymnemic acids**
- **triterpenoids**

## REFERENCES

1. Abdul, B.A.A.; Rao, M.V.; Taha, R.M. Optimization of gymnemic acid production with antidiabetic studies and regeneration of langerhans cells from *Gymnema sylvestre*. In: *4th International Conference on Biotechnology and Environment Management* (IPCBEE);

Singapore: IACSIT Press; **2014**; Vol. *75*; pp. 77–84. DOI: 10.7763/IPCBEE.2014. V75.14.

2. Agarwal, S.K.; Singh, S.S.; Verma, S.; Lakshmi, V.; Sharma, A.; Kumar, S. chemistry and medicinal uses of *Gymnema sylvestre* (Gurmar) leaves: review. *Indian Drug*, **2000**, *37*, 354–360.

3. Ahmed, A.B.A.; Rao, A.S.; Rao, M.V. Somatic embryogenesis and plant regeneration from cell suspension culture of *Gymnema sylvestre* R. Br. Ex. *KMITL Sci. Tech. J.*, **2009**, *9* (1), 18–26.

4. Ahmed, A.B.A.; Rao, A.S.; Rao, M.V.; [Taha], R.M. Production of gymnemic acid depends on medium, explants, PGRs, color lights, temperature, photoperiod and sucrose sources in batch culture of *Gymnema sylvestre*. *Sci. World J., **2012**, 897867*, 1–11.

5. Anis, M.; Sharma, M.P.; Iqbal, M. Herbal ethnomedicine of the gwalior forest division in Madhya Pradesh, India. *Pharm. Biol.*, **2000**, *38* (4), 241–253.

6. Bhansali, S.; Shafiq, N.; Pandhi.; P, Singh, A.P. Effect of deacyl gymnemic acid on glucose homeostasis and metabolic parameters in a rat model of metabolic syndrome. *Indian J. Med. Res.*, **2013**, *137*, 1174–1179.

7. Chauhan, K.; Saravanana, C.; Bajaj, G.; Chauhan, B. Therapeutic potential of *Gymnema sylvestre* leaves in streptozotocin induced diabetic rats. *IJPLS*, **2015**, *6*, 4508–4520.

8. Daisy, P.; Eliza, J.; Farook, K.A.M.M. Novel dihydroxy gymnemic triacetate isolated from *Gymnema sylvestre* possessing normoglycemic and hypolipidemic activity on STZ -induced diabetic rats. *J. Ethnopharmacol.*, **2009**, *126*, 339–344.

9. David, B.C.; Sudarsanam, G. Antimicrobial activity of *Gymnema sylvestre* (Asclepiadaceae). *J. Acute Dis.*, **2013**, *2* (3), 222–225.

10. Devi, C.S.; Srinivasan, V.M. *In vitro* propagation of *Gymnema sylvestre*. *Asian J. Plant Sci.*, **2008**, *7*, 660–665.

11. Devi, C.S.; Srinivasan, V.M. *In vitro* studies on stimulation of gymnemic acid production using fungal elicitor in suspension and bioreactor - based cell cultures of *Gymnema sylvestre* R. Br. *Recent Res. Sci. Technol.*, **2011**, *3*, 101–104.

12. Devi, C.S.; Murugesh, S.; Srinivasan V.M. Gymnemic acid production in suspension cell cultures of *Gymnema sylvestre*. *J. Appl. Sci.*, **2006**, *6* (10), 2263–2268.

13. Dholi, S.K.; Kannappan, R.R. Effect of *Gymnema sylvestre* on the Pharmacokinetics and Pharmacodynamics of Gliclazide in Diabetic Rats. *AJPCT*, **2013**, *1*, 23–36.

14. Fatani, A.J.; Al-Rejaie, S.S.; Abuohashish, H.M. Neuroprotective effects of *Gymnema sylvestre* on streptozotocin-induced diabetic neuropathy in rats. *Exp. Ther. Med.*, **2015**, *9*, 1670–1678.

15. Foster, S. *Gymnema sylvestre*. In: *Alternative Medicine Review Monographs*; Summerville, SC: Thorne Research Inc.; K. Czap (Ed.); **2002**; Vol. 1; pp. 205–207.

16. Gent, J.F.; Hettinger, T.P.; Frank, M.E.; Marks, L.E. Taste confusions following gymnemic acid rinse. *Chem. Senses.*, **1999**, *24*, 393–403.

17. Gupta, P.; Ganguly, S.; Singh, P. Miracle Fruit Plant—*Gymnema sylvestre* R. Br. (Retz). *Pharmacie Globale IJCP*, **2012**, *12*, 1–8.

18. Hazare, R. Comparing modified and relationship study of *Gymnema sylvestre* against diabetes. *J. Global Diabetes Clin. Met.*, **2018**, *3* (1), 1–3.

19. Hooper, D. Isolation and antiviral activity of gymnemic acid. *Pharm. J. Trans.*, **1887**, *17*, 867–868.

20. International Diabetes Federation (IDF); 2019; https://www.idf.org/; Accessed on June 30, 2019.

21. Isah, T. De Novo *in vitro* shoot morphogenesis from shoot tip-induced callus cultures of *Gymnema sylvestre* (Retz.) R. Br. ex Sm. *Biol. Res.*, **2019**, *52* (1), 3–19.

22. Jacob, B.; Narendhirakannan, R. T. Role of medicinal plants in the management of *Diabetes mellitus*: review. *Biotech.*, **2019**, *9* (1), 4. Epub.; doi:10.1007/s13205-018-1528-0.

23. Jung, M.; Park, M.; Lee, H.C.; Kang, Y.H. Antidiabetic agents from medicinal plants. *Curr. Med. Chem.*, **2006**, *13*, 1203–1218.

24. Kanetkar, P.V.; Singhal, R.S.; Laddha, K.S.; Kamat, M.Y. Extraction and quantification of gymnemic acids through gymnemagenin from callus cultures of *Gymnema sylvestre*. *Phytochem. Anal.*, **2006**, *17* (6), 409–413.

25. Keller, M.P.; Choi, Y.; Wang, P. Gene expression network model of type-2 diabetes links cell cycle regulation in islets with diabetes susceptibility. *Genome Res*, **2008**, *18*, 706–716.

26. Khramov, V.A.; Spasov, A.A.; Samokhina, M.P. Chemical composition of dry extracts of *Gymnema sylvestre* leaves. *Pharm. Chem. J.*, **2008**, *42*, 30–32.

27. Kiranmai, M.; Kazim, S.M.; Ibrahim, M. Combined wound healing activity of *Gymnema sylvestre* and *Tagetes erecta* Linn. *Int. J. Pharm. Appl.*, **2011**, *2* (2), 135–140.

28. Kirtikar, K.R.; Basu, B.D. *Indian Medicinal Plants*. Delhi, India: Periodicals Experts; **1975**. Vol. 3; pp. 1849–1917.

29. Kumar, H.G.A; Murthy, H.N.; Paek, K.Y. Somatic Embryogenesis and Plant Regeneration in *Gymnema sylvestre*. *Plant Cell Tissue Organ Cult.*, **2002**, *71* (1), 85–88.

30. Kumar, M.S.; Astalakshmi, N.; Arshida, P.T. Concise Review on Gurmar, *Gymnema sylvestre* R. Br. *World J. Pharm. Pharm. Sci.*, **2015**, *4* (10), 430–448.

31. Kumar, P.M.; Venkataranganna, M.V.; Manjunath, K. Methanolic leaf extract of *Gymnema sylvestre* augments glucose uptake and ameliorates insulin resistance by upregulating glucose transporter-4, peroxisome proliferator-activated receptor-Gamma, adiponectin, and leptin levels *in vitro*. *J. Intercult. Ethnopharmacol.*, **2016**, *5* (2), 146–152.

32. Kumar, U.; Singh, I.; Priyanka.; Vimala, Y. In vitro salt stress induced production of gymnemic acid in callus cultures of *Gymnema sylvestre* R. Br. *Afr. J. Biotechnol.*, **2010**, *9* (31), 4904–4909.

33. Kumar, V.H.; Nagendra Nayak, I.M.; Huilgol, S.V. Antidiabetic and hypolipidemic activity of *Gymnema sylvestre* in dexamethasone induced insulin resistance in albino rats. *Int. J. Med. Res. Health Sci.*, **2015**, *4*, 639–645.

34. Laha, S.; Paul, S. *Gymnema sylvestre* (Gurmar): potent herb with anti-diabetic and antioxidant potential. *Pharmacog. J.*, **2019**, *11* (2), 201–206.

35. Marciani, D.J.; Press, J.B.; Reynolds, R.C.; Pathak, A.K. Development of semisynthetic triterpenoid saponin derivatives with immune stimulating activity. *Vaccine.*, **2000**, *18*, 3141–3151.

36. Murakami, N.; Murakami, T.; Kadoga, M.; Matsuda, H. New hypoglycemic constituents in gymnemic acid from *Gymnema sylvestre*. *Chem. Pharm. Bull.*, **1996**, *44*, 467–471.

37. Nan, K.; Wtpsk, S. Callus induction and in vitro plantlet regeneration of *Gymnema sylvestre* R. Br. (Retz.) and the phytochemical screening of natural plants and callus cultures. *Plant Tissue Cult. Biotechnol.*, **2014**, *23* (2), 201–210.

38. Park, H.J.; Kwon, S.H.; Lee, J.H. Kalopanaxsaponin-A is a basic saponin structure for the anti-tumor activity of hederagenin monodesmosides. *Planta Med.*, **2001**, *67*, 118–121.

39. Parveen, S.; Ansari, M.H.R.; Parveen, R. Chromatography based metabolomics and *In Silico* screening of *Gymnema sylvestre* leaf extract for its antidiabetic potential. *Evid. Based Compl. Altern. Med.*, **2019**, *2019*, Article ID 7523159, 14 pages.

40. Pathan, R.A.; Bhandari, U.; Javed, S.; Nag, T.C. Anti-apoptotic potential of gymnemic acid-phospholipid complex pretreatment in wistar rats with experimental cardiomyopathy. *Ind. J. Exp. Biol.*, **2012**, *50*, 117–127.

41. Persaud, S.J.; Al-Majed, H.; Raman, A.; Jones, P.M. *Gymnema sylvestre* stimulates insulin release in vitro by increased membrane permeability. *J. Endocrinol.*, **1999**, *163*, 207–212.

42. Praveen, N.; Murthy, H.N.; Chung, I.M. Improvement of growth and gymnemic acid production by altering the macro elements concentration and nitrogen source supply in cell suspension cultures of *Gymnema sylvestre* R. Br. *Ind. Crop Prod.*, **2011**, *33* (2), 282–286.

43. Rachh, P.R.; Rachh, M.R.; Ghadiya, N.R. Anti hyperlipidemic activity of *Gymnema sylvestre* R. Br. leaf extract on rats fed with high cholesterol diet. *Int. J. Pharmacol.*, **2010**, *2010*, 138–141.

44. Reddy, P.S.; Gopal, G.R.; Sita, G.L. In vitro multiplication of *Gymnema sylvestre* R. Br., an important medicinal plant. *Curr. Sci.*, **1998**, *75* (8), 843–845.

45. Sahu, R.K.; Rajesh, T.S.; Pavithra, K. Micropropagation and *Agrobacterium*: mediated transformation of *GUS* Gene into *Gymnema sylvestre* antidiabetic plants. *J. Med. Plants Stud.*, **2016**, *4* (4), 18–24.

46. Saneja, A.; Sharma, C.; Aneja, K.R.; Pahwa, R. *Gymnema sylvestre* (Gurmar): Review. *Pharm. Lett.*, **2010**, *2*, 275–284.

47. Sastry, B.S. *Gymnema sylvestre*. Varanasi, India: Bhav Prakash Nighantu Chaukhambha; **1994**; pp. 443–444.

48. Selvam, N.T.; Hima, K.M.; Sanjayakumar, Y.R. Hypoglycaemic and antioxidant activity of SPHAG—a poly herbal formulation in alloxan induced wistar albino rats. *Int. J. Pharm. Sci. Res.*, **2015**, *6*, 767–772.

49. Shah, S.N.; Husaini, A.M.; Ansari, S.A. Micropropagation of *Gymnema sylvestre* R. Br. *Sky J. Med. Plant Res.*, **2013**, *2*(3), 18–28.

50. Shimizu, K.; Ozeki, M.; Iino, A. Structure–activity relationships of triterpenoid derivatives extracted from *Gymnema inodorum* leaves on glucose absorption. *Japan J. Pharmacol.*, **2001**, *86*, 223–229.

51. Shirugumbi, H.M.; Poornananda, M.N. Distribution of gymnemic acid in various organs of *Gymnema sylvestre. J. Forestry Res.*, **2009**, *20*, 268–270.

52. Singh, V.K.; Ansari, S.U.; Akhtar, S.; Muhammad, I. *Gymnema sylvestre* for diabetics. *J. Herbs Spices Med. Plants.*, **2008**, *14*, 88–106.

53. Singh, V.K.; Dwivedi, P.; Chaudhary, B.R.; Singh, R. Immunomodulatory effect of *Gymnema sylvestre* (R. Br.) leaf extract in rat model. *PLOS One.*, **2015**, *10* (10), 1–15. e-article ID 0139631; https://doi.org/10.1371/journal.pone.0139631.

54. Sinsheimer, J.E.; Subbarao G. Constituents from *Gymnema sylvestre* Leaves, VIII: isolation, chemistry and derivatives of gymnemagenin and gymnestrogenin. *J. Pharm. Sci.*, **1971**, *60*, 190–193.

55. Sugihara, Y.; Nojima, H.; Matsuda, H. Antihyperglycemic effects of gymnemic acid, IV, a compound derived from *Gymnema sylvestre* leaves in streptozotocin diabetic mice. *J. Asian Nat. Prod. Res.*, **2000**, *2*, 321–327.

56. Suttisri, R.; Lee, I.S.; Kinghorn, D. Plant-derived triterpenoid sweetness inhibitors. *J. Ethnopharmacol.*, **1995**, *47*, 9–26.

57. Syedy, M.; Nama, K.S. *Gymnema sylvestre*: miracle fruit for diabetes cure. *Int. J. Pure Appl. Biosci.*, **2014**, *2* (6), 318–325.

58. Syedy, M.; Nama, K.S. In vitro propagation of shoots and callus induction of *Gymnema sylvestre* R. Br. an important anti-diabetic plant. *Int. J. Curr. Pharm. Res.*, **2018**, *10* (3), 60–64.

59. Thanwar, M.; Dwivedi, D.; Gharia, A.K.; Chouhan, S. Antibacterial study of *Gymnema sylvestre* Plant. *Int. J. Chem. Stud.*, **2016**, *4* (3), 80–83.

60. Tiwari, P.; Ahmed, K.; Baig, H. *Gymnema sylvestre* for diabetes: from traditional herb to future's therapeutic. *Curr. Pharm. Des.*, **2017**, *23*, 1–10.

61. Tiwari, P.; Mishra, B.N.; Sangwan, N.S. Phytochemical and pharmacological properties of *Gymnema sylvestre*: important medicinal plant. *Biomed Res. Int.*, **2014**, *2014*, 1–18.

62. Tiwari, P.; Sangwan, R.S. Molecular cloning and biochemical characterization of a recombinant sterol 3-O-glucosyltransferase from *Gymnema sylvestre* R. Br. catalyzing biosynthesis of steryl glucosides. *Biomed Res. Int.*, **2014**, *2014*, 1–14.

63. Tiwari, P.; Sharma, P.; Khan, F. Structure activity relationship studies of gymnemic acid analogues for antidiabetic activity targeting PPARγ. *Cur. Comput. Aid Drug.*, **2015**, *11*, 57–71.

64. Tiwari, P.; Katyal, A. Lead optimization resources in drug discovery for diabetes, **2019**. https://www.ncbi.nlm.nih.gov/pubmed/30834844;

65. Tiwari, P. Recent trends in therapeutic approaches for diabetes management: a comprehensive update. *J. Diabetes Res.*, **2015**, *340838*, 1–12.

66. Usmani, S.; Amir, M.; Mujeeb M.; Ahmad, A.; Kamal, Y.T. Establishment of cell suspension culture and quantitative analysis of gymnemagenin in plant and in vitro culture of *Gymnema sylvestre*. *J. Liq. Chromatogr. Relat. Technol.*, **2013**, *36* (13), 1869–1880.

67. Vannini, S.; Villarini, M.; Levorato, S.; Salvatori, T. In vitro evaluation of cytotoxic, genotoxic and apoptotic properties of herbal products from leaves of *Gymnema sylvestre*. *Int. J. Herb. Med.*, **2017**, *5* (3), 33–38.

68. Vasi, S.; Austin, A. Effect of herbal hypoglycemics on oxidative stress and antioxidant status in diabetic rats. *Open Diabetes J.*, **2009**, *2*, 48–52.

69. Vats, S. Identification of flavonoids from plant parts and callus culture of *Gymnema sylvestre* R. Br.: antidiabetic plant. *Curr. Bioact. Compd.*, **2016**, *12*, 264–468.

70. Venkatakishore, T.; Rao, M.P.; Thulasi, B.P. Hepatoprotective activity of ethanolic extract of aerial part of *Gymnema sylvestre* against CCL4 and paracetamol induced hepatotoxicity in rats. *World J. Pharm. Pharm. Sci.*, **2016**, *5* (12), 1007–1016.

71. Vijayakumar, S.; Prabhu, S. *Gymnema sylvestre*: key for diabetes management- review. *Pharmacol. Toxicol. Res.*, **2014**, *1* (1), 1–10.

72. Vincken, J.P.; Heng, L.; deGroot, A.; Gruppen, H. Saponins, classification and occurrence in the plant kingdom. *Phytochemistry*, **2007**, *68*, 275–297.

73. World Health Organization; **2018**; (https://www.who.int/); Accessed on 19th June, 2019.

74. Xie, J.T.; Wang, A.; Mehendale, S. Anti-diabetic effects of *Gymnema yunnanense* Extract. *Pharmacol. Res.*, **2003**, *47*, 323–329.

75. Xu, R.; Yang, Y.; Zhang, Y. New pregnane glycosides from *Gymnema sylvestre*. *Molecules.*, **2015**, *20*, 3050–3066.

76. Yang, Z.; Yang, J.; Liu, W.; Wu, L.; Xing, L. T2D@ZJU: Knowledge-based integrating heterogeneous connections associated with Type-2 *Diabetes Mellitus*, Database. *J. Biol. Database Curation.*, **2013**, *2013*: article ID bat052; doi:10.1093/database/bat052.

77. Yoshikawa, K.; Amimoto, K.; Arihara, S.; Matsuura, K. Gymnemic acid V, VI and VII from gurmar, the leaves of *Gymnema sylvestre* R. Br. *Chem. Pharm. Bull.*, **1989**, *37*, 852–854.

78. Yoshikawa, K.; Amimoto, K.; Arihara, S.; Matsuura, K. structure studies of new antisweet constituents from *Gymnema sylvestre. Tetrahedron Lett*., **1989**, *30*, 1103–1116.

79. Yoshikawa, K.; Arihara, S.; Matsuura, K. New type of antisweet principles occurring in *Gymnema sylvestre. Tetrahedron Lett*., **1991**, *32*, 789–792.

80. Yoshikawa, K.; Nakagawa, M.; Yamamoto, R; Arihara, S.; Matsuura, K. Antisweet natural products: structures of gymnemic acids VIII-XII from *Gymnema sylvestre* R. Br. *Chem. Pharm. Bull*., **1992**, *40*, 1779–1782.

81. Yoshikawa, K.; Kondo, Y.; Arihara, S.; Matsuura, K. Antisweet natural products, IX: structures of gymnemic acids XV-XVIII from *Gymnema sylvestre* R. Br. *Chem. Pharm. Bull*., **1993**, *41*, 1730–1732.

82. Zarrelli, A.; Ladhari, A.; Haouala, R. New acylated oleanane and lupane triterpenes from *Gymnema sylvestre. Helv. Chim. Acta*., **2013**, *96*, 2200–2206.

83. Zhu, X.M.; Xie, P.; Di, Y.T. Two new triterpenoid saponins from *Gymnema sylvestre. J. Integ. Plant Biol*., **2008**, *50*, 589–592.

84. Zimare, S.B.; Malpathak, N.P. In vitro shoot and gymnemic acid production in *Gymnema sylvestre* (Retz.) R. Br. Ex. Sm. *Indian J. Biotechnol*., **2017**, *16*, 635–640.

# CHAPTER 4

# *PREMNA SERRATIFOLIA* L.: POTENTIAL AS NUTRACEUTICAL PANACEA

KADAKASSERIL V. GEORGE*, LEKSHMI V. BOSE,
SOLOMON HABTEMARIAM, and JOSE MATHEW

## ABSTRACT

This chapter focuses on sources of information on taxonomy, diversity, ethnobotany, and phytopharmacology of *Premna serratifolia* L. The review on the taxonomy of *P. serratifolia* revealed much perplexity due to much variability among specimens collected from different regions. The neutraceutical prospects of *P. serratifolia* are discussed from an Ayurvedic perspective. The pharmacological properties of many traditional herbal formulations of *P. serratifolia* have been explored for health benefits.

## 4.1 INTRODUCTION

The importance of traditional herbal therapy has been accepted worldwide, since many modern medicines have failed to meet the basic requirements of common people. On the other hand, herbal therapy is gaining importance as inexpensive, easily accessible, and free from side effects. The traditional herbal practitioners in different countries make use of leaves, fruits/seeds, roots/tubers, bark/wood of wild herbs, and trees either as food, food supplements, or as medicines. It is estimated that about four billion people of the world's population depend on wild edible herbs/herbal medicines for their primary healthcare requirements [139]. The Food and Agricultural Organization also pointed out the role of wild food to meet the daily nutritional requirements [17].

*Corresponding author. E-mail: kvgeorge58@yahoo.in..

The utilization of wild foods to meet the food/nutritional requirements of people living in rural areas of developing countries, where food insecurity is more pronounced, has immense significance. Hence, there is an upsurge of interests within the scientific community to evaluate the nutritional/medicinal or nutraceutical benefits of various wild edible/medicinal plants [1, 90]. Moreover, the terminology "nutraceutical" has given additional impetus to recognize the health benefits of foods and also for adopting "market-driven approach" to health foods [109]. In this context, documentation of traditional botanical information and scientific studies that validate their medicinal/ neutraceutical benefits would support further research on bioprospecting of ethnomedicinal plants.

One of the leading causes of various human ailments (such as cancer, diabetes, neuro degenerative diseases, premature ageing, cardio vascularailments, etc.) is believed to be due to heavy metal toxicity and generation of free radicals inside our body. Hence, natural antioxidants have therapeutic implications for management such diseases. Given the numerous potential unwanted effects of synthetic antioxidants (e.g., carcinogenic effects), the utility of plant-based antioxidants, in food and pharmaceutical industries have been advocated.

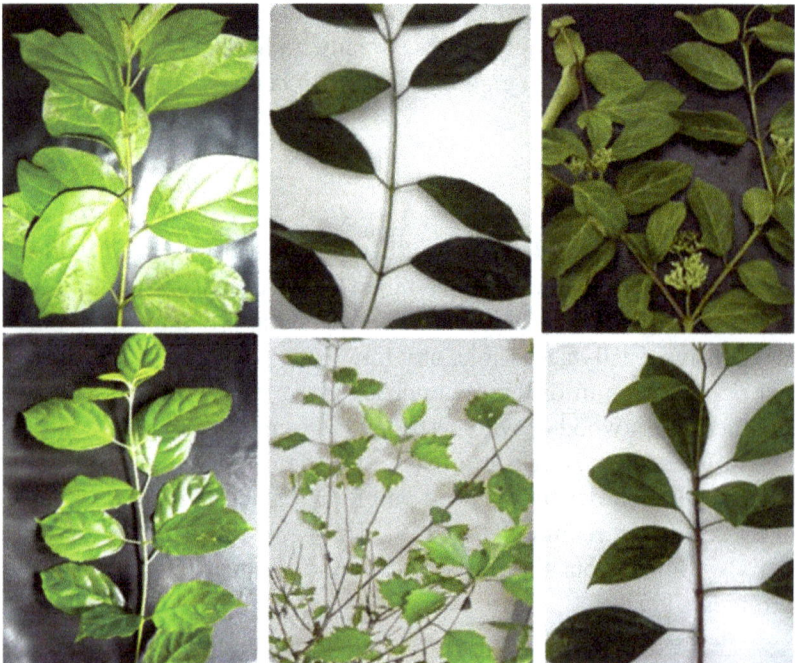

**FIGURE 4.1** Morphotypes of *Premna serratifolia*.

   *Premna serratifolia* L. (family: Lamiaceae) has broad-spectrum applications in the Indian and Asian systems of medicines. The plant is known by its trivial names, such as *Agnimantha* in Sanskrit and *Munja* in Malayalam. Its leaves, bark, and roots are essential ingredients of various Ayurvedic medicines, such as *arishtam, avaleham, kwatham, ghritham,* and *tailam* [22, 25, 27, 74, 110, 137]. In the Ayurvedic pharma industry, there is a great demand for this plant since its roots are used as an essential constituent of *Dashamoola* (a nourishing Ayurvedic muscle tonic) that is claimed to strengthen the body and calm the nerves.

   A comprehensive review of *P. serratifolia* L. is presented in this chapter to reveal its potential as a good source of active therapeutics. Comprehensive information of *P. serratifolia* collected from various sources (such as botanical literature, Indian classical texts, pharmacopoeias, Ayurvedic books, Ayurvedic practitioners, electronic databases, journals, etc.) over the last 15 years are presented in this chapter.

## 4.2   METHODOLOGY

The present study is an attempt to summarize up-to-date information and hidden potential of *P. serratifolia* L. (*Agnimanthā*: Headache tree). Relevant literature on taxonomic history, ethnobotanical, and nutritional value, therapeutic/biological activity studies, and so forth, of this plant was collected from traditional manuscripts/texts and research publications. Besides, indigenous knowledge on the plant was also collected from traditional Ayurvedic physicians of Kerala. The present comprehensive documentation would thus provide vital information for bioprospecting of *P. serratifolia.*

## 4.3   *P. SERRATIFOLIA*: AN OVERVIEW

The generic name *Premna* refers to the nature of the tree trunks of species coming under this genus. Linnaeus [77] reported *Premna* with two species (*P. serratifolia* and *Premna integrifolia*) that were collected from Ceylon. The genus *Premna* L. has more than 190 species scattered all over the world [55, 84]. The initial report on the genus *Premna* from India [77] was based on the specimen (*P. serratifolia*) collected by Konig from peninsular India. Thereafter, a revisionary work by Rajendran and Daniel [100] brought out the diversity of this genus in India with 31 species and six varieties. A comprehensive review on its systematics, geographic distribution, traditional uses, pharmacognosy, phytochemistry, and biological activity studies is described in this section.

### 4.3.1   TAXONOMIC HISTORY AND POLYMORPHIC STATUS OF P. SERRATIFOLIA

*P. serratifolia* L. shows extreme morphological variations in different geographical regions of the world. Considering the taxonomic ambiguity and complexity of species, the nomenclature and identity of this species have been debated by taxonomists [37, 82, 83]. It is a difficult species since the floral characters of different accessions (morphological variants) are little distinct contrasting their extremely variable leaves. Hence, different names (*P. integrifolia* L., *P. serratifolia* L., *Premna obtusifolia* R. Br., etc.) were given to this species complex by different taxonomists.

The polymorphic status of this species was first reported by Beer and Lam [20]. According to Bentham [21], there are many variants or interme-diate forms of *P. serratifolia/P. integrifolia* and hence detailed investigation based on authentic specimens from different geographic regions of the world is recommended. Many earlier taxonomists namely Schauer [114] and Schumann and Hollrung [115] stressed the importance of detailed studies regarding the merging of related species of *P. integrifolia*. Accepting *P. integrifolia* as a very polymorphic species, Lam et al. [76] also confirmed the existence of its various intermediate/transient types based on cross-examination of numerous specimens. According to Kok [66], *P. serratifolia* shows significant morphological variations in leaves/floral characters across wide geographical distribution.

Lam et al. [76], examining morphology/ecological features, recom-mended existence of five different morpho/ecotypes, namely, *integrifolia, abbreviata, cyclophylla, sambucina,* and *foetida* for this species. In 1919, Lam also opined the intricacy in the categorization of this species that was mostly done on the basis of the morphology of the outer floral whorls that is often changeable in different plants belonging to the same species. He also commended on the drawbacks of classical taxonomic approaches and suggested the application of novel techniques to solve the problems in systematic botany. As revealed from taxonomic literature, no valid reasons have so far been generated to explain the underlying biological process behind the species complexity.

Currently, the accepted botanical name of this medicinal plant is *P. serratifolia* L. and all other names mentioned in the literature for this is treated as its synonyms [84]. However, as revealed from the taxonomical literature, no serious attempts have been undertaken for a systematic study of this polymorphic species based on larger sample collections from different geographical locations. It is assumed that many morpho-variations might have resulted by the process of sequential evolution. In a recent study, six morphotypes of *P. serratifolia* (Figure 4.1) were collected from different parts of Kerala [22].

## 4.3.2 DISTRIBUTION

This species grows under saline and nonsaline soils. It is widely distributed in East Africa, India, Ceylon, Malaysia, Thailand, East Bengal, Southern China, Moluk islands, Japan, Indonesia, Thailand, Philippines, Java, and Australia [75]. Apart from these localities, this species is also reported from many other Asiatic regions including Ryukyu Archipelago and Melanesia.

The distribution of this species is reported from many states and union territories in India, namely, Assam, Goa, Gujarat, Maharashtra, Karnataka, Kerala, Lakshadweep, Orissa, Tamil Nadu, West Bengal, and Andaman & Nicobar Islands [62, 94, 100].

## 4.4 TRADITIONAL KNOWLEDGE OF *P. SERRATIFOLIA*

Traditional knowledge of *P. serratifolia* was collected from traditional manuscripts, Ayurvedic texts, and from traditional Ayurvedic practitioners. It was observed that the therapeutic properties of this plant were described in different manuscripts under different Sanskrit names and local names.

### 4.4.1 TERMINOLOGY OF *P. SERRATIFOLIA* IN SANSKRIT AND OTHER LANGUAGES

In traditional manuscripts, different Sanskrit names (*Agnimantha, Gani-karikaa, Jaya, Jayanthi, Jayamti, Nadeyi, Tarkari,* and *Vaijayantika*) were used as synonyms of this plant to describe its morphological and therapeutic uses. Besides, certain regional names (*Gineri, Agethu, Tekara,* or *Tankali*) have also been used instead of its original Sanskrit names. However, the most widely used terminology is *Agnimantha*, which denotes the ability of the tree stumps/sticks to produce fire when rubbed with each other [8]. This medicinal plant is also known by different following local names [6, 27, 61, 62, 65, 87, 136] in different parts of the country:

- English: Headache tree, Malbau;
- Hindi: Arani, Agetha, Ganiari;
- Kanada: Agnimandha, Naravalu, Takkila;
- Malayalam: Munja, Appel, Kozhychedy;
- Tamil: Munnai/Munney, Munni-vayz, Pasumunnai; and
- Telugu: Gabbunelli/Ghebunelli, Kanika, Karnika.

### 4.4.2 CONTROVERSIAL DRUG STATUS OF P. SERRATIFOLIA

A major drawback of the traditional systems of medicine is the difficulty in the proper identification of the genuine medicinal plants prescribed by the founders. There is much confusion in this system regarding the identity of authentic medicinal plants, since these plants are not described scientifically in the classical literature. The descriptions of the medicinal plants were given in the form of *Slokas/Mantras*, which very often lack scientific precision. Moreover, the interpretation of the Sanskrit description is often influenced by the knowledge of the commentators. Hence, very often faulty species are being used Ayurvedic drug development in different regions of the country. The medicinal plant selected in this chapter is included in the "disputed medicinal plants" of India.

A perusal of the literature revealed the controversies of this medicinal plant among the commentators of modern *Nighantus*. Experts in Ayurveda [2, 68, 88, 96, 97, 134] commented on the genuineness of the source drug of *Agnimantha*. In this respect, the opinions of different authors are summarized as follows:

In Sanskrit literature, the source drug *Agnimantha* has two varieties: (*Brihat Agnimantha* (big variety) and *Laghuagnimantha* or *Ksudragnimantha* (small variety)) that were equated by taxonomic experts to *P. integrifolia* and *Clerodendrum phlomidis*, respectively [45]. As described in *Nighantus*, these two types have identical properties. However, Charaka and Sushrutha also explained these two as different medicinal plants. *Agnimantha* mentioned in *Sushrutha Samhita* can be equated to *P. integrifolia*. However, recent researchers have equated *C. phlomidis* to small and *Premna corymbosa* to big varieties of *Agnimantha* [14, 28].

*Tarkari* and *Agnimantha* (*Arani*) are described as different plants in *Amarakosha*. According to Sodhala [128], *Tarkari* and *Agnimantha* can be equated to the botanical sources *C. phlomidis* and *P. integrifolia*, respectively. In Bhavamishra, only *Agnimantha* is mentioned and *Tarkari* is described as its synonym. In *Nighantu Ratnakara*, *Agnimantha* has *Laghu* (smaller) and *Brihat* (bigger) varieties and the former has better *sothahara* property. This property has also been mentioned in *Kaiyyadeva Nighantu*. However, in *Dhanwanthari Nighantu*, two varieties mentioned are *Kshudragnimantha* and *Agnimantha* and they are equated to *P. integrifolia* and *C. phlomidis*, respectively. Similar descriptions are also given in *Mahoushadhi Nighantu, Raja Nighantu,* and *Saligrama Nighantu*. Pandey [93] also agrees with this classification of *Agnimantha*. It should be pointed out that the dissimilarities in the properties of these two types were not recorded in *Nighantus* and *Yogas* of classical texts.

In classical Ayurvedic texts, serious defects were noted in the naming of medicinal plants. Generally in Ayurvedic system of classification, unlike scientific classification, there is no precision in the system of nomenclature. Numerous names may be found given to same plant, based on one or more characteristics of the plant. This type of cumbersome classification system followed by earlier Sanskrit scholars leads to much confusion, since the names mentioned were used to describe different plant species. Similarly, there are also cases where taxonomically unrelated plants were treated as having identical therapeutic properties, due to identical phytochemicals. In the case of *Agnimantha* too, two unrelated species *P. serratifolia* and *C. phlomidis* (Lamiaceae) were described as having similar therapeutic potential [126]. It should be noted that in most of the south Indian states including Kerala, *P. serratifolia* was used as the authentic medicinal plant. However, in North India, *C. phlomidis* is used as *Agnimantha*. In short, the properties attributed to the above-mentioned species are considered to be identical.

In earlier works, researchers have equated the source plant *Agnimantha,* to different species of the genus *Premna*, such as *P. latifolia* Roxb., *P. serratifolia* L., *P. corymbosa* Rottl., *P. spinosa* Roxb. and *Premna latifolia* Roxb. var. *mucronata* [67, 89, 119, 127, 137].

In certain classical texts excluding *Madanapala Nighantu* and *Bhavaprakasham*, two varieties of *Agnimantha* (*P. serratifolia*) were described along with their synonyms. The local names mentioned are *Kattumunja/Munja* [118], *Valiya munna, Cheriya munja, Puzhamunja,* and so forth. However, in *Dravyagunavinjan*, *C. phlomides* is equated to *Cheriya munja* or *Tarkari* and *P. mucronata* to *Valiya munja or Kattu munja* [136].

There are two schools of thoughts regarding the identity of a source drug and its alternate species. According to Chunekar [28], *C. phlomidis* is used as the source drug and *P. serratifolia* as the substitute based on identical therapeutic properties attributed to these plants. Based on the second view point [34, 64, 72, 135], researchers equate the source plant *Agnimanta* to *P. serratifolia* L.

In *Ayurvedic Formulatory of India Part 1*, two different species *P. mucronata* and *P. integrifolia* were described as substitute drugs to *C. phlomidis* Linn. f. However, in its second edition (Part I), the source plant is mentioned as *P. integrifolia*; and *C. phlomidis* and *P. mucronata* as its substitutes [10]. In Part II of the same text, *P. obtusifolia* R. Br. and *P. mucronata* Roxb. are mentioned as the substitute drugs of *C. phlomidis* Linn. f. As revealed from the above discussions, much confusion and ambiguity exist regarding the genuine botanical sources of *Agnimantha* according to Aparna [9].

In short, evidences in classical texts/*Nighantus* are not sufficient to solve the ambiguity regarding the genuineness of the source plant, *Agnimantha*. Based on comparative analysis of ethnomedicinal uses of the ascribed medicinal plants, it is quite possible that *P. serratifolia* and *C. phlomidis* might have identical medicinal properties. However, marked disagreement in phytopharmacological variables of these plants were reported in recent studies [22]. It is expected that detailed phytochemical and pharmacognostic studies will provide evidences to resolve the existing ambiguity and value addition to the source drug.

### 4.4.3 TRADITIONAL USES OF P. SERRATIFOLIA

Indegenous health benefits of *Agnimantha* (*P. serratifolia*) were mentioned in Classical Ayurvedic texts (Rig-Veda, Atharva-Veda, Astanga Sangraha, etc.). Its morphological as well as medicinal properties were also described in various *Nighantus* [6, 22]. The leaves, stems, and roots of *P. serratifolia* (*Agnimantha*) in the form of juice or decoction are used in urinary complaints, gonorrhea, and diabetes (Prameha). The traditional/folklore uses of this plant against headache, constipation, fever, heart diseases, beriberi, vaginal irritation, and neurological diseases have been reported by many researchers [25, 27, 39, 40, 61, 74, 110, 112, 137]. The candidate species is also reported to be antipyretic, diuretic, cardioprotective, stomachic, and have many other neutraceutical benefits. It overcomes *kapha* and *vata* disorders, anemia, piles, edema, poison, anasarca, abdominal diseases, and improves digestive power and is highly valued for its anti-inflammatory activity [6, 67, 72].

The whole plant decoction of *P. serratifolia* is used to strengthen the bones and related orthopedic problems, head, body, and *Vata* disorders. Aboriginal people also used this plant for wound healing and for promoting lactation. The leaves are boiled and their vapors are inhaled to relieve nasal congestion associated with fever.

*P. serratifolia* is an important constituent of Ayurvedic preparation, *Medhahara kwata,* which is used as an effective slimming agent. Sweetened decoction of the leaves with lime juice is claimed to loosen up phlegm and is effective for coughs [22]. The leaves are also useful in treating dyspepsia, flatulence, cough, fever, asthma, bronchitis, leprosy, skin diseases, constipation, diabetes, cardiac disorders, catarrah, rheumatalgia, tumors, and general debility [3, 136]. In *Hortus Malabaricus*, a decoction of the leaves of *appel* is mentioned for pains and wind in the stomach. Leaf paste is applied externally to cure piles and inflammations of the body. Hot water extract of the leaves of *P. serratifolia* is used as an antipyretic and digestive agent [129]. Leaves are boiled with water, filtered, and then used for bathing infants. Leaf paste smeared over urinary bladder may facilitate urination [22, 69]. It is also used to treat *Amavatham,* hypercholesterolemia and also to safeguard the body from heavy metal toxicity. The leaves are also used for neuralgia and rheumatism. A decoction of *Premna* leaves along with garlic, pepper, and ginger extracts is given to cure cough and colds. Infusion of the leaves is also recommended for prickly heat, indigestion, and related abdominal discomfort, in doses of 20 to 50 ml. The leaves are effective to cure headache as well as "weakness of limbs" and are also used in steam baths to cleanse the body. Its herbal tea is treatment option for fevers and coughs. Its leaf juice has certain applications in *Marma* treatment. The leaves have analgesic effects and hence used as home remedy for getting relief from backache. The potential application of its leaf extract to control the pest infestations in poultry and horti-agricultural farms can be used to develop novel biopesticides [39].

The roots of *P. serratifolia* have wider therapeutic applications in indigenous medicine as an ingredient of *dasamula* and *brahatpanchamula* [65, 92]. The roots are thermogenic, aromatic, pungent, anodyne, alexeteric, expectorant, depurative, febrifuge, and antibacterial. It is good for heart, liver and skin problems, jaundice, malaria, indigestion, kidney stones, hemorrhoids, diabetes, and general debility. In *Yunaani*, the roots are used to rectify liver complaints. Its root paste in ghee is administered for a week to treat urticaria and roseola [87]. Its root decoction twice daily is prescribed against fever, gonorrhea, gout, etc. [35]. It is also recommended for liver complaints. The roots boiled in saltwater are used externally to get relief from gout [35]. Decoction of the roots @ 50–100 mL twice daily is recommended for gonorrhea and associated intermittent fevers.

The stem bark decoction of *P. serratifolia* is a good tonic to normalize heartbeat and dilation of the pupils [27]. In certain parts of Guam, its bark is used to treat neuralgia. It enhances the production of digestive enzymes, cleanse the renal system and act as a hepatoprotective agent [51]. Stem/root bark decoction is administered in patients suffering from rheumatism, arthritis, nervine, and neuralgic complaints (*vatavyadhi*) [92]. Besides, extract from its fruits is used for nasal administration (*Nasium*) to cure sinusitis and persistent headache.

### 4.4.4   *P. SERRATIFOLIA AS A FUNCTIONAL FOOD AND MEDICINE*

A food is regarded as functional if it is beneficial for maintaining the well-being by limiting pathological infestations that lead to diseases. The presence of dietary factors (like fibers, vitamins, proteins, minerals, antioxidants, amino acids, polyphenolic compounds, etc.) in many indigenous medicinal plants boost the future prospects of these plants as functional foods. The synergy of complex combinations of botanicals in Ayurvedic system is highly relevant in this context. It is believed that many useful bioactive compounds in such herbal combinations have broad-spectrum activities as either therapeutic or as nutritional agents. Hence, whole foods with combination of many herbs are used as functional foods rather than as supplements. *P. serratifolia* is one of the medicinal plants with rich sources of bioactive constituents with proven functional attributes.

Tender leaves of *Premna* are cooked and eaten as greens in China, Malaysia, and Philippines. The leaves are also consumed by the inhabitants of the Coromandel Coast [138]. The leaves of *P. latifolia* Roxb. are eaten in curries. In the coastal areas of Karunagappally (Kollam District, Kerala), the tender leaves are used for the preparation of medicated Kanji (rice porridge) for those suffering from fever. In various parts of Indonesia, the leaves are recommended for mother to promote lactation. The leaves, combined with those of *Morinda citrifolia,* are squeezed into water and the solution is drunk twice a day to treat severe malarial fevers.

Neutraceutical benefits of *P. serratifolia* are well described in many traditional Ayurvedic texts. In Ayurvedic science, its root extract is a major ingredient of good number of Ayurvedic preparations [38]:

1. *Balarishtam* (herbal preparation for Vata/neurological disorders, heart diseases, Rhematism);
2. *Dashmoolarishtam* (general tonic/restorative tonic for women);
3. *Dashamoola Kwatha* (post-delivery tonic for women);
4. *Medhahara Kwatham, Luhunna inguru kollukwathm* (tonic for reducing excess fat/neurological system sickness);
5. Rasayana drugs (brahma rasayana and chyawanaprasha), Dashamoola Taila (oil used for sinusitis and head ache); and massage oil.

These Ayurvedic preparations are used for improving general health, vigor, and longevity. Charaka and Sushruta prescribe the entire plant for the treatment of constipation, internal obstructions and abscesses, misperistalsis, piles, urinary diseases, and calculi. According to Sushruta, its roots are excellent appetizer for disturbed digestion and dyspepsia. A decoction of *Agnimantha* is also prescribed for obesity. Besides, its leaves minced with bamboo leaves are applied externally to cure glandular enlargements and erysipelas.

### 4.4.5   *P. SERRATIFOLIA IN AYURVEDIC FORMULATIONS*

*P. serratifolia* is an essential constituent of the classical Ayurvedic drug groups: *Dasamula, Brahatpanchamula, Viratarvadi,* and so forth [92]. It is one of the 10 drugs that constitute the group *Dasamula* (10 roots), which is used for the preparations of many Ayurvedic medicines [127]. In *Ayurveda,* various drug formulations like *arishtam* (a naturally fermented herbal decoction), *rasayanam* (nutritional juices of medicinal plants), *kwatham* (coarsely powdered herbal preparation—boiled and filtered with specific proportion of water), *ghritham* (herbal extract in ghee for consumption), *thailam* (herbal extracts in oil for external applications) are practiced as a part of treatment strategy. It is to be noted that *P. serratifolia* is an essential ingredient of many such polyherbal formulations [7], such as

1. *Arishtam (Amritharishtam, Dandyarishtam, Dasamoolarishtam);*
2. *Rasayanam (Agasthya rasayana, Chyavanaprasam, Dasamoola rasayanam, Brahma rasayanam);*

3. *Kwatham* (*Indukantha kwatham, Dhanwanthara kwatham, Varanadi kwatham, Sapthasaram kwatham, Medhahara kwatham, Luhuna Kolla kwatham*);
4. *Ghritham* (*Indukanthaghritham, Dhanwanthararishtam, Sukumara ghritham, Medhaharghritham*)*;*
5. *Thailams* (*Dhanwanthara thailam, Prabhanjana thailam, Vimord-hana thailam, Sahacharadi thailam*).

Besides, it is also used for the preparation of *Agnimantha-kasaya* and *Agnimantha-mulkalka* [34].

## 4.5 PHARMACOGNOSY OF *P. SERRATIFOLIA*

The morphological and anatomical characteristics of the roots of *P. integrifolia* (Syn. *P. serratifolia*) and its common substitute, *C. phlomidis*, were investigated by earlier researchers [42]. Even though, the roots of these two species have morphological similarity, they can be distinguished from each other by noting the nature of rhytidome (outer bark, which lies external to the last formed periderm).

In *C. phlomidis,* starch deposits were noted only in xylem parenchyma and xylem rays; whereas in *P. serratifolia*, such deposits were observed in all most all tissues except cork cells. However, the presence of identical chemical compound (Clerodendrin-A) in the roots of both *C. phlomidis* and *P. serratifolia* shows their chemical affinity.

Anatomical studies on *P. serratifolia* L. were reported by earlier researchers [38, 74]. Preliminary pharmacognostic investigations based on physicochemical/phytochemical and fluorescence analysis of the officinal parts of *P. serratifolia* have also been reported [107]. Morpho-anatomical characters of the roots/root powder of another closely related species of *P. serratifolia* was also reported [131]. Pharmacognostic studies on different morphotypes of *P. serratifolia* in Kerala were conducted by the authors of this chapter [22]. Authors conducted their research using traditional *Vaidyans* of Kerala and about six morphotypes of *P. serratifolia* (Mara munja:M-1; Kozhi munja:M-2; *Chemparathi munja-* with deep leaf serrations :M-3; *Chemparathi munja-* with shallow/less leaf serrations: M-4; *Neelan munja*: M-5, and *Cheru munja*: M-6) were collected from different localities of Kerala. The existence of different morphotypes or ecotypes of candidate medicinal plant in different agro-climatic conditions of Kerala shows high degree of plasticity possessed by *P. serratifolia.*

## 4.6 MAJOR PHYTOCHEMICALS IN *P. SERRATIFOLIA*

Preliminary phytochemical studies brought to light the presence of secondary metabolities, namely, alkaloids, triterpenes, flavonoids, phenolic compounds, cardiac glycosides, iridoid glycosides, saponins, resin, tannins, carbohydrates, amino acids, and some unsaturated aromatic hydrocarbons in *P. serratifolia* [22, 26, 27, 32, 80, 87]. The presence of alkaloids was reported by Alam et al. [4].

Major alkaloids identified from this plant are premnine [18], ganikarine [19], premnazole, aphelandrine, and ganiarine [16, 50, 61]. The alkaloid premnine has been shown to decrease the heartbeat and enhances dilation of the pupils [34]. A monoterpene iridoid compound, 10-*O-trans-p*-coumaroylcatalpol (OCC: one of the major constituents of the herbal formulation "Dashmula") was reported from the stem bark of *P. integrifolia* [121]. Another active principle (diterpene compound) from the root bark of this plant was isolated and its structure (Figure 4.2) was elucidated by relevant spectroscopic analysis.

Other compounds reported from this plant are caryophellene, premnenol, premnaspirodiene, botulin and clerodendrin-A, luteolin, and linalol [11, 13, 24, 29, 30, 73, 110]. Yuasa et al. [144] also reported few novel phytoactive compounds from the related species, *P. corymbosa* var. *obtusifolia*. Among the various compounds, a compound with melting point 155 °C was very effective against Gram-positive organisms. Iridoid glycosides and their conjugates with other compounds were also detected from the leaves of *P. serratifolia* [91, 106, 108]. The leaves contain an isoxazole premnazole that shrinked granuloma formation in rats by regulating the level of adreno-corticatropic hormone and its activity was comparable to phenylbutazone [62].

Gokani and Shah [49] isolated and quantified clerodendrin-A from *P. serratifolia* that was earlier reported from *C. phlomidis*. A few novel diterpene compounds [48, 49, 113, 142] have been reported from *P. serratifolia* in recent years. Yadav et al. [141–143] identified many novel compounds namely diterpenoids, lignans, and so forth, from its stem bark. Besides, these researchers also estimated diridoid glycosides, namely, 10-*O-trans-p*-coumaroylcatalpol, 4″-hydroxy-E-globularinin (Figure 4.3) and premnosidic acid by HPTLC method [22, 140].

Antioxidant property of the methanol fractions of the root woody tissues of *P. serratifolia* was investigated by the authors of this chapter by DPPH assay [23]. The root wood fractions that displayed promising activity were subjected to further separation and purification of its active principles by flash chromatographic techniques. One of the isolated compounds, namely, acteoside (verbacoside) displayed higher antioxidant property than its crude root wood fractions. As shown in Figure 4.4, the structure of acteoside is constructed from a caffeic acid and phenethyl alcohol units; both of which bear a catechol functional moiety that have been proven to dsiplay numerous pharmacological effects. On the other hand, the two sugar units of acteoside greatly enhance water solubility that may enhance the bioavailablity of this drug in water-based medium. In another investigation, Habtemariam and George [47] isolated a novel, highly aromatic molecule with diterpene skeleton (Figure 4.2). This compound does also share with acteoside by having a catechol functional group that attributes to pharmacological effects.

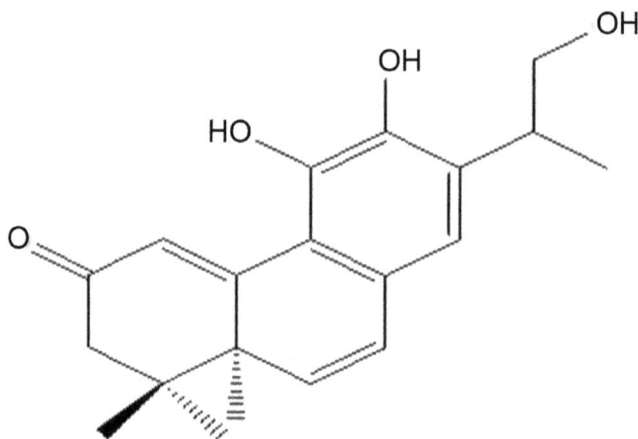

FIGURE 4.2    Structure of diterpene skeleton ($C_{20}H_{24}O_4$) isolated from the root bark of *P. serratifolia*.

Various fractionation techniques (steam/vacuum distillation, solvent extraction followed by chromatographic techniques) have frequently been used for the identification and quantification of aromatic compounds. While Teai et al. [130] identified many novel phytochemicals from the flower bud extract, Rahman et al. [98] reported only 29 compounds from the leaves of *P. serratifolia*. Singh et al. [124] reported many compounds, such as, Octasiloxane and 1,1,3,3,5,5,7,7,9,9,11,11,13,13,15,15-hexadecamethyl from the ethanolic extract of leaves and roots of *P. serratifolia*.

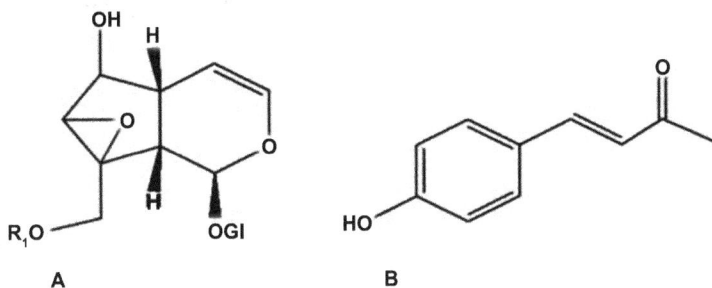

**FIGURE 4.3**   Structure of 10-*O-trans-p*-coumaroylcatalpol (10-OCC) (A) and R1 (B).

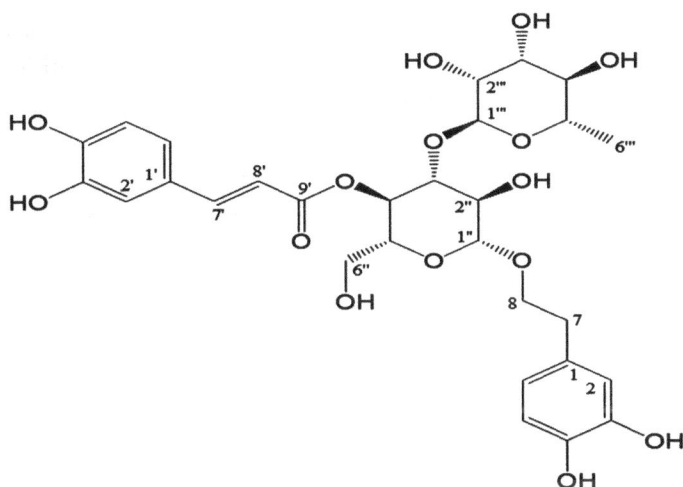

**FIGURE 4.4**   Structure of Acteoside.

Recently, George and his co-researchers extracted volatile oils by hydro-distillation from the leaves and roots of six morphotypes of *P. serratifolia* from different localities in Kerala [22]. The analysis of the essential oil fractions by GC-MS elucidated the taxonomic affinity of these morphological variants. The results were interpreted using the database of NIST Library. The study identified the presence of following similar compounds in all six morphotypes affirming these compounds as species-specific markers of *P. serratifolia* L.

1. Hydroquinone ($C_6H_6O_2$) in leaf samples;;
2. Cadinene in leaf samples;
3. Phytol ($C_{20}H_{40}O$) in leaf samples;

4.   Acetic acid (2-isopropenylcyclopentylide)–methylester $(C_{11}H_{16}O_2)$ in root samples;
5.   2-Phenannthrenol in root samples;
6.   4b,5,6,7,8,8a,9,10,-octahydro-4b,8,8-trimethyl–11-(1-methylethyl) in root samples;
7.   (4bS-*trans*)-$(C_{20}H_{30}O)$ in root samples;
8.   1,2-Benzenedicarboxylic acid in root samples; and
9.   Mono (2-ethylhexyl) ester $(C_{16}H_{22}O_4)$ in root samples.

However, restricted distribution of specific chemical compounds, namely, damascenon, tetradecanoic acid, and caryophyllene oxide in certain morpho-types shows their evolutionary advancement over other morphotypes. For example, damascenone and tetradecanoic acid were located only from the leaves of Morphotype 2; whereas caryophyllene oxide was identified only in Morphotype-6. On the other hand, wider distribution of volatile compounds (such as spathulenol, 2-pentadecanone, β-caryophyllene, isolongifolan-8-ol) was noted in four morphotypes investigated with exclusion of spathulenol in morphotype 2; 2-pentadecanone in Morphotype 2 and 6; β-caryophyllene in Morphotypes 1 and 5; Isolongifolan-8-ol in Morphotypes 1 and 3.

The cluster analysis of the GC-MS peaks showed a clustering pattern of Morphotypes 1 and 2 in one group; Morphotypes 3, 4, and 5 in second group, and the Morphotype 6 as a separate lineage [22].

### 4.6.1   DIGOXIN COMPOUND ISOLATED FROM P. SERRATIFOLIA

A cardioprotective property of the roots of this medicinal plant was also investigated [23]. As revealed in this study, the presence of cardioprotective principle digoxin, isolated from the medicinal plant *Digitalis purpurea*, was detected in the methanolic root extract of two different Morphotypes of *P. serratifolia*. The study also highlighted the significance of salinity-induced stress to enhance the metabolic synthesis of digoxin-like phytoactive compounds in the roots of *P. serratifolia*.

### 4.6.2   SYNTHESIS OF PHYTOACTIVE COMPOUNDS BY TISSUE CULTURE

Recent advances in cell culture techniques have been employed for the synthesis of natural pharma products. Synthesis of bioactive compounds by callus culture is an option for the synthesis of valuable phytoactive compounds (polyphenolic compounds, terpenoids, steroids, saponins, alka- loids, etc.) without destruction of medicinal plants in their natural habitat. In this respect, Singh [122] studied the effectiveness of the callus extract of *P. serratifolia* against selected pathogenic microbes. Researchers also investigated the efficacy of callus-induced synthesis of luteolin production and tested its bioactivity against carrageenan-induced hind paw edema in male wistar rat model experiments [123].

## 4.7 PHARMACOLOGICAL INVESTIGATION ON *P. SERRATIFOLIA*

Today, herbal drugs have tremendous therapeutic significance. *P. serratifolia* is an essential constituent of many traditional Ayurvedic preparations [38, 54] for rheumatism and arthritis, nervine/neuralgic complaints; urinary complaints, *prameha* (diabetes), digestive disorders (deranged digestion, dyspepsia, diarrhea, and constipation), piles, heapatic problems, cardiac disorders, chest pain, obesity, piles, glandular enlargement, inflammation, swelling, muscular pain (body pain, headache, backache), bronchitis, fever, skin diseases, chyluria, gonorrhea, asthma, and respiratory problems. Recent pharmacological investigations have validated the therapeutic potential of this medicinal plant. Review of various biological activities of *P. serratifolia* is presented in this section.

### 4.7.1 ANTIOXIDANT ACTIVITY

The antioxidant potential of the officinal part of this medicinal plant has been investigated by Rajendran et al. [105], Selvam et al. [116], Shilpa et al. [120], Jain et al. [52], Muthukumaran et al. [86], and Mali [79]. Aqueous and alcoholic fractions of stem bark and stem-wood were also analyzed for in vitro antioxidant activity [105]. These extracts also displayed very good free radical and nitric oxide scavenging activities. The antioxidant potential of the wood and bark of *P. serratifolia* was also determined by inducing oxidative stress in rabbits [109]. The study revealed significant antioxidant activity as evidenced from various enzyme assay techniques [22]. The study revealed significant changes in the levels of SOD, catalase, and glutathione with respect to liver, kidney, heart, and blood samples of the plant extract-treated group and was comparable with the drug "silymarin" administered group, which confirmed the potential antioxidant activity of *Agnimantha*.

Jain et al. investigated antioxidant activity of the root extracts of *P. integrifolia* in water and methanol by various antioxidant and chelation assays [52]. Satisfactory $IC_{50}$ values were reported for both aqueous and methanolic root extracts in these antioxidant assays. The antioxidant potential of its wood extract was explicated by Muthukumaran et al. [86] by various antioxidant assays. Mali [79] evaluated the beneficial effect of its root extracts, aqueous as well as Chloroform: methanol (1:1) solvent system (CMEPI), on specific human cells against $H_2O_2$-induced oxidative damage. As revealed in this study, CMEPI was more effective than aqueous root extract, probably due to higher dissolution of bioactive compounds in the latter solvent system.

As revealed from the above-mentioned in vitro antioxidant studies, entire parts of *P. serratifolia* (leaves, stem, and roots) are potential sources of natural antioxidants. These findings point to the need for bioprospecting of *P. serratifolia* as a potential therapeutic/neutaceutic agent for promoting human health and also for developing novel drugs.

### 4.7.2   CARDIOPROTECTIVE ACTIVITY

In the indigenous system of medicine, *P. serratifolia* has a prominent role to regularize the functioning of heart and circulation of blood. Anticoagulation assay of the flavonoids of this plant has been reported [46]. The cardioprotective property of this plant against isoproterenol administered experimental myocardial infarction in rats was also investigated based on ECG, electrophoresis, and biochemical analysis of relevant blood/ tissue parameters [102].

The cardiac stimulant activity of the water and ethanol extract of *P. serratifolia* was conducted by isolated frog heart perfusion technique and the result was compared with that of the drug "digoxin" [106]. The analysis of different membrane parameters ($Na^+$, $K^+$, ATPase and $Mg^{2+}$ATPase, $Ca^{2+}$ATPase, etc.) further confirmed the cardiotonic activity of this medicinal plant. As noted in the above study, ethanol extract has much pronounced cardiotonic effect than its aqueous counterpart producing β-adrenergic effect. However, further bioactivity-guided studies based fractionation of its phyto-constituents (cardiac principles) are recommended to substantiate the protective myocardial property of *P. serratifolia*.

### 4.7.3 ANTIARTHRITIC AND ANTI-INFLAMMATORY ACTIVITIES

Studies conducted by Rathore et al. [112], Barik et al. [15], Jantan et al. [53], Rajendran and Krishnakumar [103], Gokani et al. [44], and Kumari et al. [70] validate the ethno-pharmacological property of *P. serratifolia* to cure arthritis/inflammation of the joints. The toxicity activity of the ethanolic leaf extract of *P. serratifolia* was evaluated in the experimental animals [59, 60] and as suggested in these studies prolonged treatment strategy minimize the progression of chronic arthritis.

In another comparative study in Charles foster rats, *P. latifolia* leaves have shown anti-inflammatory property activity than the *P. obtusifolia* [70]. In another animal model study, the alkaloid compound of *P. serratifolia* has shown positive results to reduce granuloma formation [15] and the results were comparable to that of phenylbutazone. Gokani et al. [44] investigated the anti-inflammatory and in vitro antioxidant potential of the roots of *P. serratifolia* in various experimental models. The luteolin concentration and anti-inflammatory activity of the root as well as root callus extract of *P. serratifolia* against carrageenan-induced paw edema was also investigated [123].

### 4.7.4 ANTIMICROBIAL ACTIVITY

The root bark [56, 71], stem wood and stem bark [101, 104], and essential oil fractions [98] of *P. serratifolia* were subjected to antimicrobial screening. Its root bark extract in ethanol is active against *Streptococcus hemolyticus* and inactive against *Escherichia coli* and *Shigella dysenteria*. Kapoor [56] substantiated the antibacterial activity of the phenolic compounds of the root bark of this medicinal plant against *Staphylococcus aureus, Bacillus subtilis,* and *Streptococcus hemolytics*.

In another study, Rahman et al. [98] examined antibacterial potential of the essential oil and various organic extracts of *P. integrifolia and these fractions* were effective against *Sarcinalutea, B. subtilis, E. coli, Pseudomonas* sp., *Klebsiella pneumoniae* and *Xanthomonas campestries*. Rajendran studied the broad-spectrum antimicrobial activity of its stem wood/bark extracts in different solvents against certain bacteria and fungi and the results were compared to ciprofloxacin and amphotericin-B [101]. The plant material was also screened against selected Gram +ve/Gram -ve bacterial organisms and fungi [104].

Singh [122] evaluated the antimicrobial property of the extracts of callus derived from different explants (leaves and roots) and their live materials against selected human pathogens. The results revealed better inhibitory property for the callus-derived extracts compared to natural plant material extracts. As suggested in this study, the secondary metabolities derived from various callus tissues of *P. serratifolia* can be employed as potential antimicrobial agents in food, pharmaceutical, and agro industries.

### 4.7.5   ANTIDIABETIC ACTIVITY

The efficacy of different species of *Premna* to reduce serum glucose level was reported by Alamgir et al. [5], Kar et al. [57], Dash et al. [31], and Majumdar [78]. Alamgir et al. [5] reported the effect of *P. integrifolia* against blood glucose in stretozotocin-induced diabetic rats. Kar et al. [57] investigated the hypoglycaemic activity of this medicinal plant. Similarly, antihyperglycemic activity of *P. corymbosa* root extracts in rat model experiments was also reported [31]. As revealed in this study, the extract at 400 mg/kg dose level produced significant reduction of blood glucose at the 8th h of administration in normoglycemic animals. Studies conducted by Thiruvenkata and Jayakar [132] and Majumdar [78] further substantiated the antidiabetic, antihyperlipidaemic, and antioxidant properties of *P. corymbosa* and *P. integrifolia*, respectively.

### 4.7.6   ANTIOBESITY/HYPOLIDEMIC ACTIVITY

Ghosh and Sukumar [41] studied the efficacy of *P. obtusifolia* R. Br. (syn. *P. serratifolia* L.) as an antiobesity drug among 26 over-weight subjects. The results of their study revealed remarkable decrease in body mass index, midtriceps skin-fold thickness of the treated group. Studies conducted by Mali et al. [81] substantiate the results of Ghosh and Sukumar [41] confirming the antiobesity property of *Premna* species in mice model experiments. Antihyperlipidaemic activity of *P. integrifolia* on nicotine-induced hyperlipidaemia in male albino rats was also evaluated [95].

### 4.7.7   GASTROPROTECTIVE POTENTIAL

In *Ayurveda*, the drug *Agnimantha* is one of the specific drugs prescribed to enhance the digestive power eliminating the ill effects of *kapha* and *vata*.

Studies reported by Jothi et al. [54] and Rajathi et al. [99] highlight gastro-protective potential of the leaves and bark extract of *P. serratifolia* L. against Aspirin-induced ulcer in rats. According to these studies, leaves/bark extract of *P. serratifolia* has antiulcer property. The results revealed dose-dependent decrease in ulcer index, gastric acid secretion, free acidity, and total acidity in aspirin and extract-treated group of animals. Histopathological investigations further confirmed the efficacy of the leaf extract in preventing ulcer formation.

### 4.7.8   TUMOR CELL SUPPRESSION/CYTOTOXICITY STUDIES

Selvam et al. [117] evaluated the antioxidant and cytotoxic potential of the methanolic leaf extract of *P. serratifolia* in various in vitro model systems. The leaf extract was screened by SRB assay agaist selected breast, liver, and lung cancer lines and was very effective against MCF7, HepG2, A549 cell lines. In a recent investigation, Habtemariam and George [47] screened the cytotoxicity of the leaves, root wood, and root bark extracts of *P. serratifolia* against neuroblastoma and melanoma cancer cell lines. In this study, they isolated an aromatic diterpene compound from the root bark extract with promising cytotoxicity against SHSY-5Y and B16 cell lines.

### 4.7.9   HEPATOPROTECTIVE ACTIVITY

Hepatoprotective activity of the leaf and root extract of *P. serratifolia* L. (500 mg/kg) was tested in albino rats by comparing the levels of various hepatic enzymes (ALP, ACP, SGPT, and SGOT) in the blood serum and liver of normal group with that of the treatment groups ($CCl_4$ group and $CCl_4$ + *P. serratifolia* leaf/bark extract groups) [38]. The study revealed the effectiveness of its leaves and roots to normalize the level of heapatic enzymes. Muthukumaran et al. [85] examined the effectiveness of the aqueous extract of this medicinal plant against $CCl_4$ and paracetamol-induced experimental liver damage in rats. Studies conducted by Vadivu et al. [133] substantiated the hepatoprotective/in vitro cytotoxic properties of its leaves. Singh et al. [125] examined the hepatic activity of its root and root callus extract of in relation to silymarine, a proven hepatoprotective drug molecule. Histopatho-logical examinations confirmed the efficiency of root /root callus extract in preventing the development of chronic hepatic damage.

### 4.7.10   IMMUNOMODULATORY, ANTINOCICEPTIVE, NEUROPHARMACOLOGICAL, ANTICONVULSANT, AND ANTIPARASITIC ACTIVITIES

Pharmacological properties of *P. serratifolia* with special reference to PAF receptor binding, cell growth suppression, antiparasitic activities, and so forth, were investigated in recent years.

Gokani et al. [43, 44] investigated anti-inflammatory, antioxidant, and immunomodulatory potential of the methanolic extracts of *Agnimantha* drugs (*P. integrifolia* and its substitute *C. phlomidis*) in mice. Root extracts of these plants (300 mg kg⁻¹ × 7 days) were administered orally to mice prior to immunization with sheep red blood cells (SRBC). In response to specific immune activity, the substitute drug *C. phlomidis* showed better activity. However, with reference to nonspecific immune activity, the roots of both *P. integrifolia* and *C. phlomidis* have shown almost equal responses.

Karthikeyan and Deepa [61, 62] evaluated the anti-inflammatory, toxicity, and antinociceptive activity of the leaf extract of *P. corymbosa* in Wistar albino rats. The study confirmed the pain-relieving property of this medicinal plant. It was noted that the toxicity evaluation of this drug has not shown any clinical manifestation of mortality even at high doses. The property of *P. serratifolia* leaves to reduce pain has been reported by the traditional Ayurvedic and Marma practitioners of Kerala. In folklore medicine, *P. serratifolia* is recommended as an analgesic to relieve body pain, backache, and headache. In this backdrop, Karmakar et al. [58] assessed the analgesic property of the ethanolic leaves extract of this medicinal plant in mice employing acetic acid-induced writhing model experiments. However, further studies are needed to isolate and characterize bioactive compounds that show antinociceptive activity.

Shukla et al. [121] isolated an active principle from *P. serratifolia* that delays the process of aging and its efficacy was demonstrated in an animal model, *Caenorhabditis elegans*. The delayed aging process is often linked with the level fat and reactive oxygen species in the worms. This study thus highlights the prospects of developing suitable geriatric medicine from *P. serratifolia* to delay aging process. Neuropharmacological, anti-inflammatory, and analgesic properties of the bark extract of *P. integrifolia* were also investigated [63].

Its methanolic bark extract (200 mg/kg) has shown remarkable anti-inflammatory property in rats. Anticonvulsant property of *Premna* species against Pentylenetetrazole/electroshock-induced convulsions in mice was also evaluated [12]. Besides, antiparasitic activity of *P. serratifolia* was reported against *Leishmania donovanim* [33]. Based on the above findings, it is assumed that bioactivity-guided fractionation of lead molecules in *P. serratifolia* and related species may serve to develop suitable products to fight againstmany age-related health issues.

## 4.8   FUTURE PROSPECTS

In the Ayurvedic traditional system of medicine, *P. serratifolia* has a signifi-cant position. However, the current ambiguity and dispute regarding the taxo-nomic and Ayurvedic status of the genuine drug "Agnimantha" as described in classical Ayurvedic texts should be resolved by subjecting the different morphological variants of *P. serratifolia* and their substitute species, namely, *C. phlomidis* for detailed pharmacognostic and pharmacological evaluation.

It is expected that the current review on traditional knowledge, pharma-cognostic, and pharmacological studies of *P. serratifolia* would provide a means for bioprospecting of this species as a neutraceutcal food supplement considering its proven broad-spectrum biological activity as antiarthritic, anti-inflammatory/anticancerous, antiobesity, cardioprotective, gastropro-tective, hepatoprotective, immune-modulatory, and longevity-promoting agent.

The prospect of developing value-added products like "herbal tea" from *P. serratifoia* can be explored since its tender leaves are rich sources of natural antioxidants viz., polyphenolic compounds. However, detailed studies on toxicological as well as nutritional aspects of its leaves at different stages of leaf development are suggested to bring forth the "food value" of this underutilized ethnomedicinal plant species.

## 4.9   SUMMARY

The leaves, bark, and roots of *P. serratifolia* L. are indispensable for the preparation of different Ayurvedic formulations like *arishtam, avaleham, kwatham, ghritham,* and *tailam.* The major aim of the present investigation is to bring out the hidden potential of this medicinal plant as an excellent source of active therapeutics. Relevant literature on taxonomic history, ethnobotanical and nutritional value, therapeutic/biological activity studies, and so forth of the plant was collected from traditional manuscripts/texts, pharmacopoeias, traditional Ayurvedic physicians, and research publications.

The present status of *P. serratifolia* with special reference to its taxonomy, ethnobotanical knowledge, Ayurvedic drug status, indigenous uses as food/medicines/Ayurvedic formulations, pharmacognostic, pharmacological studies, and so forth is presented in this chapter.

## ACKNOWLEDGMENT

This chapter is partially based on, *"Bose, Lekshmi, V.; George, K. V. Pharmacognostic and Phytochemical Studies on P. serratifolia in Kerala. PhD Dissertation; Kottayam—Kerala: Mahatma Gandhi University; 2014; pages 215."*

## KEYWORDS

- **antiarthritic**
- **antidiabetic**
- **anti-inflammatory**
- **antimicrobial**
- **antiobesity**
- **antioxidant**
- **cardioprotective**
- *Premna serratifolia*

## REFERENCES

1. Aberoumand, A.; Deokule, S.S. Studies on nutritional values of some wild edible plants from Iran and India. *Pak. J. Nutr.*, **2009**, *8* (1), 26–31.
2. Acharya, Y.T. *Dravyaguna Vijnanam, II.* Bombay: Nirnaya Sagar Press; **1950**; p. 300.
3. Agarwal, V.S. *Drug Plants of India.* New Delhi: Kalyani Publishers; **1977**; vol. 2; p. 584.
4. Alam, M.; Rukmani, B.; Meenakshi, N.; Dasan, K.S.; Bhima, R.R. Standardization studies of some *dasamula* containing formulations. *J. Res. Ayur. Siddha*, **1993**, *4* (1), 68–73.
5. Alamgir, M.; Rokeya, B.; Hannan, J.M.; Choudhuri, M.S. The effect of *Premna integrifolia* Linn. (Verbenaceae) on blood glucose in stretozotocin induced type 1 and type 2 diabetic rats. *Pharmazie.*, **2001**, *56*, 903–904.

6. Anonymous. *Pharmacognosy of Ayurvedic Drugs.* Series I, No: 2; Pharmacognosy Department, Ayurveda College, Trivandrum; **1978**; pp. 23–30.

7. Anonymous. *The Ayurvedic Pharmacopoeia of India.* Part 1, Volume III; New Delhi: Government of India, Ministry of Health and Family Welfare, Department of ISM and Homoeopathy; **2001**; pp. 3–4.

8. Anonymous. *The Wealth of India: Dictionary of Indian Raw Materials and Industrial Products—Raw Materials.* New Delhi: Government of India, Ministry of Health and Family Welfare, Department of ISM and Homoeopathy; **1972**; p. 240.

9. Aparna, S.; Ved, D.K.; Lalitha, S.; Venkatasubramanian, P. Botanical identity of plant sources of *Daśamūla drugs* through an analysis of published literature. *Anc. Sci. Life*, **2012**, *32*, 3–10.

10. *Ayurvedic Formulary of India.* Part I, 2nd ed.; New Delhi: Government of India, Ministry of Health and Family Welfare Department of Indian Systems of Medicine and Homoeopathy; **2000**; pp. 307–330.

11. *Ayurvedic Formulary of India.* New Delhi: Government of India, Ministry of Health and Family Welfare, Department of Indian Systems of Medicine and Homoeopathy; **1978**; pp. 241–259.

12. Baby, D.A.; Pothen, N.; Kurian, D.S.; Jose, J.; James, T.S.; Amal, D. Evaluation of Anticonvulsant activity of *Premna corymbosa* in experimental mice. *Int. J. Exp. Pharmacol.*, **2011**, *1* (2), 37–41.

13. Bagchi, C.; Tripathi, S.K.; Hazra, A.; Bhattacharya, D. Evaluation of hypolipidemic activity of *P. integrifolia* Linn. bark in rabbit model. *PHARBIT*, **2008**, *18*, 149–153.

14. Bapalal, Vaidya. *Some Controversial Drugs in Indian Medicine.* Varanasi, UP: Chaukhambha Orientalia; **1982**; pp. 267–270.

15. Barik, B. R.; Bhowmik, T.; Dey, A. K.; Patra, A. Premnazole, an isoxazole alkaloid of *Premna integrifolia* and *Gmelina arborea* with anti-inflammatory activity. *Fitoterapia*, **1992**, *63* (3), 290–295.

16. Barik, B.R.; Bhowmik, T.; Dey, A.K. Premnazole, an isoxazole alkaloid of *Premna integrifolia* and *Gmelina arborea* with anti-inflammatory activity. *Fitoterapia*, **1992**, *63* (4), 296–299.

17. Barlingame, B. Comparison of total lipids, fatty acids, sugars and nonvolatile organic acids in nuts from Castanea species. *J. Food Comp. Anal.*, **2000**, *13*, 99–100.

18. Basu, N.K.; Dandiya, P.C. Chemical investigation of *Premna integrifolia. J. Am. Pharm. Ass. Sci. Educ.*, **1947**, *36*, 389–391.

19. Basu, N.K.; Joneja, A.N. Chemical investigation of *Premna integrifolia. Indian J. Pharm.*, **1949**, *11*, 191–193.

20. Beer, E.; Lam, H.J. The Verbenaceae collected in Papua by L. J. Brass for the Archbold Expedition. *Blumea*, **1936**, *2*, 221–228.

21. Bentham, G. *Verbenaceae: Flora Australiensis.* London: L. Reeve and Co.; **1870**; vol. 5; pp. 31–70.

22. Bose, L.V. *The Pharmacognostic and Phytochemical Studies on Premna serratifolia L. in Kerala.* PhD Thesis; Mahatma Gandhi University, Kerala; **2014**; p. 219.

23. Bose, L.V.; George, K.V.; Iyer, R.S.; Deepa, T.D. Identification of novel cardiac principle in the roots of *Premna serratifolia* L. *J. Pharm. Res.*, **2012**, *5*, 3261–3264.

24. Caldecott, T.; Tierra, M. *Ayurveda: The Divine Science of life.* New York: Elsevier Health Sciences; **2006**; p. 316.

25. Chopra, R.N. *Drugs of India.* Chennai, TN: Orient Longman Ltd.; **1969**; p. 116.

26. Chopra, R.N.; Chopra, I.C. *A Review of Work on Indian Medicinal Plants*. New Delhi: Indian Council of Medical Research; **1955**; p. 45.

27. Chopra, R.N.; Nayar, S.L.; Chopra, I.C. *Glossary of Indian Medicinal Plants*. New Delhi: Council of Scientific and Industrial Research; **1956**; p. 203.

28. Chunekar, K.C. *Bhavaprakashanighantu of Sri Bhavamisra*. Varanasi, UP: Choukamba Orientalia; **1982**; p. 281.

29. Chunekar, K.C. *Illustrated Dravyaguna Vijnana*. 2nd ed. Varanasi, UP: Vhaukhambha Orientalia; **2005**; vol. 2, p. 117.

30. Dasgupta, B.; Sinha, N.K.; Pandey, V.B.; Ray, A.B. Major alkaloid and flavonoid of *Premna integrifolia*. *Planta Medica,* **1984**, *50* (3), 278–281.

31. Dash, G.K.; Patrolm, C.P.; Maiti, A.K. A study on the anti-hyperglycaemic effect of roots of *Premna corymbosa* Rottl. *J. Nat. Rem.,* **2005**, *5*, 31–34.

32. Debelmas, A.M.; Dobremez, J.F.; Srivastava, M.; Benarroche, L. Medicinal plants of Nepal. *Plant Med. Phytotherapy,* **1973**, *7*, 104–105.

33. Desrivot, J.; Waikedre, J.; Cabalion, P. Anti-parasitic activity of some New Caledonian medicinal plants. *J. Ethnopharmacol.,* **2007**, *112* (1), 7–12.

34. Dey, A.C. *Indian Medicinal Plants used in Ayurvedic Preparations*. Dehradun, UP: Bishen Singh Mahendra Pal Singh; **1980**; p. 11.

35. Drury, H. *Useful Plants of India*. Madras: Thomas W.M. Asyulum, Mount Road; **1858**; pp. 365–366.

36. Etkin, N.L.; Ross, P.J. (Eds.). *Pharmafood and Nutraceuticals: paradigm shifts in biotherapeutics, Joint Meeting of the Society for Economic Botany and the International Society for Ethnopharmacology: Plants for Food and Medicine*; Kew, UK: Royal Botanic Gardens; **1996**; pp. 3–16.

37. Fletcher, H.R. Nomenclature of *Premna obtusifolia* R. Br. *Taxon,* **1938**, *2*, 88–89.

38. George, K.V. *Ethnobotanical, Phytochemical and Pharmacognostic Studies on Premna serratifolia* L. Kottayam, India: Research Project, C.M.S. College; **2006**; p. 107.

39. George, K.V.; Mathew, B.D.; Thomas, R.P. Pharmacognostic Studies on *Agnimantha*. *Int. Congress on Science and Technology for Sustainable Development*; **2006**; pp. 33–35.

40. George, K.V.; Samuel, K.A. Phytochemical investigations on *P. serratifolia* L. *Aryavaidyan,* **2003**, *16* (4), 234–239.

41. Ghosh, R.; Sukumar, G. Therapeutic efficacy of *Agnimantha* (*Premna obtusifolia*) in obesity. *J. Trad. Knowl.,* **2009**, *3*, 369–371.

42. Gokani, R.H.; Kapadia, N.S.; Shah, M.B. Comparative pharmacognostic study of *Clerodendrum phlomidis* and *Premna integrifolia*. *J. Nat. Remed.,* **2008**, *8*, 222–231.

43. Gokani, R.H.; Lahiri, S.K.; Santani, D.D.; Shah, M.B. Evaluation of immunomodulatory activity of *Clerodendrum phlomidis* and *Premna integrifolia* roots. *Int. J. Pharmacol.,* **2007**, *3*, 352–356.

44. Gokani, R.H.; Lahiri, S.K.; Santani, D.D.; Shah, M.B. Evaluation of anti-inflammatory and antioxidant activity of *Premna integrifolia* roots. *J. Compl. Integr. Med.,* **2011**, *8* (1), 1553–3840.

45. Gokani, R.H.; Shah, M.B. Isolation and estimation of *Clerodendrum phlomidis* and *P. integrifolia* roots. *J. Pharm. Res.,* **2009**, *8*, 9–11.

46. Gopal, R.H.; Purushothaman, K.K. Effect of plant isolates on coagulation of blood: An *in vitro* study. *Bull. Med. Ethnobot. Res.,* **1984**, *5*, 171–177.

47. Habtemariam, S.; George, K.V. A novel diterpene skelton: Identification of a highly aromatic, cytotoxic and antioxidant 5-Methyl-10-demethyl-abietane type diterpene from *Premna serratifolia*. *Phytoth. Res.,* **2015**, *29* (1), 80–85.

48. Habtemariam, S.; Gray, A.l.; Halbert, G.W.; Waterman, P.G. A novel antibacterial diterpene from *Premna schimperi. Planta Med.*, **1990**, *56*, 187–189.
49. Habtemariam, S.; Gray, Al.; Waterman, P.G. Flavonoids from three Ethiopian species of *Premna. Z. Naturforsch.*, **1991**, *47*, 144–147.
50. Hang, N.T.; Ky, P.T. Study on the chemical constituents of *Premna integrifolia* L. *Nat. Prod. Commun.*, **2008**, *3*, 1449–1452.
51. Hussain, A.; Virmani, O.P.; Popli, S.P. *Dictionary of Indian Medicinal Plants.* New Delhi: Central Institute of Medicinal and Aromatic Plants; **1992**; p. 375.
52. Jain, S.; Singh, M.; Barik, R.; Malviya, N. *In-vitro* antioxidant activity of *Premna integrifolia* Linn. roots. *Res. J. Pharmacol. Pharmacodyn.*, **2013,** *5* (5), 293–296.
53. Jantan, I.B.; Kang, Y.H.; Suh, D.Y.; Han, B.H. Inhibitory effects of Malaysian medicinal plants on platelet activating factor receptor binding. *Nat. Prod. Sci.*, **1996**, *2* (2), 86–89.
54. Jothi, E.T.; Karthikeyan, R.; Suryalakshmi, P.V.; Srinivasababu, P. Gastro protective potetial of *Premna serratifolia* L. leaves against aspirin induced ulcer in albino rats. *Pharmacology,* **2010**, *3*, 189–198.
55. Kadareit, J.W. *Flowering Plants—Dicotyledons, the Families and Genera of Vascular Plants.* Volume 7; Berlin, Heidelberg: Springer-Verlag; **2004**; p. 478.
56. Kapoor, L.D. *CRC Handbook of Ayurvedic Medicinal Plants: Herbal Reference Library.* Boca Raton, FL: CRC Press; **2001**; p. 70.
57. Kar, A.; Choudhary, B.K.; Bandyopadhyay, N.G. Comparative evaluation of hypoglycaemic activity of some Indian medicinal plants in alloxan diabetic rats. *J. Ethnopharmacol.*, **2003**, *84* (1), 105–108.
58. Karmakar, U.K.; Pramanik, S.; Sadhu, S.K.; Shill, M.C.; Biswas, S.K. Assessment of analgesic and antibacterial activity of *P. integrifolia* Linn. (Family: Verbenaceae) leaves. *Int. J. Pharm. Sci. Res.*, **2011**, *2* (6), 1430–1435.
59. Karthikeyan, M.; Deepa, M.K. Anti-inflammatory activity of *Premna corymbosa* (Burm.f.) Rottl. & Willd. leaves extracts in Wistar albino rats. *Asian Pac. J. Trop. Med.*, **2011**, *4* (7), 510–513.
60. Karthikeyan, M.; Deepa, M.K. Effect of ethanolic extract of *Premna corymbosa* (Burm. f.) Rottl. & Willd. leaves in complete Freund's adjuvant-induced arthritis in Wistar albino rats. *J. Basic Clin. Physiol. Pharmacol.*, 2010, *21* (1), 15–26
61. Kartick, C.B. *Pharmacopoeia Indica.* Dehra Dun: Bishen Singh Mahendra Pal Singh; **1984**; p. 17.
62. Khare, C.P. *Indian Medicinal Plants - An Illustrated Dictionary.* Berlin, Heidelberg: Springer-Verlag; 2007; p. 516.
63. Khatun, H.; Majumder, R.; Mamun, A. Preliminary pharmacological activity of the methanolic extract of *Premna integrifolia* barks in rats. *Avicenna J. Phytomed.*, **2014***, 4* (3), 215–224.
64. Kirtikar, K.R.; Basu, B.D. *Indian Medicinal Plants.* Allahabad, Allahabad Sharma Publisher; **1918**; p. 992.
65. Kirtikar, K.R.; Basu, L.M. *Indian Medicinal Plants.* New Delhi: Periodical Experts Book Agency, Vivek Vihar; **1992**; vol. 3, pp. 1926–1928.
66. Kok, R. The genus *Premna* L. (Lamiaceae) in the flora Malesiana area. *Kew Bull.*, **2013**, *68,* 1–30.
67. Kolammal, M. *Pharmacognosy of Ayurvedic drugs.* Bulletin 10; Trivandrum: Pharmacognosy Department, Ayurveda College; **1979**; pp. 2–23.

68. Krishnamurthy, K.H.; Masilamoney, P.; Govindraj, N. The nature of the confusion in the botanical identity of *Agnimantha* and pharmacology of one claimant viz., *Clerodendron phlomides* L. *J. Res. Indian Med.*, **1972**, *7* (1), 27–36.
69. Kumar, V.; Jain, S.K. Plant products in some tribal markets of Central India. *Econ. Botany*, **2002**, *56* (3), 242–245.
70. Kumari, H.; Shrikanth, P.; Chaithra, P.R.; Nishteswar, K. A comparative experimental evaluation of anti-inflammatory activity of *Premna obtusifolia* Linn. and *Premna latifolia* Roxb. leaves in Charles foster rats. *Anc. Sci. Life*, **2011**, *31* (2), 58–61.
71. Kurup, P. A. Antibiotic substance from the root bark of *Premna integrifolia*. *Die Naturwissenschaften* (Natural Sciences), **1964**, *1964*, 480–484.
72. Kurup, P.N.V.; Ramdas, V.N.K.; Joshi, P. *Handbook of Medicinal Plants*. New Delhi: Government of India, Ministry of Health and Family Welfare Department of Indian Systems of Medicine and Homoeopathy; **1979**; pp. 2–8.
73. Ky, P.T.; Hang, N.T.; My, T.T. Preliminary study on the chemical components in flowers of *Premna integrifolia* L. *Tap. Chi. Duoc. Hoc.,* **2005**, *12*, 9–10.
74. Lalithamma, K. *Pharmacopoeia.* Thiruvananthapuram. Kerala: Publication Division, Ayurveda College; **1996**; p. 218.
75. Lam, H.J. *The Verbenaceae of the Malayan Archipelago*. Groningen: M. De. Waal; **1919**; p. 87.
76. Lam, H.J.; Brink, R.C. Revision of the Verbenaceae of the Dutch East- Indies and surrounding countries. *Bull. Jard. Bot. Buitenz. III.,* **1921**, *3*, 1–116.
77. Linnaeus, C. *Mantissa Plantarum Altera Genrum editionis VI & Specierum editionis II* (Species Plantarum genre Version 6 and Version 2 of Species); Stockholm: Laurentius Salvius; **1971**; p. 75.
78. Majumder, R.; Akter, S.; Naim, Z.; Al-Amin; Adam, B. Antioxidant and anti-diabetic activities of the methanolic extract of *Premna integrifolia* bark. *Adv. Biol. Res.*, **2014**, *8* (1), 29–36.
79. Mali, P.Y. Beneficial effect of extracts of *Premna integrifolia* root on human leucocytes and erythrocytes against hydrogen peroxide induced oxidative damage. *Chronicles Young Sci.*, **2014**, *5* (1), 53–58.
80. Mali, P.Y.; Bhadane, V.V. Comparative account of screening of bioactive ingredients of *Premna integrifolia* Linn. with special reference to root by using various solvents. *J. Pharm. Res.*, **2010**, *3*, 1677–1679.
81. Mali, P.Y.; Bigoniya, P.; Panchal, S.S.; Muchhandi, I.S. Anti-obesity activity of chloroform-methanol extract of *Premna integrifolia* in mice fed with cafeteria diet. *J. Pharm. Bioallied Sci.*, **2013**, *5* (3), 229–236.
82. Meeuse, A.D.J. *Notes of Japanese Verbenaceae. Blumea*, 1942, *5*, 66–80.
83. Merrill, E.D. *Verbenaceae. An Interpretation of Rumphius's Herbarium Amboinense.* Manila: Bureau of Printing; **1917**; pp. 448–456.
84. Munir, A.A. Taxonomic revision of the genus *Premna* L. (Verbenaceae) in Australia. *J. Adelaide Bot. Gard.*, **1984**, *7*, 1–44.
85. Muthukumaran, P.; Pattabiraman, K. Hepatoprotective activity of *P. serratifolia* Linn. on experimental liver damage in rats. *Asian J. Sci. Technol.*, **2010**, *6*, 105–107.
86. Muthukumaran, P.; Salomi, S.; Umamaheshwari, R. *In vitro* antioxidant activity of *Premna serratifolia* Linn. *Asian J. Res. Pharm. Sci.,* **2013**, *3* (1), 15–18.
87. Nadkarni, K.M. *Indian Materia Medicawith Ayurvedic, Unani and Home remedies.* Mumbai: Popular Prakashan Pvt. Ltd.; **2007**; vol. 1, pp. 1009–1010.

88. Nadkarni, K.M.; Nadkarni, A.K.; Chopra, R.N. *Indian Materia Medica*. Bombay: Popular Prakashan Pvt Ltd.; **1954**; vol. 1, p. 353.

89. Nair, R.V. *Controversial Drug Plants*. Hyderabad: Orient Longman Pvt. Ltd.; **2004**; pp. 8–9.

90. Nazarudeen, A. Nutritional composition of some lesser known fruits used by the ethnic communities and local folks of Kerala. *Ind. J. Trad. Knowl.*, **2010**, *9* (2), 398–402.

91. Otsuka, H.; Watanabe, E.; Yusana, K. A verbascoside iridoid glucoside conjugate form *Premna corymbosa* Rott. *Phytochem.*, **1993**, *32* (4), 983–986.

92. Pandey, G. *Dravyaguna Vijnana*. Varanasi: A-J Krishnadas Academy; **1998**; pp. 60–65.

93. Pandey, G. *Dravyaguna Vijnana* (Materia Medica: Vegetable Drugs), Part -1. Varanasi: A-J Krishnadas Academy; **2002**; pp. 72–76.

94. Parkinson, C. E. *Forest Flora of the Andaman Islands*. Dehradun: Bishen Singh Mahendra Pal Singh; **1922**; p. 218.

95. Patel, M.J.; Patel, J.K. Evaluation of the anti-hyperlipidaemic activity of *Premna integrifolia* on nicotine induced hyperlipidaemia in rats. *Int. J. Pharma Biosci.*, **2012**, *3* (2), 220–226.

96. Purandare, N.V. *Rajanighantu Sahito Dhanvantariya Nighantu* (Dhanvantari Dictionary with Rajani Ghantu). Poona: Anand Asram Press; **1896**; pp. 27–28.

97. Puri, H.S. *Rasayana*: *Ayurvedic Herbs for Longevity and Rejuvenation*. Boca Raton, FL: CRC Press; **2002**; pp. 34–37.

98. Rahman, A.; Shantaa, Z.S.; Rashida, M.A.; Parvina, T. *In vitro* antibacterial properties of essential oil and organic extracts of *P. integrifolia* Linn. *Arab. J. Chem.*, **2016**, *9*, 475–479.

99. Rajathi, K.; Indhumathi, T. Antiulcer activity of *Premna serratifolia* against aspirin induced gastric ulcer model. *Int. Res. J. Pharm.*, **2013**, *4* (6), 171–176.

100. Rajendran, R.; Daniel, P. *The Indian Verbenaceae: a Taxonomic Revision*. Dehradun, Uttarakhand*: Bishen Singh Mahendra Pal Singh,* 23-A New Cannaught Place, Chakrata Road; **2002**; pp. 67–71.

101. Rajendran, R. Antimicrobial activity of different bark and wood of *Premna serratifolia* Lin. *Int. J. Pharma Biosci.*, **2010**, *1* (1), 1–9.

102. Rajendran, R.; Basha, S.N. Cardioprotective effect of ethanol extract of stem-bark and stem-wood of *Premna serratifolia* L., (Verbenaceae). *Res. J. Pharm. Tech.*, **2008**, *1* (4), 487-491.

103. Rajendran, R.; Krishnakumar, E. Anti-arthritic activity of *Premna serratifolia* Linn., wood against adjuvant induced arthritis. *Avicenna J. Med. Biotechnol.*, **2010**, *2* (2), 101–106.

104. Rajendran, R.; Saleem, B.N.Antimicrobial activity of crude extracts and fractions of *Premna serratifolia* Linn. roots. *Med. Plants Int. J. Phytomed. Rel. Indus.*, **2010**, *2* (1), 1–5.

105. Rajendran, R.; Srinivasan, M.; Bavan, S.; Sundharajan, R. *In-vivo* antioxidant activity of *Premna serratifolia* Linn. in high fat diet fed rabbits. *Biosci., Biotechnol. Res. Asia*, **2009**, *6* (2), 785–789.

106. Rajendran, R.; Suseela, L.; Meenakshi, S.R.; Basha S.N. Cardiac stimulant activity of bark and wood of *Premna serratifolia*. *Bangl. J. Pharmacol.*, **2008**, *3*, 107–113.

107. Rajendran, R.; Susheela, L. Pharmacognostical studies on *Premna serratifolia* Lin. (Verbenaceae). *Med. Plants- Int. J. Phytomed. Rel. Ind.*, **2010**, *2* (2), 169–174.

108. Rao, C.B.; Krishna, P.G.; Suseela, K. Chemical examination of *Premna* species, Part X: New isoprenoids from the root bark of *Premna integrifolia* Linn. and *P. latifolia* var. *Mollissima. Indian J. Chem.*, **1985**, *24*, 403–407.

109. Rapport, L.; Lockwood, G.B. *Nutraceuticals.* London: Pharmaceutical Press; 2003; pp. 20–25.

110. Rastogi, R.P.; Mehrotra, B.N. *Compendium of Indian Medicinal Plants.* Lucknow, UP: Central Drug Research Institute; **1991**; vol. 2, p. 560.

111. Rastogi, R.P.; Mehrotra, B.N. *Compendium of Indian Medicinal Plants.* Lucknow, UP: Central Drug Research Institute; **1990**; vol. 1, p. 327.

112. Rathore, R.S.; Prakash, A.; Singh, P.P. Preliminary study of anti-inflammatory and anti arthritic activity. *Rheumatism*, **1977**, *12*, 130–134.

113. Salae, A.W.; Boonnak, N. Obtusinones D and E, linear and angular fused dimeric icetexane diterpenoides from *Premna obtusifolia* roots. *Tetrahedron Lett.*, **2013**, *54*, 1356–1359.

114. Schauer, J.C. Verbenaceae. In: *Prodromus Systematis Naturalis Regni Vegetabilis* (Vegetable Kingdom Natural History System); De Candolle, A. (Ed.); Paris: Victoris Masson; **1847**; vol. 2; pp. 522–700.

115. Schumann, K., Hollrung, M. *Verbenaceae.* In: *Die Flora von Kaiser Wilhelms Land* (The Flora of *Kaiser Wilhelms Land*). Berlin: Asher and Co.; **1889**; pp. 118–122.

116. Selvam, N.T.; Vengatakrishnan, V.; Damodar, K.S.; Murugesan, S. Evaluation of tissue level antioxidant activity of *Premna serratifolia* leaf in paracetamol intoxicated Wistar albino rats. *Int. J. Pharm. Life Sci.*, **2010**, *1*, 86–90.

117. Selvam, N.T.; Venkatakrishnan, V.; Damodar, K.S. Antioxidant and tumor cell suppression potential of *Premna serratifolia* Linn. leaf. *Toxicol. Int.*, **2012**, *19* (1), 31–34.

118. Sharma, P.V. *Dravyaguna Vijnan.* Varanasi: Choukamba Bharati Academy; **1998**; vol. 4, pp. 30–37.

119. Sharma, P.V. *Dravyaguna Vijnana.* Varanasi: Choukamba Bharati Academy; **2006**; vol. 2, pp. 60–67.

120. Shilpa, V.N.; Rajasekaran, N.; Gopalakrishnan, V.K.; Devaki, K. *In-vivo* antioxidant activity of *Premna corymbosa* (Rottl.) against streptozotocin induced oxidative stress in Wistar albino mice. *J. Appl. Pharm. Sci.*, **2012**, *2* (10), 60–65.

121. Shukla, V.; Phulara, SC.; Yadav, D.; Tiwari, S.; Kaur, S. Iridoid compound 10-*O-trans-p*-coumaroylcatalpol extends longevity and reduces alpha synuclein aggregation in *Caenorhabditis elegans. CNS & Neurol. Disorders Drug Targets*, **2012**, *11*, 984–992.

122. Singh, C.R. Antimicrobial effect of callus and natural plant extracts of *Premna serratifolia* L. *Int. J. Pharm. Biomed. Res.*, **2011**, *2* (1), 17–20.

123. Singh, C.R.; Nelson, P.; Boopathy, N.S. *In-vitro* conservation and protective effect of *Premna serratifolia* Linn.—An important medicinal tree. *Int. J. Pharm. Appl.*, **2012**, *3*, 332–343.

124. Singh, C.R.; Nelson, P.; Muthu, K.; Pargavi, B. Identification of volatile constituents from *Premna serratifolia* L. through GC-MS. *Int. J. Pharm. Tech. Res.*, **2011**, *3*, 1050–1058.

125. Singh, C.R.; Nelson, R.; Krishnan, P.M.; Mahesh, K. Hepatoprotective and anti-oxidant effect of root and root callus extract of *Premna serratifolia* L. in paracetamol induced liver damage in male albino rats. *Int. J. Pharma. Biosci.*, **2011,** *2*, 244–252.

126. Singh, T.B.; Chunekar, K.C.; Sharma, P.S. *Glossary of Vegetable Drugs in Brihattrayi.* Varanasi: Chowkhamba Sanskrit Series; **1972**; pp. 4–5.

127. Sivarajan, V.V.; Indira, B. *Ayurvedic Drugs and their Plant Sources.* New Delhi: Oxford and IBH publishing Co. Pvt. Ltd.; **1996**; p. 21.

128. Sodhala.*Gadanigraha,* Part 2. 3rd ed.; Varanasi: Chaukambha Sanskrit Samsthana; **1994**; pp. 30–36.

129. Sturtevant, E.L. *Sturtevant's Edible Plants of the World.* New York: Dover; **1972**; p. 216.

130. Teai, T.; Bianchini, J.P.; Cambon, A. Volatile constituents of flower buds concrete of *Premna serratifolia* L. *J. Essent Oil Res.,* **1998**, *10*, 307–309.

131. Thirumalai, D.; Paridhavi, M.; Gowtham, M. Evaluation of physiochemical, pharmacognostical and phytochemical parameters of *Premna herbacea. Asian J. Pharm. Clin. Res.,* **2013**, *6* (1), 173–181.

132. Thiruvenkata, S.R.; Jayakar, B. Antihyperglycemic and antihyperlipidemic activities of *Premna corymbosa* (Burm. F.) Rottl. on Streptozotocin induced diabetic rats. *Der Pharm. Lett.,* **2010**, *2*, 505–509.

133. Vadivu, R.; Jerad, S.; Girinath, K. Evaluation of hepatoprotective and in-vitro cytotoxic activity of leaves of *Premna serratifolia* Linn. *J. Sci. Res.,* **2009**, *1*, 145–52.

134. Vaidya, B.G. *Nighantu Adarsh* (Uttarardh). Surat: Shri Swami Atamanand Sarasavati Ayurvedic, Government Pharmacy Ltd.; **1965**; 815–820.

135. Vaidya, K.M. *The Ashtangahridayakosha with the Hridayaprakasha Commentary* (Ashtanga Hridakosha with the heartbreak Commentary). Trichur; **1936**; p. 5.

136. Warier, P.K. *Indian Medicinal Plants- a Compendium of 500 Species.* Anna Salai, Madras: Orient Longman Ltd.; **1995**; vol. 4, pp. 348–352.

137. Warrier, P.K.; Nambiar, N.K.K.; Ramankutty, C. *Indian Medicinal Plants - A Compendium of 500 Species.* Anna Salai, Madras: Orient Longman Ltd.; **1994**; vol. 3, pp. 110–114.

138. Whitelaw, A. *Materia Indica.* New Delhi: Neeraj Publishing House, Ashok Vihar; **1984**; p. 210.

139. *WHO Guidelines on Safety Monitoring of Herbal Medicines in Pharmaco Vigilance Systems.* Geneva, Switzerland: World Health Organization; **2004**; pp. 10–15.

140. Yadav, D.; Gupta, M.M. Isolation and HPTLC analysis of iridoids in *Premna integrifolia,* an important ingredient of Ayurvedic drug Dashmool. *J. Planar Chromat.,* **2013**, *26* (3), 260–266.

141. Yadav, D.; Masood, N.; Luqman, S.; Brindha, P.; Gupta, M.M. Antioxidant furofuran lignans from *Premna integrifolia. Ind. Crops Prod.,* **2013**, *41*, 397–402.

142. Yadav, D.; Tiwari, N.; Gupta, M.M. Diterpenoids from *Premna integrifolia. Phytochem. Lett.,* **2010**, *3*, 143–147.

143. Yadav, D.; Tiwari, N.; Gupta, M.M. Simultaneous quantification of diterpenoids in *Premna integrifolia* using a validated HPTLC method. *J. Sep. Sci.,* **2011**, *34*, 286–291.

144. Yuasa, K.; Ide, T.; Otsuka, H.; Takeda, Y. Chemical examination of stems of *Premna corymbosa* var. *obtusifolia. J. Nat. Prod.,* **1993**, *56* (10), 1695–1699.

# CHAPTER 5

# SURVEY OF INDIGENOUS KNOWLEDGE OF MEDICINAL PLANTS IN INDIA

ACHARAYA BALKRISHNA, NISHANT GUPTA, DEEPAK K. GOND,
ISHWAR P. SHARMA, RACHANA BHANDARI, and VEDPRIYA ARYA*

## ABSTRACT

The forest ranges in Morni Hills and Raipur Rani from Haryana, India were selected for ethnobotanical and medicinal studies. The local people in these regions treat most of their ailments using medicinal plants due to their inherent traditional knowledge. Many of the common health problems (viz., cough and cold, bleeding, wounding, various kinds of fever, pain) and many other diseases (stone, piles, cancer, etc.) are cured by traditional herbal remedies. Salty water has great importance for locals and nearby people, who use it to cure stones, urinary diseases, skin diseases, digestive tract disorders, and cancer. Several medicinal plants have been used to cure different genito-urinary ailments (including infertility, gynecological disorders, urinary disorders, menstrual problems, etc.). This chapter focuses on the evaluation and exploration of traditional medicine knowledge in India. However, further studies related to their efficacy and clinical trials are still demanded.

## 5.1 INTRODUCTION

The people dwelling in interior regions in India usually depend on the forests, which have rich biodiversity to meet their livelihood and health care [9, 16, 25, 36, 37]. Natural herbal medicines from forest resources are being

---

*Corresponding author. E-mail: vedpriya.arya@prft.co.in.

used by them for which scientific evidences must be validated, because least information is available in the literature on their usage. Recent scientific studies have shown that forest plants are important for scientific research for validation and development of noble herbal medicines and also to explore the traditional knowledge in developing countries [10, 39].

India is a hotspot of traditional culture with more than 427 tribal communities, which utilize herbal products, but the information base of traditional knowledge and practices have not been explored due to various reasons [37]. Several researchers have initiated and explored this knowledge throughout India [2, 6, 35]. Several ethnobotanical and medicinal studies have been conducted in various parts of India. However, these are still for a specific region [28, 33, 34].

The survey in this chapter focuses on the access and documentation of ethnobotanical and medicinal plants with their traditional medicinal practices in Morni and Raipur Rani Ranges. Therefore, the documentation of indigenous knowledge might be useful for the conservation of biodiversity and traditional knowledge.

## 5.2  MATERIALS AND METHODS

### 5.2.1  STUDY AREA

Morni Hills range and Raipur Rani range were selected for the survey due to great historical importance. It is believed that the name Morni came after Queen Morni, who once ruled this area perhaps before the British era in India. The Raipur Rani; however, had a different story, according to a tale The King and Queen of Nahan (Himachal Pradesh) were child-less until a *Vaidh* (traditional doctor) treated them for infertility; consequently, they were blessed by a baby boy after several years of marriage. The king hailed and praised to *Vaidh* for their successful treatment and donated him several villages of the Raipur Rani region as a reward. The fort of *Vaidh* exists today in Raipur Rani's compartment-30 in decayed conditions (Figure 5.1).

Morni Hills range lies between 650 and 1330 m elevation; 30° 42′ 21.48″ N latitude and 76° 58′ 32.99″ E longitude, while Raipur Rani range ranges between 450 and 780 m elevation; 30° 34′ 54.48″ N latitude and 77° 01′ 13.87″ E longitude (Figure 5.2).

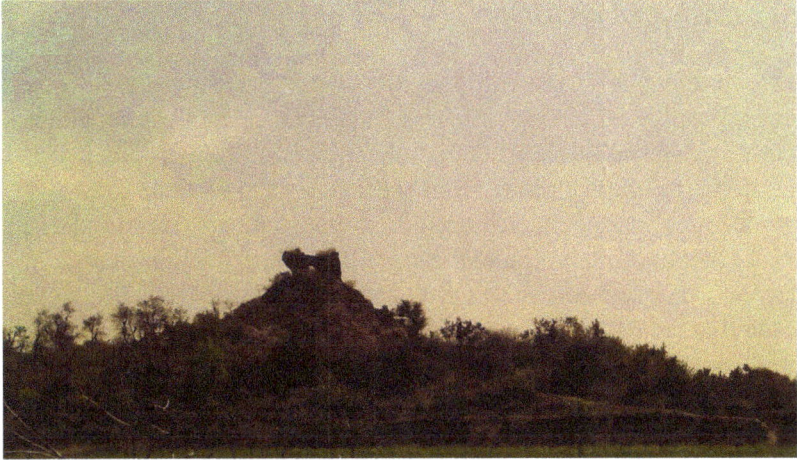

**FIGURE 5.1**  Panoramic view of almost decayed fort of *Vaidh*.

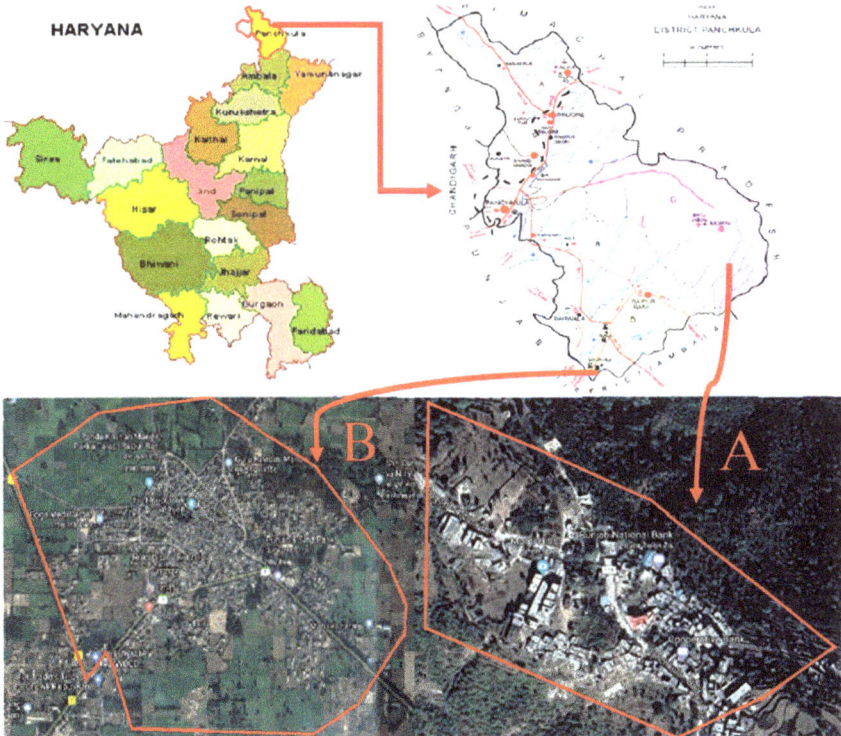

**FIGURE 5.2**  Aerial view of Morni hills (A) and Raipur Rani range (B).

## 5.2.2   DATA COLLECTION

The study area was thoroughly surveyed for information on the usages of medicinal plant by tribal practitioners. This investigation was conducted for 1 month in March of 2017. To analyze the traditional knowledge of medicinal herbs, numerous native plants from selected ranges were investigated. The plant specimens were collected, identified, and authenticated with the help of previous literature review, nomenclature, and correct author citation for all collections validated through POWO (2018 database) [23] that was further submitted to the Patanjali Research Institute, Haridwar (India).

The information was taken from resource informants and traditional healers to get ethnobotanical and medicinal information through direct interviews and oral conversations. Information gathered from traditional people on local name, plant part used, plant using method, medicine preparation method, other uses, so forth, were collected for the traditional plant. All medicinal herbs were also verified for vernacular name and medicinal uses by natives and Rakhas (local forest caretaker).

Based on the information obtained from the traditional practitioners, medicinal uses are divided into 24 different categories: (1) infertility, (2) piles, (3) stone, (4) pain, (5) cancer, (6) fevers, (7) cough and cold, (8) repellent, (9) dysentery, (10) skin problems, (11) cardiac ailments, (12) antidiabetic, (13) antitode, (14) various digestive disorders, (15) memory and nervous, (16) respiratory, (17) urinary, (18) gynecological, (19) gastrointestinal; and (20) other uses: edible, (21) abortifacient, (22) sacred, (23) dye, and (24) fumitories and masticatories.

## 5.3   RESULTS

### 5.3.1   DOCUMENTATION OF INDIGENOUS ETHNOBOTANICAL AND MEDICINAL KNOWLEDGE

The Morni Hills and Raipur Rani Forest ranges belong dominantly to dry deciduous forest. The study area remains arid throughout the year. However, rivers (Ghaggar, Beghna, and Dangarwali) are life-lines for the selected regions. During the study, a total of 860 plants species were collected and identified that have been submitted to Patanjali Herbarium, Patanjali Research foundation, Haridwar in India. Out of the collected plant species, 77 plants were identified for ethnobotany and medicines that are being frequently used by the natives. Table 5.1 indicates all information such as scientific name, local name, life form, plant part in use, and their applications.

**TABLE 5.1**   List of Commonly Used Medicinal Plants in Morni Hills and Raipur Rani Forest Ranges

| Botanical Name (Family) | Local Name | Life Form | Range* | Part of Plant Used** | Applications |
|---|---|---|---|---|---|
| *Abrus precatorius* L. (Fabaceae) | Ratti | Climber | RR | Rt, Sd | Nervous disorder |
| *Achyranthes aspera* L. (Amaranthaceae) | Charchita | – | – | – | Gynecological disorders, liver pain |
| *Aegle marmelos* (L.) Corrêa (Rutaceae) | Beli | Tree | MH, RR | Fr | Dysentery and diarrhea |
| *Agave cantala* (Haw.) Roxb. ex Salm-Dyck (Asparagaceae) | Ram Bans | Herb | MH | Wp | Fever |
| *Artemisia* | Dona | Herb | MH | Lv | Laxative and insect repellent |
| *Asparagus racemosus* Willd. (Asparagaceae) | Shatawari | Shrub | MH, RR | Rt | Abdominal pain, nervous disorders. |
| *Azadirachta indica* A. Juss. (Meliaceae) | Neem, Bkain | Tree | RR | Lv | Edible |
| *Bacopa monnieri* (L.) Wettst. (Plantaginaceae) | Jangali Brahmi | Herb | MH, RR | Wp | – |
| *Barleria cristata* L. (Acanthaceae) | Bansla | Shrub | MH | Rt, Lv | Respiratory disorders |
| *Bauhinia purpurea* L. (Fabaceae) | Kachnari | – | – | – | Repellant, edible |
| *Bauhinia vahlii* Wight and Arn. (Fabaceae) | Maljan | Shrub | MH | Lv | Edible |
| *Berberis* (Berberidaceae) | Kasmodo | Shrub | MH | Wp | Gastrointestinal disorders |

**TABLE 5.1** *(Continued)*

| Botanical Name (Family) | Local Name | Life Form | Range* | Part of Plant Used** | Applications |
|---|---|---|---|---|---|
| *Berberis aristata* DC. (Berberidaceae) | Kashmal, Daruhaldi | Shrub | MH | Rt, St, Fr | Fever |
| *Boerhavia diffusa* L. (Nyctaginaceae) | Punarnava | Herb | RR | Rt | Antidote, Jaundice |
| *Bryophyllum pinnatum* (Lam.) Oken (Crassulaceae) | Patherchata | Herb | MH, RR | Lv | Stone |
| *Butea monosperma* (Lam.) Kuntze (Fabaceae) | Dhak | Tree | RR | Lv, Fl | Dye |
| *Calotropis gigantea* (L.) Dryand. (Apocynaceae) | Aak | Shrub | RR | Lt | Piles |
| *Cannabis sativa* L. (Cannabaceae) | Bhaang | Herb | RR | Rt | – |
| *Cassia fistula* L. (Fabaceae) | Amalthash | Tree | MH | Br, Fr | Skin disease |
| *Celastrus paniculatus* Willd. (Celastraceae) | Mal Kangni | Climber | MH, RR | Sd, Lv | Edible, joint pain |
| *Celastrus paniculatus* Willd. (Celastraceae) | Besharm, Behaya | Shrub | RR | Lv | Laxative and insect repellent |
| *Centella asiatica* (L.) Urb. (Apiaceae) | Mandukparni | Herb | MH | Lv | Neurological disorders |
| *Cissampelos pareira* L. (Menispermaceae) | Path | Climber | RR | Lv | Piles |
| *Citrus limon* (L.) Osbeck (Rutaceae) | Galgal | Shrub | MH | Fr | Edible |
| *Colebrookea oppositifolia* Sm. (Lamiaceae) | Bindda | Shrub | MH | Lv | Edible |
| *Crateva magna* (Lour.) DC. (Capparaceae) | Barna, Varun | Herb | MH | Br | Kidney stones, skin disease |

**TABLE 5.1** *(Continued)*

| Botanical Name (Family) | Local Name | Life Form | Range* | Part of Plant Used** | Applications |
|---|---|---|---|---|---|
| *Datura innoxia* Mill. (Solanaceae) | Safed Datura | Herb | RR | Rt, Sd | – |
| *Datura metel* L. (Solanaceae) | Kala Datura | Herb | RR | Rt, Sd | – |
| *Digera* (L.) Mart. (Amaranthaceae) | Taandla | Herb | MH, RR | St | Urinary disorders |
| *Dioscorea belophylla* (Prain) Voigt ex Haines (Dioscoreaceae) | Turar | Climber | MH, RR | Rt, Lv | Abortifacient |
| *Diospyros melanoxylon* Roxb. (Ebenaceae) | Kendu | Tree | MH, RR | Fr | Repellent, fish poison |
| *Diplocyclos* (Cucurbitaceae) | Shivlingi | Climber | MH | Sd | Female infertility |
| *Eclipta prostrata* (L.) L. (Asteraceae) | | | | | Hair dye, antiseptic (repellent) |
| *Euphorbia hirta* L. (Euphorbiaceae) | Dudhi | Herb | MH | Lv | Piles, dysentery, and diarrhea |
| *Euphorbia royleana* Boiss. (Euphorbiaceae) | Siyuri | Shrub | MH | Wp | Infertility |
| *Ficus benghalensis* L. (Moraceae) | Burgud | Tree | RR | Rt, Br | Infertility, sacred |
| *Ficus mollis* Vahl (Moraceae) | Dudhala | Tree | MH | Lv | Fodder |
| *Ficus racemosa* L. (Moraceae) | Goolar | Tree | MH | Fr, Lt | Piles, edible |
| *Ficus religiosa* L. (Moraceae) | Peepal | Tree | RR | Rt, Br | Infertility, sacred |
| *Flacourtia indica* (Burm.f.) Merr. (Salicaceae) | Kandai, Panyala | Shrub | MH | Lv, Rt | Dysentery and diarrhea |
| *Helicteres isora* L. (Malvaceae) | Marorphali | Tree | MH | | Dysentery and diarrhea, Abdominal pain |

**TABLE 5.1** *(Continued)*

| Botanical Name (Family) | Local Name | Life Form | Range* | Part of Plant Used** | Applications |
|---|---|---|---|---|---|
| *Hellenia speciosa* (J.Koenig) (Costaceae) | Keu, Kushta | Herb | MH | Rh | Leprosy, skin disease |
| *Hemidesmus indicus* (L.) R.Br. (Apocynaceae) | Anantmool | Herb | MH | Rt | – |
| *Holoptelea integrifolia* (Roxb.) Planch. (Urticaceae) | Chilbil, Papadi | Tree | MH, RR | Br | Antidiabetic |
| *Justicia adhatoda* L. (Acanthaceae) | Bassa | Shrub | MH, RR | Lv | Cough and cold |
| *Kigelia africana* (Lam.) Benth. (Bignoniaceae) | Balamkhira | Tree | RR | Fr | Gastrointestinal disorder |
| *Lannea coromandelica* (Houtt.) Merr. (Anacardiaceae) | Jhingan | Tree | MH, RR | Lv | Edible |
| *Mallotus* (Lam.) Müll. Arg. (Euphorbiaceae) | Kamila | Herb | MH | Br, Fr | Skin diseases |
| *Martynia annua* L. (Martyniaceae) | | Herb | MH | Fr, Rt | Antidote, inflammations |
| *Moringa oleifera* Lam. (Moringaceae) | Shejan | Tree | MH | – | Edible |
| *Morus alba* L. (Moraceae) | Shahatut | Tree | MH, RR | Fr | Edible |
| *Morus indica* L. (Moraceae) | Tut | Tree | RR | Fr | Edible |
| *Murraya koenigii* (L.) Spreng. (Rutaceae) | Curry Patta | Shrub | MH, RR | Lv | Pain |
| *Nyctanthes aculeata* Craib (Oleaceae) | Harshingar | Shrub | MH, RR | Lv | Edible |
| *Phoenix acaulis* Roxb. (Arecaceae) | Khajuri | Shrub | RR | Fr | Edible |

**TABLE 5.1** *(Continued)*

| Botanical Name (Family) | Local Name | Life Form | Range* | Part of Plant Used** | Applications |
|---|---|---|---|---|---|
| *Phyllanthus emblica* L. (Phyllanthaceae) | Amla | Tree | RR | Fr | Diuretic, hair dyes, edible |
| *Phyllanthus niruri* L. (Phyllanthaceae) | Hajar Dana | Herb | RR | Sd | Infertility |
| *Physalis angulata* L. (Solanaceae) | Rasbhari, Papotan, Bambholan | Herb | MH, RR | Fr | Tonic, appetizer, edible |
| *Prosopis cineraria* (L.) Druce (Fabaceae) | Jund | Tree | RR | St, Br | Sacred wood |
| *Prosopis juliflora* (Sw.) DC. (Fabaceae) | Vilayati Kikkar | Tree | MH, RR | St | Pain |
| *Psidium guajava* L. (Myrtaceae) | Amrood | Tree | MH, RR | Fr, Lv | Edible, cough and cold |
| *Punica granatum* L. (Lythraceae) | Daadma, Anar | Shrub | MH | Fr | Edible, digestive disorders |
| *Senegalia catechu* (L.f.) P.J.H.Hurter and Mabb. (Fabaceae) | Kher | Tree | RR | Br | Pain, cough and cold |
| *Senna tora* (L.) Roxb. (Fabaceae) | Panwar | Shrub | MH | Lv | Insect repellent |
| *Solanum erianthum* D. Don (Solanaceae) | Ban Tamakhoo | Herb | MH | Rt, Lv | Fumitories and masticatories |
| *Solanum nigrum* L. (Solanaceae) | – | – | – | – | Edible, pain |
| *Syzygium cumini* (L.) Skeels (Myrtaceae) | Jammun | Tree | RR | Fr, Lv | Antidiabetic |
| *Terminalia arjuna* (Roxb. ex DC.) Wight and Arn. (Combretaceae) | Arjun | Tree | MH | Br, Fr | Cardiac ailments |
| *Terminalia bellirica* (Gaertn.) Roxb. (Combretaceae) | Baheda | Tree | MH, RR | Fr | Digestive disorders |

**TABLE 5.1** *(Continued)*

| Botanical Name (Family) | Local Name | Life Form | Range* | Part of Plant Used** | Applications |
|---|---|---|---|---|---|
| *Terminalia chebula* Retz. (Combretaceae) | Harad | Tree | MH, RR | Fr | Digestive disorders |
| *Tinospora cordifolia* (Willd.) (Menispermaceae) | Climber | Herb | MH, RR | St, Lv | – |
| *Vachellia nilotica* (L.) (Fabaceae) | Kikkar | Tree | – | St | Toothache, pain |
| *Vernonia anthelmintica* (L.) Willd. (Asteraceae) | Kali Jiri | Herb | MH | Fr | Repellant |
| *Withania somnifera* (L.) Dunal (Solanaceae) | Asgandha | Herb | RR | – | Fever |
| *Woodfordia* (L.) Kurz (Lythraceae) | Dhau | Tree | MH | Br, Fl | Dysentery and diarrhea |
| *Zanthoxylum armatum* DC. (Rutaceae) | Timur | Tree | MH | St, Fr | Pain, Fever |
| *Zingiber officinale* Roscoe (Zingiberaceae) | Adraak, Sonth | Herb | MH | Rh | Pain, digestive disorder |

Br  Branches
Fr  Flowers
Lv  Leaves
MH        Morni Hills
Rh  Rhizome
RR Raipur Rani
Rt  Root
Sd  Seed
St  Stem
Wp Whole plant

Unique methods to treating various health ailments by local natives have been documented. A local *Vaidh* claimed to treat various serious disorders including cancer, especially gall bladder and kidney cancer. Another *vaidh* (Mr. Indrajeet Gaur) shared his experience and knowledge to treat 17 chronic to lethal diseases. In our documentation, a salty water body was reported in Raipur Rani forest range, which is geographically located at 550–600 m elevation; 36°33′4.2″ N latitude and 77°8′34.7″ E longitude (Figure 5.3) and is quite popular among the natives for medicinal purposes. However, there is no scientific evidence for these logics. Hence, it is a challenge to researchers for finding main bioconstituents and prove these scientifically.

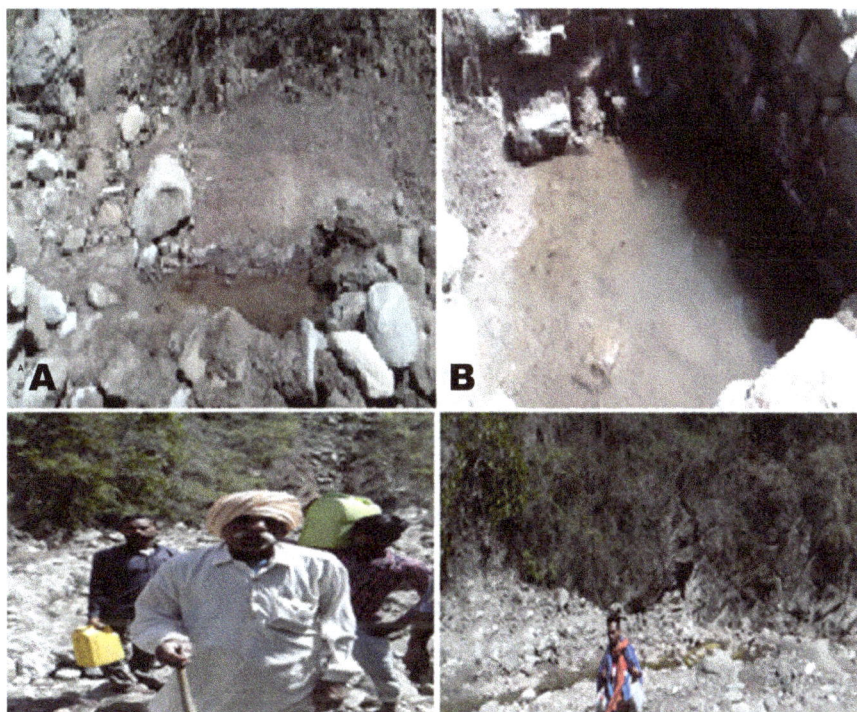

**FIGURE 5.3**    Salty water bodies (A, B); persons carrying salty water in plastic vessels (C, D).

During this survey, 77 angiospermic plants species were important ethnobotanically and medicinally for several uses. Among these 26 were herbs, 18 shrubs, 28 trees, and 5 climbers (Figure 5.4). All these plants species were reported for their enumerated ethnobotanical and medicinal importance, except *Zingiber officinale* (Zingiberaceae) and *Phoenix acaulis* (Arecaceae). For plant family analysis, authors observed a total of 39 plant families, out of which fabaceae (10 plant species) was the most dominant family followed by solanaceae (6 plants species) and moraceae (6 plants species); while another species had few number of plants species (Figure 5.5). Moreover, some plants are being used for many diseases, namely, *Achyranthes aspera* (gynecological disorders, liver pain), *Asparagus racemosus* (abdominal pain, nervous disorders), *Cannabis sativa* (abdominal pain, digestive disorders), *Crateva magna* (kidney stones, skin disease), *Euphorbia hirta* (piles, dysentery, and diarrhea), *Helicteres isora* (dysentery and diarrhea, Abdominal pain), *Hemidesmus indicus* (urinary problems, skin problems), and *Senegalia catechu* (various pain, cough, and cold).

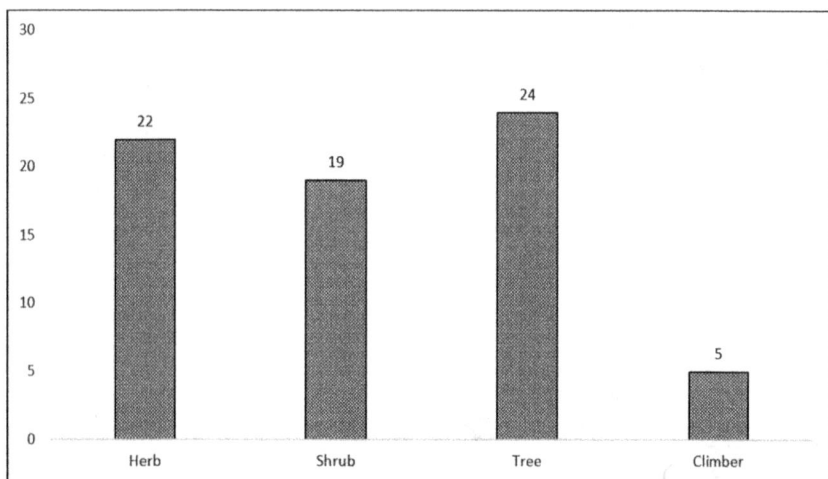

**FIGURE 5.4**　Habit analysis for different species.

Many of the plants reported for serious disease are:

- *Achyranthes aspera* for gynecological disorders;
- *Berberis lyceum* and *Kigelia africana* for gastrointestinal disorder;
- *Calotropis gigantean, Cissampelos pareira, Euphorbia hirta* and *Ficus racemosa* for piles;
- *Datura metel* and *Datura innoxia* for cancer;
- *Helicteres isora, Aegle marmelos, Euphorbia hirta, Woodfordia fruticose,* and *Flacourtia indica* for dysentery and diarrhea, etc.

## 5.3.2　PARTS OF PLANT USED

In this study, nearly all plant parts from various plant species were reported as ethnobotanically and medicinally important. Most of the plants reported were economically important with their fruits (27 plants) and leaves (27 plants) followed by root (18 plants), bark (11 plants), stem (7 plants), and seeds (6 plants). Among these (Figure 5.6)

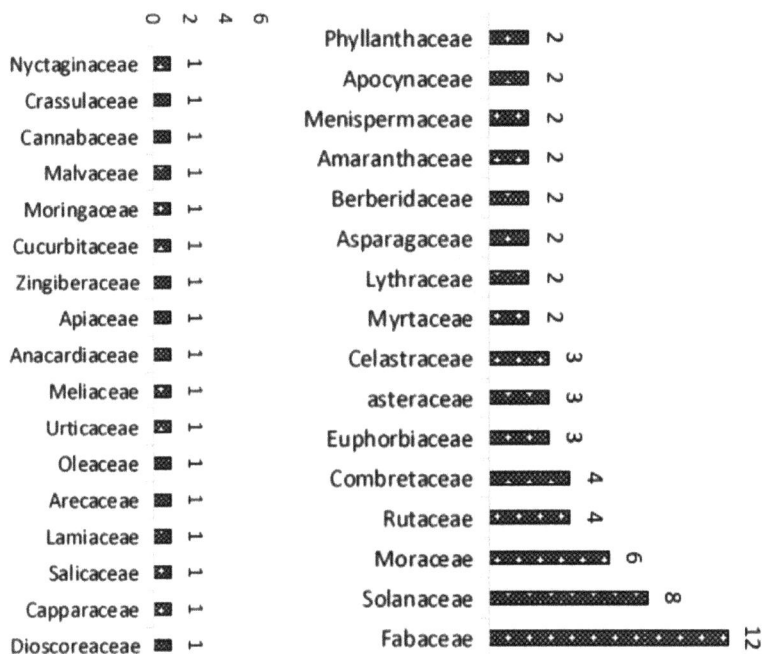

**FIGURE 5.5** Family analysis for number of species.

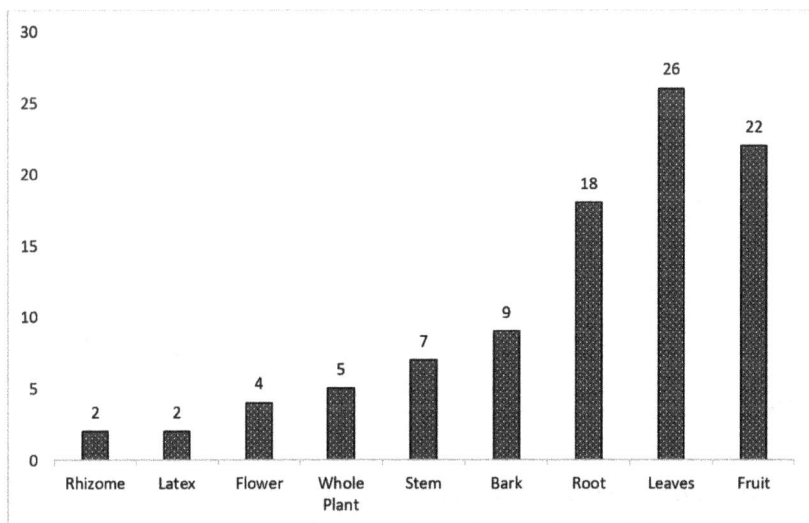

**FIGURE 5.6** Use of different parts of plant for a number of species.

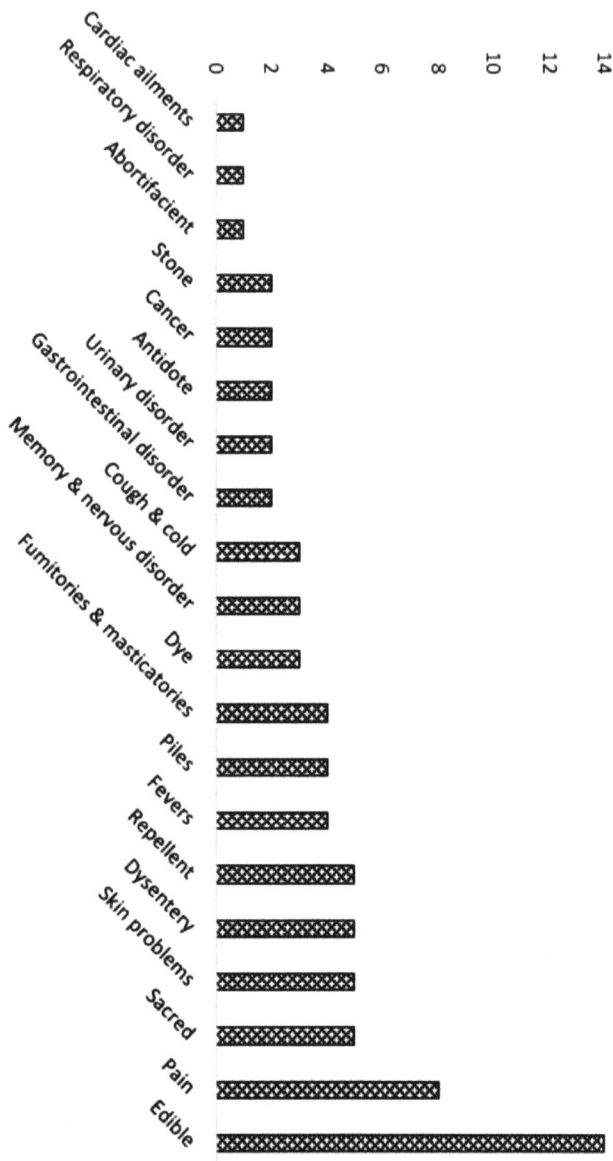

**FIGURE 5.7**  Various uses of plant species.

1. five plant species were reported to be important completely (*Achyranthes aspera, Berberis lyceum, Agave cantala, Bacopa monnieri,* and *Euphorbia royleana*);

2.  four plant species were reported important for their flowers (*Bauhinia purpurea, Woodfordia fruticose, Butea monosperma,* and *Moringa oleifera*);

3.  *Calotropis gigantean* and *Ficus racemose* are important for their milky latex and

4.  two plants for their rhizome (*Hellenia speciose* and *Zingiber officinale*).

A total of 24 uses were identified. Of these maximum number of plants were reported for their edible value along with various diseases; a maximum of 12 plants were used by natives for relief from various types of pain, while many other plants were used in various other uses (Figure 5.7).

## 5.4   DISCUSSIONS

The local practitioners used the medicinal plants for treatment of common diseases as well as other major ailments, such as various types of fever, pain, and various disorders. Due to modernization, these local herbal remedies are disappearing. In this study, *Boerhavia diffusa* was found useful for jaundice. Similarly, Samvatsar and Diwanji [37] reported 13 plants from western Madhya Pradesh (India), Muthu et al. [9] reported *Phyllanthus amarus* from Kancheepuram district of Tamil Nadu (India) and reported various remedies from five plants by Kani tribes of Kerala (India) for jaundice treatment. Many of the previous studies investigated the use of natural plants to treat jaundice [5, 8, 11, 27]. Fever, cough, and cold are common natural ailments. Therefore, these are treated at the household level [1, 9, 13, 17].

*Datura metel* and *Datura innoxia* are used by natives for treatment of cancer in the selected study areas. In other previous studies, *Helicteres isora* [13–15] was reported for cancer treatment. Various herbal remedies have been studied for different genito-urinary ailments (such as infertility, gynecological disorders, urinary disorders, sexual weakness, menstrual problems, etc.) [8, 9, 24, 29].

Four plant species (*Calotropis gigantean, Cissampelos pareira, Euphorbia hirta,* and *Ficus racemosa*) were identified for pile treatment by the natives of Morni Hills and Raipur Rani forest ranges. *Boerhavia diffusa, Artemisia scoparia, Bauhinia purpurea, Vernonia anthelmintica, Eclipta prostrata, Diospyros melanoxylon,* and *Celastrus paniculatus* were identified as repellent to many undesirable elements [5, 11, 19, 20, 38].

In some previous studies performed at Bhiwani district [3, 4], *Bryophyllum pinnatum* and *Crateva magna* were reported useful in stone-related problems. *Scoparia dulcis* was reported from different study areas [8]. Similar ethnobotanical and medicinal practices have previously been studied in different localities of Haryana, such as

- Jhajjar district [18],
- Central Haryana [4, 7],
- Gurugram district [21],
- Hisar district [40],
- Karnal district [26],
- Mahendergarh district [30, 31, 32],
- Plains of Yamuna Nagar district [22],
- Whole Haryana [3, 12].

## 5.5  SUMMARY

This survey demonstrated different herbal medicines, which are ethnobotanically and medicinally important. It was found that the salty lake water is highly medicinal; however, its chemical constitutions and scientific evidences further need to be studied. On the other hand, the *Vaidh* (traditional doctor) practices need to be explored for protecting traditional knowledge and well-being of mankind through easily available natural resources. Overall, the efficacy and safety of all the reported important plants are the subject of ongoing investigation by authors. The *Vaidh* and other natives have a strong belief that the plant would vanish and become useless if the mystery about the therapeutic properties of a particular plant is disclosed. This study may be a new addition in traditional knowledge on the unexplored locals of Haryana and also help to conserve the rich biodiversity of this region.

## ACKNOWLEDGMENTS

Authors express sincere gratitude to honorable Swami Ramdev Ji for his continuous blessings and regular guidance and also thankful to Haryana Forest Department, Panchkula, for funding and survey proposal. Special thanks to M. P. Sharma (Chief Conservator of Forests), forest guards, and Rakhas (Shadi Ram and Raghuveer) for their valuable contributions.

## KEYWORDS

- **Morni hills**
- **Raipur Rani**
- **salty water**
- **traditional knowledge**

## REFERENCES

1. Alluri, V. Krishnaraju; Rao, V.N.; Sundararaju, D.; Vanisree, M.; Sheng Tsay, H.; Subbaraju, V. Biological screening of medicinal plants collected from eastern ghats of India using artemiasalina (brine shrimp test). *Int. J. Appl. Sci. Eng.* **2006**, *4* (2), 115–125.
2. Anil-Kumar, J.; Patole, S.N. Less known medicinal values of plants among some tribal and rural communities of pachmarchi forest (M.P). *Ethnobotany,* **2001**, *13*, 96–100.
3. Anup, S. ethnobotanical study of medicinal plants in Bhiwani district of Haryana, India: Part I. *J. Med. Plants Studies.* **2016**, *4* (2), 212–215.
4. Anup, S.; Tak, H.S.; Singh, L.; Kumar, A.; Kumar. S. Ethnobotanical survey of common medicinal plants in Bhiwani, Haryana, India. *World J. Pharm. Sci.* **2015**, *3* (3), 492–499
5. Arun, V.; Liju, V.B.; John, J.V.; Parthipan, B.; Renuka, C. Traditional remedies of kani tribes of kottoor reserve forest in Agasthyavanum, Thiruvananthapuram, Kerala. *Indian J. Tradit. Knowl.,* **2007**, *6* (4), 589–594.
6. B. Sandhya; Thomas, S.; Isabel, W.; Shenbagarathai, R. 2006. Ethnomedicinal plants used by valaiyan community of Piranmalai hills, Tamil Nadu, India: pilot study. *Altern. Med.* **2006**, *3* (1), 101–114.
7. Balkar, S.; Singh, J. Ethnobotanical uses of some plants from Central Haryana, India. *Phytodiversity.* **2014**, *1* (1&2), 7–24.
8. Binu, T.; Rajendran, A. Less known ethnomedicinal plants used by kurichar tribe of Wayanad district southern western ghats, Kerala, India. *Bot. Res. Int.* **2013**, *6* (2), 32–35.
9. Chellaiah, M.; Ayyanar, M.; Raja, N.; Ignacimuthu, S. Medicinal plants used by traditional healers in Kancheepuram District of Tamil Nadu, India. *J. Ethnobiol. Ethnomed.,* **2006**, *2*(1), 43–46.
10. Cleber, S.; Fronza, M.; Goettert, F.; Luik, S.; Flores, E.M.; Bittencourt, C.F. Biological studies on Brazilian plants used in wound healing. *J. Ethnopharmacol.* **2009**, *122* (3), 523–532.
11. Devi-Prasad, A.G; Shyma, T.B.; Raghavendra, M.P. Plants used by tribes for treatment of digestive system disorders in Wayanad District, Kerala. *J. Appl. Pharm. Sci.* 2013, *3* (8), 171–175.
12. Gitika; Kumar, M. Ethnobotanical study of some medicinal plants of Haryana, India. *World J. Pharma. Pharmace. Sci.* **2016**, *5* (8), 1717–1736.
13. Govindamenon, J.; Ajithabai, M.D. Ethnobotanical survey of plants used in the treatment of diabetes. *Indian J. Tradit. Knowl.* **2010**, *9* (1), 100–104.

14. Jagmahender, S.; Singh, N.; Satpal, S.K.; Singh, B. Observations on plant formulations for paediatric use in Haryana, India. *J. Global Biosci.* **2016**, *5* (2), 3656–3664.

15. K. Kadhirvel; Ramya, S.; Sathya, T.; Veera Ravi, A. Ethnobotanical survey of plants used by tribals in Chitteri hills. *Environ. Int. J. Sci. Tech.* **2010**, *5,* 35–46.

16. Kennedy, F.; Chah; K.F.; Eze, C.A.; Emuelosi, C.E.; Esimone, C.O. Antibacterial and wound healing properties of methanolic extracts of some Nigerian medicinal plants. *J. Ethnopharmacol.* **2006**, *104,* 164–167.

17. Kofi, B. Medical provision in Africa: past and present. *Photother. Res.* 2005, *19,* 919–923.

18. Manju, P.; Arya, V.; Yadav, S.; Kumar, S.; Yadav, J.P. Indigenous knowledge of medicinal plants used by saperas community of Khetawas, Jhajjar District, Haryana, India. *J. Ethnobiol. Ethnomed* **2010**, *6* (4), 2–11.

19. Muniappan, A.; Ignacimuthu, S. Ethnobotanical survey of medicinal plants commonly used by Kani Tribals in Tirunelveli hills of Western Ghats, India. *J. Ethnopharmacol.* **2011**, *134,* 851–864.

20. Muniappan, Ayyanar; Ignacimuthu, S. Traditional Knowledge of Kani Tribals in Kouthalai of Tirunelveli hills, Tamil Nadu, India. *J. Ethnopharmacol.,* 2005, *102,* 246–255.

21. Naveena, Dinodia; Nisha, V. Ethnobotanical study of medicinal plant in Gurgaon District. *Bull. Pure Appl. Scie. Bot.* **2015**, *34* (1&2), 13–24.

22. Parul, B.V. Ethnobotanical study of plains of Yamuna Nagar District. *Int. J. Innov. Res. Sci. Eng. Technol.,* **2015**, *4* (1), 18600–18607.

23. Plants of the World Online. Royal Botanic Gardens, Kew; http://powo.science.kew.org/; Accessed on October 31, 2019.

24. R., Venkatasamy; Mohammad Mubarack, H.; Doss, A. Ethnobotanical study of medicinal plants used by malasar tribals in Coimbatore district of Tamil Nadu. *Asian J. Exper. Biolog. Sci.,* **2010**, *1* (2), 387–392.

25. Ram Nath, C.; Nayar, S.L.; Chopra, I.C. *Glossary of Indian Medicinal Plants.* New Delhi, India: Council of Scientific and Industrial Research, Government of India; 1986; p. 329.

26. Ravinder, K.; Vashistha, B.D. Ethnobotanical studies in Karnal District, Haryana, India. *Int. Res. J. Biol. Sci.* **2014**, *3* (8), 46–55.

27. Revathi, P.; Parimelazhagan, T. Traditional knowledge of medicinal plants used by the Irula tribe of Hasanur hills, Erode District of Tamil Nadu, India. *Ethnobot. Leafl.* **2010**, *14,* 136–160.

28. S. Ignacimuthu; Ayyanar, M.; Sankarasivaraman, K. Ethnobotanical investigations among tribes in Madurai district of Tamil Nadu, India. *J. Ethnobiol. Ethnomed.* 2006, 2–25.

29. Saba, I.; Singh, J.; Jain, S.P.; Khanuja, S.P.S. *Curculigo orchioides* Gaertn (Kali Musali): endangered medicinal plant of commercial value. *Nat. Prod. Radiance.* **2006**, *5* (5), 369–372.30.

30. Sanjay, Yadav; Arya, V.; Kumar, S.; Yadav, M.; Yadav, J.P. Ethnomedicinal flora of dosi hills of Mahendergarh district (Haryana), India. *Ann. Biol.* 2010, *28* (2), 152–157.

31. Sanjay, Y.; Bhandoria, M.S. Ethnobotanical exploration in Mahendergarh district of Haryana *(India). J. Med. Plants Res.* **2013**, *7* (18), 1263–1271.

32. Sanjay, Y.; Yadav, J.P.; Arya, V.; Panghal, M. Sacred groves in conservation of plant biodiversity in Mahendergarh district of Haryana. *Indian J. Trad. Knowl.* **2010**, *9* (4), 693–700.

33. Sevugaperumal, Ganesan; Suresh, N.; Kesavan, L. Ethnomedicinal survey of lower palani hills of Tamil Nadu. *Indian J. Tradit. Knowl.* **2004**, *3* (3), 299–304.
34. Sheelu, R.; Sethuraman, M.; Mukerjee, P.K. Ethnobiology of Nilgiri Hills, India. *Phytother. Res.* **2002**, *16*, 98–116.
35. Subramanyam, R.; Newmaster, S.G. Valorizing the irulas traditional knowledge of medicinal plants in the Kodiakkarai reserve forest, India. *J. Ethnobiol. Ethnomed.,* **2009**, *5*, 10–13.
36. Subramanyam, R.; Steven, N.G. Consensus of the malasars traditional aboriginal knowledge of medicinal plants in the Velliangiri Holy Hills, India. *J. Ethnobiol. Ethnomed.* **2008**, *4*, 8–10.
37. Swati, S.; Diwanji, V.B. Plant sources for the treatment of jaundice in the tribals of western Madhya Pradesh of India. *J. Ethnopharmacol.* **2000**, *73*, 313–316.
38. Thangaraj, F.X.; Kannan, M. Ethnobotanical study of Kani Tribes in Thoduhills of Kerala, India. *J. Ethnopharmacol.* **2014**, *152*, 78–90.
39. V. H. Harsha; Hebbar, S.S., Shripathi, V., Hegde, G.R.. Ethnomedicobotany of Uttara Kannada District in Karnataka, India plants in treatment of skin diseases. *J. Ethnopharmacol.* **2003**, 84, 37–40.
40. Veni, B.; Bhardwaj, A.; Kiran; Vasudeva, N. Ethnobotanical survey of medicinal plants having food value in Hisar District. *Am. J. Pharm Tech. Res.* **2013**, *3* (1), 699–709.

# CHAPTER 6

# CONSUMER VIEWS ON HEALTH ISSUES ARISING FROM FOOD PRODUCTS

HARITA R. DESAI and MURLIDHAR MEGHWAL*

## ABSTRACT

This chapter discusses the importance of health risks arising from contaminated foods that may cause several illnesses and can be fatal to human health. Food contamination can occur at any phase of food chain from crop cultivation to its arrival on the kitchen table. USFDA, ISO, and *Codex Alimentarius Commission* have come up with recommendations, regulations, and safety standards to avoid food contamination. The chapter also includes agents (chemical/physical/biological) that can boost or promote this contamination due to contaminated resources, such as soil, water, and air.

## 6.1 INTRODUCTION

Food, water, and air are three major sources of energy for human survival. Food in various forms (natural and processed) is consumed in varying amounts owing to its nutritional value. The nutritional value of a food item mainly depends on its source and processing method [39]. From the soil to the fork, the food is exposed to various stages, where it becomes vulnerable to changes in its quality either by external addition of contaminants, internal changes of the food components, or effect of external stresses on the food impacting its final safety. "You are what you eat": the growth and development conferred by a food item depends on the extent to which it can supply the claimed nutritional content in the desired form without any undue modification.

*Corresponding author. E-mail: murli.murthi@gmail.com.

Our primary motivation for food consumption is due to the provision of nutrients to our body and the taste/pleasure. Healthy food is defined as the food, which on consumption in an ordinary amount provides the person with one-sixth of that person's daily requirement of minimal nutrients without supplementing any amount of harmful substance [95]. The value of a health food enhances significantly as the number of components providing nutritional value to the food are increased and the amount of contaminating elements decreases.

The enormous improvement in food production due to advancements in food technology also raises sources, which can enhance the contamination profile of the final food product. The importance of a robust quality control system cannot be undermined by the fact that the final food product available to consumer can be a harbor of components causing health ailments and diseases, if a strict quality control mechanism is not followed. The tremendous competition to produce new food products enhances the tendency of manufacturers to incorporate artificial flavors and tastemakers into the food in larger amounts, thus enhancing the hazards possible to consumer health [88].

Industrial agriculture and chemical synthesis are two main sources by which various food items are produced. Industrial agriculture resorts to cultivation of foods with different nutritional contents using natural resources of soil, seeds, and chemicals (such as pesticides, insecticides, herbicides, fungicides). These chemicals may cause various health hazards and risks, for example, endocrine disruptions and cancer. Exposure to antibiotic-resistant microbes through contaminated food items also forms one of the many ways that pose health hazards to us. The effectivity of known treatment methods has declined by consumption of food contaminated with antibiotic-resistant microbes [74].

The nutritional value of food is directly associated with the technology of food growth techniques and processing conditions. The conventional methods of food growth comprise of means of sustainable agriculture, which comprises of using means of farming that can enhance the quality of environment by ensuring the use of environmentally compatible sources. This method of food growth aids indirectly to affect the quality of life and well-being of the society.

The outbreak of the industrial revolution has led to the sudden transition of agricultural means from sustainable agriculture to industrial agriculture. Industrial methods comprise of utilizing chemicals, hormones, additives, preservatives, and antibiotics to enhance the rate of food production. The need to produce larger quantities of food has led to the decreased use of sustainable agricultural techniques. Industrial agriculture on the other hand leads to the production of copious quantities of food at decreased costs [92]. The food grown by Industrial agricultural techniques can be hazardous to human health. Synthetic compounds (such as pesticides, insecticides, herbicides, fungicides, antimicrobials, hormones, etc.) show an inherent tendency of causing intracellular damage and can be carcinogenic and mutagenic on long-term use [52, 55, 59].

The indiscriminate use of antibiotics to livestock health is responsible for causing antibiotic resistance in humans. The use of synthetic hormones to increase the rate of growth in livestock has caused adverse effects on the naturally occurring levels of hormones in humans [69, 107].

This chapter focuses on (1) recommendations, regulations, and safety standards for a food product; (2) agents causing food contamination; (3) perception, role, and views of consumers on health risks; and (4) responsibilities of consumers to avoid health risks due to intake of contaminated food.

## 6.2   NUTRITION VERSUS HUMAN HEALTH

A well-balanced enriched diet plays a key role in imparting health to us. A well-balanced and effective functioning and productivity of human beings are mainly driven by healthy body. Individual health is composed of versatile interactive complex components that are strongly influenced by nutritional status, availability of appropriate means of healthcare, social economy, relationships, personal influences, habits, lifestyle, etc. In addition to environmental and social influences on human mind, fulfillment of desirable nutritional requirements of human body has a major impact on the effective functioning of human mind.

The importance of food for desirable nutritional benefits depends on the pattern of utilization of the food in our body. Different people from different age groups and cultures exhibit diverse needs of food in terms of nutritional value due to inter-individual variations [12].

Nutritional malpractices and food safety hazards form a major concern in the industrialized countries; and have major impact on human health making it vulnerable to a host of infectious diseases. About 30% of the population in the industrialized countries (e.g., United States) has been affected by food-borne illnesses. Age and presence of chronic immunosuppressive conditions can enhance the susceptibility of population to food-borne diseases [19].

Frequent occurrences of conditions, such as Bovine Serum Encephalopathy, hoof and mouth disease, and avian influenza have made it essential to come up with strict food safety standards by national and international food regulatory bodies [5].

## 6.3 IMPACT OF FOODS ON HUMAN BODY

Good human health is a consequence of intake of a balanced nutritious diet. Therefore, the knowledge of the interplay of several nutritional factors contributing to human health is a must. Human health is mainly affected by several intermingling factors, such as access to nutrients, social and economic status, genetic composition, social relationships with family and community, personal habits and choices, social exposure, etc. Availability and use of versatile aspects of novel agricultural practices also play a significant role in human health [108].

### 6.3.1 ORGANIC FOOD: IMPACT ON HUMAN HEALTH

Currently, cultivation and utilization of food of organic origin are being extensively promoted owing to health benefits exhibited by such foods. Innumerable animal and human studies on benefits of organic food versus conventional food have shown positive results indicating wide-scale bioavailability and health effects due to presence of large amount of dry matter and low amount of nitrates and lower percentage of pesticide residues [15].

Organic farming is an eco-friendly farming that is conducted without harmful chemicals in food production thus aiding to maintain a balance in the ecosystem [24, 75]. With the advent of agricultural boom, the exorbitant utilization of fertilizers and pesticides has become a way of agricultural trend worldwide. The setting up of the "International Federation of Organic Agricultural Movement" has led to the government regulations on organic farming since 1972 [72, 73].

The concept of organic farming utilizes natural modes of organic processing over extended periods. Thus by adopting a holistic approach toward farming, it aids in enhancing the soil health by minimalizing the use of hazardous insecticides and pesticides. Some approaches of organic farming comprise of (Figure 6.1): (1) effective maintenance of soil structure and fertility; (2) timely control of pests, diseases, and weeds; and (3) careful utilization of available water and soil resources.

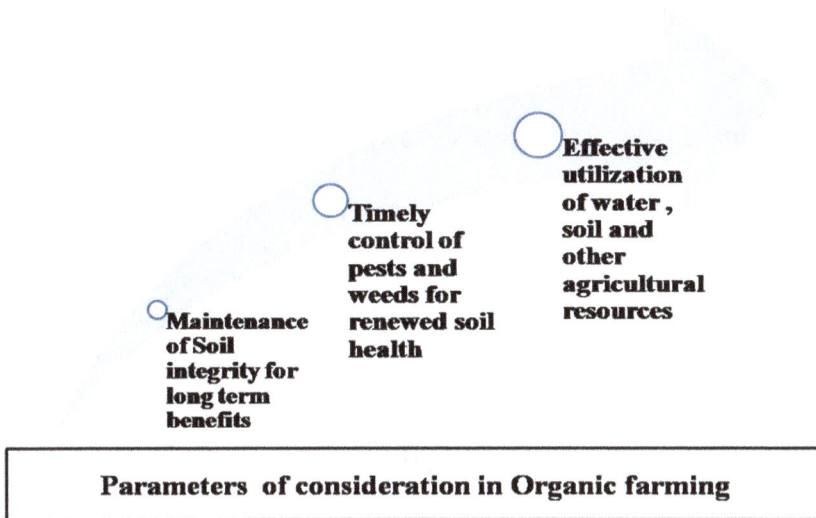

**FIGURE 6.1**  Factors for consideration in organic farming.

1.  *Effective maintenance of soil structure and fertility*: The natural quality of soil can be maintained by timely cultivation, recycling and composting of crop wastes and animal resources, crop rotation, utilization of green manures, legumes, and mulching.
2.  *Timely control of growth of pests and weeds*: The growth of unwanted pests can be controlled by careful planning of crop choice and growth, adopting good ecofriendly cultivation practices, increasing genetic diversity, and encouraging use of predators that eat pest.
3.  *Careful utilization of available water and soil resources*: Organic farming also aims at making effective utilization and conservation of available water and soil long-term productivity.

Organic farming comprises of adopting a combination of traditional methods with modern scientific techniques and skills. It involves understanding and harnessing natural elements and utilizing nature in harmony with advanced scientific techniques. Thus a healthy balance between nature and agricultural development can be maintained [20, 22].

The growing population, technological advancements, and growing needs have further led to the enhancement in the use of such artificial growth promoters that inadvertently affect the soil ecosystems. Organic food has found to be rich in vitamin C. Organic farming involves the use of nature-based wastes of animal, farm, and aquatic origin along with biofertil-izers that minimize the use of synthetic fertilizers, antibiotics, etc. [53, 109].

## 6.3.2 PRINCIPLES OF ORGANIC FARMING

The organic farming is based on the principle of maintaining healthy balance among natural resources, farming practices to produce eco-friendly food with least harmful contaminants. The agriculturists and farmers are culturally and socially bound to manage all natural resources (such as soil, air, water, plants, and animals) to yield food of high quality with optimum utilization of the resources at least environmental hazards and risks [110]. According to the International Federation for Organic Agriculture Movement, organic farming includes several aspects of principles of ecology, health, care, and fairness [10].

The objective of Organic Agriculture is to render the society sustainable agricultural production system based on the backbone of natural processes. Organic farming has proved to be highly beneficial to small scale and marginal farmers [14].

## 6.4 RISK FACTORS ASSOCIATED WITH FOOD MICROBIOLOGICAL HAZARDS

Severe health hazards have been associated with food-borne pathogenic microorganisms. Pathogenic elements form the major causative factor causing food-borne ailments. Serious health perils have been caused by agents like *Campylobacter jejuni*, members of the Salmonella species, Listeria monocytogenes; *Escherichia coli*. Currently, Prion (a protein-based infectious agent) has been identified as a risk factor causing hazardous conditions in humans. The Bovine Spongiform Encephalopathy and variant Creutzfeldt–Jakob diseases in humans have been caused due to prions [100, 116].

### 6.4.1 COMMON MICROBIAL SPECIES ASSOCIATED WITH FOOD HAZARDS

Microbial contamination in food can be assessed based on Hazard Analysis and Critical Control Points (HACCP) system, which is based on several risk factors, management, and control of contamination by micro-organisms [90]. Utilization of effective microbial indicators can help to identify the contaminant microbes. An overall reduction in shelf-life of products is due to indiscriminate use of such indicators. Such common microbial indicators include aerobic mesophilic bacteria, total coliforms, *Enterobacteriaceae*, *Staphylococcus aureus*, *E. coli*, etc. *Listeria monocytogenes* is widely recommended and has been included as safety criteria for the processed marketed foodstuffs by the current EU regulations, No. 1441/2007 [25].

## 6.4.1.1 AEROBIC MESOPHILIC MICROORGANISMS

Bacteria, yeasts, fungi, etc. growing in aerobic environment are being used in fresh foods as indicators of safety measures that are undertaken during several steps of manufacturing of such processed food. The toxicity of microbially contaminated food mainly depends on the concentration levels rather than the extent of pathogenicity. Foods contaminated with higher levels of aerobic mesophilic microbes may be cause of severe toxicity instead of low pathogenicity of the species. The recommended concentration for the use of aerobic mesophilic microorganisms in packaged foods is 5.0 log cfu/g [66, 98].

## 6.4.1.2 LACTIC ACID PRODUCING BACTERIA

Lactic acid bacteria production encompasses several species of microorganisms, such as Streptococcus species, Pediococcus species, Leuconostoc species, *Lactobacillus* species, and Lactococcus species. These have been widely used as starter cultures in the manufacturing of fermented foods, such as cheese, yoghurt, and fermented meats. Some commonly utilized species are *Lactobacillus sakei, Lactobacillus pentosus, Pediococcus acidilactici, Lactobacillus plantarum, and Pediococcus pentasaceus*. Along with their beneficial role, these microbes produce metabolites causing deterioration of food quality and decrease in shelf-life. Depending on the storage conditions (such as temperature, humidity, packaging), different *Lactobacillus* species may show different final levels in food. The undesirable changes in food due to these species can be easily detected by smell, taste, color, gas production, etc. [61, 86].

## 6.4.1.3  ENTEROBACTERIACEAE

The presence of enterobacterial species in food has been associated with food contamination due to inefficient handling, inefficient cooking, cross contamination, contaminated equipments, insufficient holding time, and temperature. These species comprise of bacteria belonging to Gram negative, aerobic, or facultative anaerobic class comprising of *Salmonella enterica*, *Edwardsiella* species, *Hafnia* species, *Morganella* species, *Enterobacter* species, *Serratia* species, *Klebsiella* species, and *Erwinia* species. The presence of these species in food is associated with elevated levels of morbidity and mortality due to the production of thermolabile and thermostable endotoxins, exotoxins, verotoxins, and shigatoxins. These are widely found in food products, such as processed meat, fresh vegetables, and products containing milk [106, 117].

## 6.4.1.4  TOTAL AND FECAL COLIFORMS

Organisms belonging to *Klebsiella* species, *Citrobacter* species, *E. coli* are specific groups within Enterobacteriaceae family. These organisms grow at 35 °C–40 °C. Total coliforms ferment the lactose at 44 °C–45 °C. *E. coli*, *Citrobacter*, *Klebsiella*, etc., belong to these groups. Fecal contamination of food may be indicated by presence of coliforms. However, the contamination may also be contributed to contamination of equipments and utensils. Processed foodstuffs contaminated by coliforms will indicate contamination due to environmental factors, insufficient hygiene, fluctuations in storage conditions (such as temperature and humidity) [79, 112].

## 6.4.1.5  E. COLI

Different serotypes of enteropathogenic *E. coli* may contaminate food by producing Shiga-like toxins, Verocell toxins, or other such thermolabile/thermostable toxins causing diarrhea. The VTEC serotypes are highly infectious and severe; however, the outbreaks of illnesses due to the serotypes are less frequent. Foods originating from catering services and restaurants have been found to be contaminated by *E. coli* serotypes. Foods of animal origin (such as pork, poultry, beef) or plants (such as cabbage, lettuce, spinach, etc.) may also be contaminated by *E. coli*. Irrigation of plants with contaminated water may cause contamination by certain *E. coli* serotypes. Out of several

*E. coli* serotypes, the *E. coli* 015:H7 serotype is found to cause severe disease conditions at low infective dose [23, 41].

### 6.4.1.6   S. AUREUS

Ready-to-eat cooked or cured meals are considered as foods with reduced water activity and are commonly associated with use of *S. aureus* as a microbial indicator. Accidental contamination of food sources due to mishandling or during storage and processing may introduce *S. aureus* as a contaminant in the food. Food poisoning is mainly caused due to consumption of food containing enterotoxins belonging to Staphylococcal species in concentration of 20–100 ng.

Some common factors causing microbial contamination of food are food handling practices, availability of cleaning resources, food storage and processing conditions, intervention measures, etc. [6, 91].

### 6.4.2   CHEMICAL HAZARDS

Several foodborne conditions and ailments may be associated with the chemical hazards, which are difficult to identify and appear long after consumption. The chemical quality of food is compromised due to use of pesticides resulting into entry of unwanted toxic residues and contaminants into the food chain. Many chemical hazards have been found to be linked with processing of high profile foods, which cause alerts, withdrawals, and other such serious issues on long-term basis. A keen attempt to identify such chemical hazards at the risk assessment stage should be made by the food industry to avoid the chain of complications arriving in the long-term.

Understanding of the chemical hazard is an important aspect to identify the toxicological issues associated with a specific food hazard. Chemical hazard identification for food safety involves study of extent of exposure on daily intake. Development of robust HACCP plans for chemical hazard control requires assessment of inherent possible chemical hazards associated with processing of a specific food product followed by study of the related toxicological issues together [44]. Some of the common sources of chemical hazards associated with food safety are [34]:

1.  Hazards introduced during regular food manufacturing and processing,

2.  Hazards introduced from environmental sources,
3.  Hazards caused due to sources inherent in food,
4.  Contamination introduced in food raw materials during raw material processing.

**TABLE 6.1**  Some Common Sources of Chemical Hazards

| Source of Chemical Hazard | Details |
|---|---|
| **Synthetic contaminants**: Polycyclic aromatic hydrocarbons, benzene, furans, acrylamide, chloropropanol, bisphenol, acrylates | These are commonly found in processed foods as end-products of processing conditions, such as temperature, pH changes, chemical interactions between food raw materials, chemical interactions by contact of food contact with container surface or packaging surface, etc. |
| **Chemicals from environmental sources**: Dioxins, heavy metals, Perchlorates, etc. | **Dioxins**: These chemicals are introduced from the environment, mainly, soil, plant surface, animal tissues, etc. These have severe toxicogenic and carcinogenic effects on human body. They also become a part of the food chain and exist in the food chain for prolonged period. |
| | **Heavy metals**: Metals like arsenic, cadmium, etc., form part of the soil and have severe toxicological effects even at very low residual levels. |
| **Toxins** | **Fungal toxins**: Mycotoxins, Ochratoxins, Aflatoxins, etc. |
| | **Plant toxins**: Lectins, Cucurbitacins, Furocoumarins, and Glycoalkaloids occur naturally. |
| | **Fish-based toxins** include Tetrodo-toxins. Diet of certain molluscs, like Shellfish, comprise of a toxin Domoic acid, which shows strong allergenicity. |
| **Naturally occurring**: Allergens | Substances having allergenic potential and derived from plants, animals and other natural sources exist during any time before or after harvest; and form part of raw material of processed foods. Some common sources include certain fish species, such as tuna, mahi, whose spoilage can show potential of immunogenic reactions. Sea corns contaminated with mold growth may act as natural immunogenic agents [87]. |

Toxicological studies on human and animal volunteers for short-term and long-term exposure can aid to arrive at Dose-Response Data, which can help to extrapolate the minimum and maximum tolerable exposures. Processing of Pharmacodynamic data from these studies also aid to arrive at the mechanism of action by which such chemical exposures can affect our body [30]. Preparation and reference of detailed "Material Safety Data Sheets" can help in easy identification of health hazards. Some common chemical hazards identified with food are indicated in Table 6.1.

### 6.4.3 PHYSICAL HAZARDS

Physical hazards in food product manufacturing are mainly caused by either accidental introduction of extraneous particulate matter or as part of raw material used in processing/manufacturing of a food [54]. The extent of risks posed by physical hazards in food depends on several factors, such as size of contaminant, consumer age, product type, contaminant type/concentration/characteristics, and portal of entry . Any contaminant sizing up to or greater than 2 mm may pose a threat to the consumer health. Adversity of consumption of such accidentally introduced contaminants is of higher degree, if the consumer is an elderly or an infant [2, 31]. Some common sources of contamination in food due to physical hazards include:

1. glass from food containers,
2. light sources,
3. metallic particulates from manufacturing vessels,
4. stirrers, etc.,
5. plastic contaminants from packaging materials,
6. wooden impurities from storage cases used for transportation,
7. components that are inherently present as part of food material, such as bones and calciferous shells.

The risk level posed by such contaminants enhances, if the product is in beverage-form, where uptake tendency of the contaminant by the circulation system increases. The adversity is also influenced by size, sharpness, and hardness of physical contaminants, for example, metals, glass, and wood. Such contaminants may affect the consumer health by causing choking, injury, or blockage of important blood vessels. The injury induced by such physical hazards is immediate and the source can be easily identified [56].

## 6.5   RISK FACTORS ASSOCIATED WITH TECHNOLOGY-BASED HAZARDS

### 6.5.1   IMPACT OF GENETIC MODIFICATION OF FOODS

Genetic modification using varied technology as a means to obtain novel strains of plants has been currently overrated. A change in the nutritional status of the plant is most predicted outcome of genetic modification. However, this change is accompanied by several adverse outcomes on the therapeutic effects of plant on our body [62]. Currently, no allergic reactions have been contributed to the utilization of genetic modification in improving the plant nutritional status. Usage of plant viral DNA sequences in induction of genetic change in the plant strain has currently posed a concern for human health. The incorporation of genes in the genetic makeup of the consumer can lead to several hazardous changes in the phenotype and genotype of the following generations; thus contradicting the basic purpose of using the technology [83].

The use of genetically modified plants has several advantages, such as food quantity and quality, nutrition, health, and agricultural practice [94]. However, the use of genetically modified food (GMF) has been associated with the safety concerns of general public. Genetic modification in plants is achieved by deliberate insertion of specific genetic material into plants using recombinant DNA technique [96].

Genetic modification allows development of a crop at faster rate with induction of desirable characteristics by insertion of genetic material from varied species. The technique of genetic modification makes it possible to insert a single gene and achieve enhancement of or introduction of new traits in the existing plant species. Varied plant features (such as resistance to insects and pests, development of tolerance to specific herbicides, etc.) can be introduced into a plant, which is not possible by use of conventional technique. The plant growth yield and tolerance to stressful elements can also be targeted using genetic modification techniques [60, 70].

### 6.5.1.1   SUBSTANTIAL EQUIVALENCE AND EVALUATION OF SAFETY OF GMF

The underlying concept of substantial equivalence mainly emphasizes that GMF exhibits composition and safety equivalent to an existing conventional

[104]. This principle was further highlighted by the Joint Food and Agriculture Organization (FAO)/World Health Organization (WHO) group in 1996, which identified some inherent facts that food comprising of highly complex components and entailed composition will have its nutritional value dependent on invariable factors, such as climate, harvest conditions, and growth factors [80].

It also emphasizes that evaluation of whole food is difficult compared to the food additives due to difficulty in ingestion in sufficient quantities because of bulkiness of food components. Application of such evaluation tests to conventionally is regarded as safe foodstuffs thus giving false results [119].

### 6.5.2   FOOD COMPONENTS WITH NEGATIVE EFFECTS ON OUR HEALTH: ADDITIVES AND PRESERVATIVES

The addition of additives and preservatives to food can increase food stability for a longer period mainly during storage and transportation of foods. Preservatives prevent the microbial degradation of the food substances thus aiding in maintaining the flavor and quality of the food. Thus, they help to prevent the decline of nutritional value of the food that is claimed on the labels of the food packages [18]. An additive is any component added to food to impart a desirable property to the food item [33].

Additives that impart a specific property to the food products are classified as direct additives; and substances to which the food gets exposed unintentionally during storage and transportation are classified as indirect additives [89]. The vulnerability of adults and children to additives used in varied processed foods was highlighted by Dr. Ben Feingold. Based on research reports, food additives >3000 has been approved by the USFDA comprising of preservatives, processing agents, taste enhancers and modifiers, color enhancers, nutritional agents, etc. [51]. Food additives exhibit pathologies, such as skin allergic events, disorders to respiratory and gastrointestinal system, asthmatic events, conjunctivitis, and migraine headache [120]. The absence of an exhaustive listing of ingredients on the food label as regulated by food law makes it difficult for the consumer to identify the causative agents for adverse anatomical events.

One of the major classes of additives is artificial flavors, which act as flavor enhancers to impart specific taste to the food product or complement the flavor of an existing component of the final food product. Examples are artificial sugars, vanilla, etc. Synthetic flavors include benzaldehyde, mono-sodium glutamate (MSG), and nitrites [13].

### 6.5.2.1   IMPACT OF DYES AND COLORANTS AS FOOD ADDITIVES

The colorant Tartarazine (E102: an azo dye by nature) has been frequently used in beverage industry. The reduction of this dye in the intestine and liver causes production of antigenic compounds by metabolism. The observed reactions for this dye are asthma, urticarial, and rhinitis. An interaction study of the dye in 122 patients @ 50 mg evoked adverse reactions, such as palpitation, weakness, heat sensation, suffocation, urticarial, pruritus, and rhinorrhea. The dye has also been frequently associated with hyperactivity in children. The possible mechanism for the adverse event has been chelation of zinc metal by the dye, causing zinc depletion [35]. Few examples are as follows:

1. *Amaranth* (E123): Toxicity studies of Amaranth (E123) in laboratory animals have been found to exhibit cancer, birth defects, sterility, fetal deaths, etc. [58].
2. *Caramel* (E150): It has been widely used as a coloring agent in Cola drinks industry, alcohol industry, and in several food products such as crisps, breads, and sauces. The presence of 4-methylimidazole has been associated with convulsions, inhibition of absorption of vitamin B6 and fluctuations in levels of white blood cells in toxicity studies in rats, mice, and chicks [16].
3. *Curcumin* (E100): Use of Curcumin E100 in flour confectionary, margarine, etc. has been linked to the bacterial mutations. Toxicity and interaction studies at high doses in pigs have shown severe inci-dences of thyroid damage [114].
4. *Erythrosine* (E127): Use of Erythrosine (E127) as a coloring agent in sweets and confectionaries exhibited inhibitory action in neurotransmitters and reduced dopamine turnover leading to hyper-activity in children. Erythrosine use has shown carcinogenicity in lab animals [37].
5. *Sunset Yellow* (E110): An administration of biscuits containing Sunset Yellow (E110) to laboratory rats has been associated with renal and adrenal damages and carcinogenic outcomes [113].

## 6.5.2.2   EFFECT OF PRESERVATIVES AND ANTIOXIDANTS

1.  Benzoates (E210–E219): Food products like jams, salads, creams, and marinated fish have been found to contain benzoic acid and its salts as additives. Use of these synthetic food additives has been associated with symptoms of angioedema, asthma, urticarial, and behavioral hyperactivity in children [36].
2.  *Butylated Hydroxyl Anisole* (BHA E320): It is used as an antioxidant compound in cheese products. The readymade soup mixtures have shown tumorigenic and allergenic effects [65].
3.  MSG: Snacks, sauces, savoring foods, and meat products have been found to contain MSG as a flavoring agent. Excessive use of this agent has caused severe symptoms, such as burning sensations, gripping headache, and asthma in susceptible individuals. It has also been linked to epileptic attacks and brain damage in young rodents [38].
4.  Sulfites (E220–E227): Sulfities have been used widely in fruit-based products, such as packaged juices, syrups, and deserts. The consumption of sulfities has been associated to conditions, such as pruritus, angioedema, and asthma [118].

## 6.5.2.3   EFFECTS OF SYNTHETIC SWEETENERS

1.  *Aspartame*: It comprises of amino acid phenyl alanine and has been widely utilized as an artificial sweetening agent in soft drink and sweet food industries. Toxicity studies of aspartame in rats have shown a rise in phenyl alanine levels in brain. The phenyl alanine levels in brain were raised when consumed with carbohydrates. Significant rise in brain tyrosine levels was observed by synergistic use of Aspartame leading to a reduction in brain tryptophan levels that caused aggressive behavior. Reduced brain tryptophan levels reduced the brain serotonin levels furthermore aggravating the hyperactivity [64].
2.  *Processed sucrose*: Excessive consumption of sucrose/table sugar has been found to be associated with criminal and antisocial behavioral patterns [102].
3.  *Saccharin*: It is used as an artificial sweetening agent in sweet and beverage industry; and has exhibited mutagenicity, carcinogenicity and congenital malformations in rodent studies [9].

### 6.5.3   IMPACT OF USE OF PESTICIDES ON FOOD SAFETY

Insecticides, herbicides, and fungicides are some common classes of pesticides frequently used in agriculture. Organophosphates (such as Malathion and Chlorpyrifo) are used as pesticides for growth of fruits, vegetables, cereals, etc. [3]. The use of pesticides in food has been regulated and assessed. Pesticides are unique set of chemicals with selective toxicity and effects on biological targets. A specific pesticide is allowed to be used in growth of a plant only after assessing the effect of the residual amount of pesticide present in the final food product [76].

The ALARA (As Low as Reasonably Achievable) principle is adopted to regulate the residual levels of pesticide in a crop harvest. A maximum level (MRL) is set for the potential residue, which is used as a trading standard and in the assessment of correct applications of a particular pesticide. The use of a pesticide above the MRL level indicates the inappropriate usage of the pesticide but does not indicate a concern to consumer health. Food products exhibiting pesticide residues above the MRL level are exempted from marketing. To restrict the level of pesticide in a particular food product below the MRL level, a farmer is required to use the pesticide as per good agricultural practices and according to the instructions on the pesticide package label [122].

Infants, children, and adults are exposed to hazards of pesticide by consuming food containing pesticides. Agricultural workers working in farms are exposed to pesticides, while on work and thus are exposed to acute and chronic poisoning [7]. Some of the symptoms of pesticide poisoning are nausea, anxiety, abdominal cramps, confusion, dizziness, etc. Effect of exposure involves adverse effects on memory, birth disorders, Parkinson's disorder, cancer, skin disorders, depression, miscarriage, etc. [71]. Hazardous effects have been observed due to exposure of pesticides on children compared to adults, due to consumption of more food with respect to body weight. The probability of occurrence of adverse events enhances, when children are exposed to pesticides during vulnerable stages of development [40].

Innovations in the field of pesticide delivery have helped to reduce the chemical load induced by conventional pesticide delivery on plants. Use of air-assisted electrostatic nozzle-based spray driers has been found to enhance the deposition efficiency of the pesticide and the bio-efficacy [77].

## 6.6 GLOBAL CONSIDERATIONS IN FOOD SAFETY

### 6.6.1 *ASSESSMENT OF SAFETY OF FOOD ADDITIVES: FDA PERSPECTIVE*

Use of food additives generally regarded as safe can be permitted to be used in processed food products only after establishment of general safety to consumers. For this, a general precaution is to ensure that the amount taken does not exceed daily intake limit established by competent authorities [43].

For evaluation of the general safety of such chemicals to be used as food additives, the Food and Drug Administration (US FDA) has defined certain assessment parameters. Two important parameters that aid to gauge the safety of food additives are: determination of Acceptable Daily Intake (ADI) and Estimated Daily Intake (EDI). These two assessments are affected by several factors, such as consumer preferences, changes in consumer choice over changing health conditions, growing technological advances on food processing industry, changing diet plan with age and region, advancement in toxicological studies [49]. The US Food and Drug Act of 1906 prohibits food adulteration by toxic unsafe products [11]. As per code of US Federal Regulations, safety is defined as "an assurance in the observation of food scientists that the food sample under study does not show any unwanted effects for the proposed use."

Three parameters to be considered by the FDA in safety assessment of a food product are probability factors, factors related to consumption, and safety factors [32]. The FDA participates in safety assessment at the premarket stage, when a manufacturer requests FDA review on the safety of the manufactured food. The FDA may initiate safety assessment of a food product of a manufacturer as a self-initiative at a post-market level if it identifies a health concern at the public level [28]. The evaluation of the ADI and EDI of a food additive is the major parameter defined by FDA for processed foods.

The calculation of ADI is based on chemical nature and toxicological assessment data. ADI can be expressed as milligrams per kilogram body weight per day (mg/kg of bw/day). The ADI is calculated by application of safety factors to the lowest important *No-Observed Adverse Effect Level* and evaluating the chemical nature of the compound. ADI mainly measures the maximum concentration of food additive that a consumer can consume daily throughout his lifetime without experiencing health risk. The WHO defines dietary exposure assessment as "measuring the probable consumption of chemicals comprised in foods, supplements, beverages, drinking water", etc.

The EDI of a substance can be calculated from frequency of food intake, portion size, and concentration present. The calculation of EDI is based on assessment of routine dietary exposure to a food additive. A lower EDI compared to ADI is expected for a food additive to comply with the specified food standards. A higher EDI compared to ADI is indicative that a food additive may not be allowed into the market [47].

The RedBook provides guidance to food manufacturers regarding various aspects of toxicological evaluation of food products. The first edition comprises of US-FDA criteria for assessment of food safety. It comprises of principles to establish safety of a food additive after its entry into the market and thus safeguarding the consumer health. The safety recommendations of FDA are based mainly on evaluation of pharmacokinetic parameters, such as absorption, distribution, metabolism, and excretion properties of a food additive [58].

## 6.6.2 ASSESSMENT OF SAFETY OF A FOOD: CODEX ALIMENTARIUS COMMISSION (CAC)

The general discussions on various assets of continuous improvisation of food products were held in the 1950s and 1960s. Both the WHO and United Nations FAO participated in the discussions and played an important role to lay out guidelines for the same. Important points essentially discussed in the forum comprised of exorbitant use of food additives to improvise food features, utilization of pesticides in agricultural practice and storage of food, worldwide difference in food standards and all associated food-related issues, such as labeling criteria, food hygiene, food contamination by insects, rodents, bird, filth, and pathogens.

The agenda of FAO/WHO discussing various aspects of food standards, safety, and quality issues was laid down in the conference held at Hot Springs—Virginia in June of 1943. The conference mainly addressed issues related to food and agriculture exacerbated by war [42].

The CAC comprises of a governmental organization regulating food standards at the international platform. Its two crucial functions are ensuring implementation of fair practices in food supply and ensuring consumer health. Furthermore, it composes several international rules and criteria for a wide range of foodstuffs, such as food additives, pesticide residues, and food contaminants. The recommendations laid down by this commission are followed as guidelines by the government to lay down regulations for safeguarding food quality. One of the prime steps of CAC is the identification of microbiological hazards in food products. Several activities conducted by CAC have been instrumental in creating global awareness on safety and quality of food.

*Codex Alimentarius* comprises of an amalgamation of food standards represented in a systematic codified manner. All regulations associated with principal foodstuffs of different nature (such as processed, semiprocessed) are found in the "Codex Alimentarius", which comprises of 300 standards in 13 volumes associated with properties and safety profile of food products.

The CAC regulates the quality of food based on risk analysis. Conduct of risk analysis of food consists of aspects, such as assessment, management, and communication. Risk assessment of a food includes identification of hazard, characterization of hazard, assessment of exposure, and characterization of risk. Risk management comprises of consideration of alternatives in policy making and uptake of suitable preventive and control steps. Risk communication comprises of exchange of information among risk assessors, managers, industry, consumer, etc.

The Joint Conference on Food Standards, Chemicals in Foods and Food Trade held at Rome, Italy by the FAO/WHO recommended to the important committees to evaluate food products scientifically for consistent risk assessments. Some of the changes affecting food control include establishments of food standards.

The food standards defined in Codex help to identify the product giving the composition and quality factors. The basic theme of each standard is the protection of consumer health and provisions on food additives, contaminants, and food-related hygiene necessities. Supplementary informative documents are referred as supportive documents to the standards and codes prescribed in *Codex* [48, 121].

## 6.6.2.1   IMPACT OF CODEX STANDARDS ON CONSUMERS

By setting up of various standards and food regulations related to food safety, *Codex* has been a vehicle in safeguarding the health of consumers. The Guidelines for Consumer Protection was published in 1986 by the United Nations Bodies as a step toward the same. Several conferences were held in the early 1990s to promote consumer health and safety associated with use of food products [97]. The 1991 FAO/WHO conference in cooperation with GATT was based on standards in chemicals and food trade and gave several recommendations associated with enhancement of consumer role in making policies and guidelines for food products. One such recommendation given at the 1st FAO/WHO International conference in 1992 indicated enhancement in food quality and safety to ensure consumer protection [45].

### 6.6.3  ASSESSMENT OF SAFETY OF FOOD: ISO STANDARDS

ISO stands for International Organization of Standardization. ISO food standards are mainly laid down to establish confidence in consumer regarding the carefree utilization of the specific foodstuff. The standards help to ensure the security of all food product manufacturers regarding the performance of specific food product by establishing a food validating system [93]. A critical task to be executed by all members of food chain includes: establishing food quality and maintaining quality of a food product till it reaches the consumer. The presence of ISO standards helps to develop an assurance to the consumer on quality of the food product [111].

The quality of processed food has been timely controlled by various quality management systems. The ISO 9001-2000 established a robust quality system. It contains several clauses providing guidance for management of food quality at the manufacturing level [103]. The ISO system has been used inadvertently with the HACCP system as a quality assurance system. The ISO standards ensure that all food products reaching the consumer possess same standardized-recipe thus ensuring final food product quality. By adopting to ISO standards, several industries become competent to remain updated and incorporate innovative solutions with the latest know-hows without entering costly innovative developments [21].

### 6.7  GENERAL PRINCIPLES OF FOOD HYGIENE

As per European regulations, hygiene can be defined as "steps and measures essential for controlling hazards and ensuring the suitability of a foodstuff for human consumption. Food hygiene mainly comprises of two assets: food safety and food suitability [50, 81]".

### 6.7.1  HAZARD ANALYSIS IN FOOD SAFETY AND IMPLEMENTATION MEASURES

As a means to prevent contamination in food catering outlets, the unit of the HACCP has been developed. An important function of the HACCP system is the identification and regulation of the varied steps involved in ensuring food product safety in a cost-effective manner. It mainly aims at controlling the food quality and safety based on a preventive approach [26]. There are seven steps in hazard identification and analysis, for example

1. Conducting the hazard analysis.
2. Identification of the CCP.
3. Establishment of critical levels and limits.
4. Establishment of a robust regulating system.
5. Undertaking corrective measures.
6. Verification of steps taken.
7. Documentation.

One of the recommendations of the various assets of HACCP system include improvement of food service centers [82]. One of the primary steps to be taken while overtaking food safety measures includes conducting training of food handlers and working on the hygienic parameters affecting food quality. Most of the food-borne illnesses and conditions have been associated to catering [67]. People most frequently fall vulnerable to food-borne ailments at places like hospitals, school canteens, general eateries.

Some of the major factors causing microbial contamination of food include: processing and preparation methods, sanitation measures undertaken at catering venues including food handling. A special attention should be given to service centers and catering venues serving susceptible population, such as children, elderly, and immunocompromised persons. In recent times, the changing trends of consumer habits and choices have caused enhancement in application of technological innovations in catering practices [8, 29].

Catering ventures and food service outlets are business and associations undertaken to serve food preparations. Some of the several outlets are restaraunts, cafeterias and other such small and big scale establishments. While serving food as a part of business at such establishments, food is often transported, stored, distributed by different means making it vulnerable to get contaminated with disease-causing microorganisms [85].

## 6.8 CONSUMER PERCEPTION OF A HEALTH RISK: ROLE AND VIEWS

Consumer forms the prime factor of a concern for the food manufacturer. The entire food processing by a manufacturer is done with regards to end result of consumer satisfaction. Just as food safety is a matter of concern for a consumer, vis-à-vis consumer satisfaction is a matter of concern for a food manufacturer [68]. Food nutritional factors, food contamination, food sources, food processing mechanism, food preservation, resultant impact, etc. are some of the critical points of concern for food consumer [78]. Appropriate food labeling comprising of contents like calorie count, food additives added (concentration, quality, suitability), sources, manufacturing details, storage information can help to provide maximum information to consumers [57]. However, the information invariably is not enough to satisfy the inquisitive mindset of consumers toward food safety and the associated health effects.

The genuine concerns of consumer regarding food safety can be addressed only when the food industry works in collaboration with government and academic institutes and educational communities. In order to understand the consumer needs and concerns regarding the food, it becomes essential to conduct a thorough research on the consumer perceptions. The product purchase is dependent on the financial, social, performance, and health associated risk perceptions of consumer [105]. The food safety attitudes of consumers can be determined by measuring the confidence with which a consumer buys a food product thus indicating no observed food-related health risks. The measurement of such confidence levels and consumer attitudes can be achieved by conducting of surveys and seminars [115].

Consumer perception of a health risk associated with a given processed food product is influenced by nature of technology utilized and several variables influencing the technology [27]. Health risk perception can be determined as the probability of loss of a valuable component. Measurement of consumer perception of health risk requires defining of parameters, for example, nature of health hazard and to what context the exposure to food hazard occurs. The well-planned surveys aid to determine the confidence levels of consumers. The growing consumer awareness makes it necessary to keep the consumer well-informed about the processing parameters of a food [101]. Unusual care has to be taken while labeling the food by application of novel advanced technology to conventional processes.

Food crises and observed adverse events in food products have become a major reason to lower the extent of utility of the food product by a consumer. In such cases, a complete transparency from the manufacturer to the consumer may play a vital role in reviving consumer faith in a product. Utilization of scientific principles along with regulations need not to offer complete assurance toward safety and declined risk of a food product [46].

While considering the issue of food safety, it also becomes necessary that the consumer is aware of the major parameters affecting food safety and the do's and don'ts of handling the food. Maintenance of cleanliness during food preparation and during food consumption is of utmost importance. Some simple steps to enhance the food safety are:

1. *Maintaining cleanliness while food preparation*: Washing hands, cleaning the surfaces of table, using cleaned utensils and apparatus, etc., can prove very beneficial and enhance food safety.
2. *Separation of food components*: It is always preferable to separate the raw materials in food preparation from the finally prepared food-stuff. Prevention of cross-contamination of prepared foodstuffs with raw materials can prove to be derogatory for general food safety. This care should be taken especially, when use of perishable foodstuffs like meat, poultry, seafood are used as raw materials.
3. *Maintainance of processing temperatures*: "The temperature at which the food preparation is processed and the temperature at which the raw material is used for food preparation" is a crucial role in imparting safety to final processed food. The processing temperature affects the safety of final food preparation in two ways, namely: (1) Controlling the growth of hazardous pathogens and destroying the already existing pathogens; (2) Maintaining the quality of a final food product thus preventing the production of harmful and toxicogenic ingredients introduced in the food due to erroneous food processing methods.
4. *Adequate and timely refrigeration*: Safety of a food can be ensured by refrigeration irrespective of the type of foodstuff. Timely refrigeration of raw materials (like milk, meat, and other degradable food components) has been found to affect food quality and enhance it for long periods of time. Storing the food in refrigerators has found to enhance the utility of the foodstuffs for longer durations [17].

Consumers are also required to possess basic general knowledge regarding the varied food-borne illnesses associated with the consumption of contaminated or deteriorated food stuff. Information regarding the storage conditions is of utmost importance for packaged processed foods [69]. The consumer should ensure that the canned and packaged foodstuff is stored in a cool dry place protected from temperature and humidity extremes. Exceptional care should be taken while storing foods with acid contents [1]. Canned food is found to exhibit higher signs of contamination by Clostridium botulinum.

Hence, consumer should exhibit general awareness on the signs of Clostridial contamination of food, also known as botulism [84].

Consumers should be well versed in identifying the signs of accidental or intentional contamination. A thorough understanding on the identification of intact or tampered seals is of paramount importance in case of use of canned processed raw materials or prepared foodstuffs [4]. Consumption of food available at food outlets (like restaurants, cafeterias, etc.) has been mainly associated with frequent occurrences of food-borne illnesses. However, consumption of preparations processed at home has been found to be a routing cause of food-borne conditions at a much higher level [99].

Consumer knowledge, participation, and satisfaction are the three important parameters to determine the success of a food product. A manufacturer assuring the fulfillment of these three parameters can ensure a successful product to be established.

## 6.9  SUMMARY

An important consideration to be made while evaluating the degree of food safety includes the various aspects of role played by technology, manufacturer, and consumer. It is the responsibility of a food manufacturer to assess and confirm food safety bearing in mind consumer knowledge. Advancement in technology enhances the number of critical parameters affecting food safety thus enhancing the responsibility of manufacturer to maintain more stringent measures in food processing, thus aiding in imparting higher confidence levels for the output of a food product.

## KEYWORDS

- consumer
- contaminants
- food safety
- genetic modification
- hazard
- organic farming
- refrigeration

# REFERENCES

1. Ababio, P.F.; Adi, D.D.; Amoah, M. Evaluating the awareness and importance of food labelling information among consumers in the Kumasi Metropolis of Ghana. *Food Control*, **2012**, *26*, 571–574.

2. Akanele, E.; Chukwu, S.M.; Chukwu, M.A. Microbiological contamination of food: the mechanism, impact and prevention. *International Journal of Scientific and Technology Research*, **2016**, *5* (3), 65–78.

3. Aktar, M.W.; Sengupta, D.; Chowdhury, A. Impact of pesticides use in agriculture: their benefits and hazards. *Interdisciplinary Toxicology*, **2009**, *2* (1), 1–12. doi: 10.2478/v10102-009-0001-7.

4. Altekruse, S.F.; Street, D.A.; Fein, S.B. Consumer knowledge of foodborne microbial hazards and food-handling practices. *Journal of Food Protection*, **1996**, *59*, 287–294.

5. Arnoldi J.M. *Foreign Animal Diseases: The Gray Book*. Committee on Foreign Animal Diseases of the United States Animal Health Association (USAHA); 1998; www.usaha.org; Accessed on November 4, **2019**.

6. Asao, T. Extensive outbreak of staphylococcal food poisoning due to low-fat milk in Japan: estimation of enterotoxin-A in the incriminated milk and powdered skim milk. *Epidemiology and Infection*. **2003**, *130*, 33–40. DOI: 10.1017/S0950268802007951.

7. Baker, B.P.; Benbrook, C.M. Pesticide residues in conventional, integrated pest management (IPM)-grown and organic foods: insights from three US data sets. *Food Additives* & Contaminants, **2002**, *19*, 427–446.

8. Baluka, S.A.; Miller, R.; Kaneene, J.B. Hygiene practices and food contamination in managed food service facilities in Uganda. *African Journal of Food Sciences*, **2015**, *9*(1), 31–42.

9. Bandyopadhyay, A.; Ghoshal, S.; Mukherjee, A. (2008) Genotoxicity testing of low-calorie sweeteners: aspartame, acesulfame-K, and saccharin. *Drug and Chemical Toxicology*, **2008**, *31*, 447–457

10. Barar, M. Organic agriculture: conceptual approach for sustainable environment: review. *International Journal of TechnoChem Research*, **2015**, *1*(3), 156–164.

11. Barkan, I.D. Industry invites regulation: the passage of the pure food and drug act of 1906. *American Journal of Public Health*; **1985**, *75* (1), 18–26; PMC ID: 1646146.

12. Basiotis P.P.; Lino, M.; Dinkins, J.M. Consumption of Food Group Servings: People's Perceptions vs. Reality, Nutrition Insights. USDA Center for Nutrition Policy and Promotion; **2000**. https://www.cnpp.usda.gov/sites/default/files/nutrition_insights_uploads/Insight20.pdf; accessed on November 4, **2019**.

13. Bearth, A.; Cousin, M.E.; Siegrist, M. The consumer's perception of artificial food additives: influences on acceptance, risk and benefit perceptions. *Food Quality and Preferences*, **2014**, *38*, 14–23.

14. Bhattacharya, P.; Chakraborty, G. Current status of organic farming in India and other countries. *Indian Journal of Fertilizers*, **2005**, *1* (9), 111–123.

15. Birkhofer, K. Long-term organic farming fosters below and aboveground biota: implications for soil quality, biological control and productivity. *Soil Biology & Biochemistry*, **2008**, *40*, 2297–2308.

16. Brecher, S. (2007) Toxicology and Carcinogenesis Studies of 4-Methylimidazole in F344/N Rats and B6c3f1 Mice. National Toxicology Program (NTP), Technical Report

TR-535, NIH Publication 07-4471; Washington, DC: National Institute of Health; **2004**; 56.

17. Byrd-Bredbenner, C.; Berning, J.; Martin-Biggers, J.; Quick, V. food safety in home kitchens: literature review. *International Journal of Environmental Research* and *Public Health*, **2013**, *10*, 4060–4085. doi:10.3390/ijerph10094060

18. Carocho, M.; Barreiro, M.F.; Morales, P.; Ferreira, I. adding molecules to food, pros and cons: review on synthetic and natural food additive. *Comprehensive Reviews in Food Science and Food Safety*, **2014**, *13*, 377–399. doi:10.1111/1541-4337.12065

19. Centers for Disease Control and Prevention (CDCP). Surveillance for Foodborne Disease Outbreaks: United States, 1998–2008. *Morbidity and Mortality Weekly Report*, **2013**, *62* (2), 1–34; https://www.cdc.gov/mmwr/pdf/ss/ss6202.pdf; accessed on November 4, **2019**.

20. Chhonkar, P. K. Organic farming myth and reality. In: *Proceedings of the FAI Seminar on Fertilizer and Agriculture Challenges*; New Delhi, India; December **2002**; pp. 85–88.

21. Chivandi, A. Evaluation of ISO: 22000 Food safety standards awareness and implementation in zimbabwean branded fast food outlets: customer, employee and management perspectives. *African Journal of Hospitality, Tourism and Leisure*, **2017**, *6* (2), 1–24.

22. Choudhary, R.S.; Das, A.; Patnaik, U.S. (2003) Organic farming for vegetable production using vermicompost and FYM in kokriguda watershed of Orissa. *Indian Journal of Soil Conservation*, **2003**, *31* (2), 203–206.

23. Chu, P.; Hemphill, R.R. Acquired hemolytic anemia. In: *Emergency Medicine: A Comprehensive Study Guide*; Judith Tintinalli (Ed. General); 9th Edition; NY: McGraw-Hill Education; **2020**; pp. 1490–1494.

24. Cicia, G.; Del-Giudice, T.; Scarpa, R. (2002) Consumers' perception of quality in organic food: random utility model under preference heterogeneity and choice correlation from rank-orderings. *British Food Journal*, **2002**, *104* (3), 200–213.

25. Cordier, J. L. Microbiological Criteria and Indicator Microorganisms. Chapter 4; In: *Food Microbiology: Fundamentals and Frontiers*; M. P. Doyle (Ed.); Washington, DC: ASM Press; **2013**; pp. 81–90.

26. Cusato, S.; Tavolaro, P. Implementation of Hazard Analysis and Critical Control Points System in the Food Industry: Impact on Safety and the Environment. Chapter 7; In: *Novel Technologies in Food Science-Integrating Food Science and Engineering Knowledge into the Food Chain*; McElhatton, A. and Sobral, P.J.A. (Eds.); **2012**; pp. 21–35; DOI 10.1007/978-1-4419-7880-6_2,

27. da Costa, M.C.; Deliza, R.; Rosenthal, A. non-conventional technologies and impact on consumer behavior. *Trends in Food Science & Technology*, **2000**, *11*, 188–193.

28. Darrow, J.J.; Avorn, J.; Kesselhiem, A.S. New FDA breakthrough - drug category: implications for patients. *The New England Journal of Medicine*, **2014**, *370* (13), 1252–1258

29. Djekic, I.; Smijic, N.; Kalogianni, E. Food hygiene practices in different food establishments. *Food Control*, **2014**, *39*, 34–40.

30. Donoghue, D.J. Antibiotic residues in poultry tissues and eggs: human health concerns. *Poultry Science*, **2003**, *82*, 618–621.

31. Dougherty, C. dietary exposures to food contaminants across the United States. *Environmental Research Section A*, **2000**, *84*, 170–185; doi:10.1006/enrs.2000.4027.

32. EAFUS. Food and Drug Administration: Everything Added to Food in the United States. Version **2002**; http://www.accessdata.fda.gov/scripts/fcn/fcnnavigation. cfm?rpt=eafuslisting; accessed on November 4, 2019.
33. EAFUS. Food and Drug Administration: Everything Added to Food in the United States. Version **2013**; http://www.accessdata.fda.gov/scripts/fcn/fcnnavigation. cfm?rpt=eafuslisting; accessed on November 4, 2019.
34. Edgar, J. Future impact of food safety issues on animal production and trade: implications for research. *Australian Journal of Experimental Agriculture*, **2004**, *44*, 1073–1078.
35. EFSA Panel on Dietetic Products, Nutrition and Allergies (NDA). Scientific Opinion on the Appropriateness of the Food Azo-Colors: Tartrazine (E 102), Sunset Yellow FCF (E 110), Carmoisine (E 122), Amaranth (E 123), Ponceau 4R (E 124), Allura Red AC (E 129), Brilliant Black BN (E 151), Brown FK (E 154), Brown HT (E 155) and Litholrubine BK (E 180) for Inclusion in the List of Food Ingredients in Annex - IIIa of Directive 2000/13/EC. *EFSA Journal*, **2010**, *8* (10), 1778; p. 11; DOI: 10.2903/j.efsa.2010.1778
36. EFSA Panel on Food Additives and Nutrient Sources (ANS). Scientific Opinion on the Re-evaluation of Benzoic Acid (E 210), Sodium Benzoate (E 211), Potassium Benzoate (E 212) and Calcium Benzoate (E 213) as Food Additives. *EFSA Journal*, **2016**, *14* (3), 4433–4440; DOI: 10.2903/j.efsa.2016.4433
37. EFSA Panel on Food Additives and Nutrient Sources (ANS). Scientific Opinion on the re-evaluation of Erythrosine (E 127) as a food additive. *EFSA Journal*, **2011**, *9* (1), Online article ID: **1854**; p. 9; DOI: 10.2903/j.efsa.2011.1854
38. Egbuonu, A.C.C.; Obidoa, O.; Ezeokonkwo, C.A. Hepatotoxic effects of low dose oral administration of monosodium glutamate in male albino rats. *African Journal of Biotechnology*, **2009**, *8* (13), 3031–3035.
39. Elmadfa, I.; Meyer, A.L. Importance of food composition data to nutrition and public health. *European Journal* of *Clinical Nutrition*, **2010**, *64* (3), S4–S7. DOI: 10.1038/ ejcn.2010.202.
40. Eskenazi, B.; Bradman, A.; Castorina, R. Exposure of children to organophosphate pesticides and their potential adverse health effects. *Environmental Health Perspectives*, **1999**, *107* (3), 409–419.
41. European Food Safety Authority (EFSA). The European Union (EU) Summary Report on Trends and Sources of Zoonoses, Zoonotic Agents and Foodborne Outbreaks in 2009. *The EFSA Journal*, **2010**, *8* (1), Online article ID: **1496**; p. 10; DOI:10.2903/j.efsa.2010.1496
42. FAO - Committee on World Food Security. *Report CFS 2012/39/4*; **2012**; p. 47; http:// www.fao.org/docrep/meeting/026/MD776E.pdf; accessed on November 4, 2019.
43. FAO/WHO. Dietary Exposure assessment of chemicals in food. Chapter 6; In: *Environmental Health Criteria-240: Principles and Methods for the Risk Assessment of Chemicals in Food*; Rome, Italy: Food & Agricultural Organization; **2009**; p. 98; http:// www.inchem.org/documents/ehc/ehc/ehc240_chapter6.pdf; accessed on November 4, 2019.
44. FAO/WHO. *Food Safety Risk Analysis: A Guide for National Food Safety Authorities*. Food and Nutrition Paper 87. Rome, Italy: World Health Organization and Food and Agricultural Organization of United Nations; **2006**; p. 119; http://www.fao.org/3/a-a0822e.pdf; accessed on November 4, 2019.
45. FAO/WHO. General Agreement on Tariffs and Trade (GATT). FAO/WHO Conference on Food Standards, Chemicals in Food and Food Trade-1; Rome, Italy: World Health

Organization and Food and Agricultural Organization of United Nations; **1991**; p. 119; http://www.fao.org/3/u5900t/u5900t09.htm; accessed on November 4, 2019.

46. FAO/WHO. *Assuring Food Safety and Quality: Guidelines for Strengthening National Food Control Systems*. FAO Food and Nutrition Paper 76; Rome, Italy: World Health Organization and Food and Agricultural Organization of United Nations; **2003**; pp. 1–73, http://www.fao.org/docrep/006/y8705e/y8705e00.htm; accessed on November 4, 2019.

47. FAO/WHO. Dietary Exposure Assessment of Chemicals in Food. In: *Principles and Methods for the Risk Assessment of Chemicals in Foods*; Rome, Italy: World Health Organization and Food and Agricultural Organization of United Nations; **2009**; pp. 1–92; https://apps.who.int/iris/bitstream/handle/10665/44065/WHO_EHC_240_eng.pdf;js essionid=C8ECD0C8A0AC417631970FA4D6292D9A?sequence=152; accessed on November 4, 2019.

48. FAO/WHO. Codex Alimentarius Commission, Joint FAO/WHO Food Standards Programme 21st Edition; Rome, Italy: World Health Organization and Food and Agricultural Organization of United Nations; **2013**; p. 214; http://www.fao.org/3/a-i3243e.pdf; accessed on November 4, 2019.

49. FAO/WHO. *Safety Evaluation of Certain Food Additives*. WHO Food Additive Series 70; Prepared by 79th meeting of the Joint FAO/WHO Expert Committee on Food Additives (JECFA); Rome, Italy: World Health Organization and Food and Agricultural Organization of United Nations; **2015**; p. 378; http://apps.who.int/iris/bits tream/10665/171781/3/9789240693982_eng.pdf; accessed on November 4, 2019.

50. FAO/WHO. *Codex Alimentarius Commission, REP 16/FH*. Report of the 47th Session of the Codex Committee on Food Hygiene, Joint FAO/WHO Food Standards Programme; Rome, Italy: World Health Organization and Food and Agricultural Organization of United Nations; **2016**; p. 96; http://www.fao.org/fao-who-codexalimentarius/sh-proxy/ en/?lnk=1&url=https%253A%252F%252Fworkspace.fao.org%252Fsites%252Fcodex %252FMeetings%252FCX-712-47%252FReport%252FREP16_FHe.pdf; accessed on November 4, 2019.

51. Feingold, B. *Why Your Child is Hyperactive*. New York: Random House; **1975**; p. 211.

52. Fores, J. Feeding the world today and tomorrow: the importance of food science and technology. *Comprehensive Review in Food Science and Safety*, **2010**, *9* (5), 572–599; https://onlinelibrary.wiley.com/doi/full/10.1111/j.1541-4337.2010.00127.x; accessed on November 4, 2019.

53. Gaur, A.C. Handbook of Organic Farming and Biofertilizers. Jaipur, India: Ambica Book Agency; Vedams eBooks (P) Ltd. (New Delhi, India); **2006**; p. 318.

54. Gil, F.; Hernandez, A.; Martin-Domingo, M.C. Toxic Contamination of Nutraceuticals and Food Ingredients, Nutraceuticals. 2016; pp. 825–836; DOI: http://dx.doi.org/10.1016/ B978-0-12-802147-7.00058-9; accessed on November 4, 2019.

55. Gill, H.; Garg, H. (Eds.). Pesticides: Environmental Impacts and Management Strategies, Pesticides-Toxic Aspects. IntechOpen.com; **2014**; online open access book; pp.187–230; DOI:10.5772/57399

56. Gorham, T.R.; Zarek, L. Filth and Other Foreign Objects in Foods: Review of Analytical Methods and Health Significance. Chapter 4; In: *Handwork of Food Science Tech and Engineering, Four Volume Set*; Hui, Y. (Ed.); Boca Raton, FL: CRC Press; **2006**; volume 2; pp. 224–267.

57. Grujic, S.; Grujic, R.; Petrovic, D.; Gajic, J. The importance of consumers' knowledge about food quality, labeling and safety in food choice. *Journal of Food Research*, **2013**, *2* (5), 57–65; DOI:10.5539/jfr.v2n5p57

58. Gungormus, C.; Kilic, A. The Safety Assessment of Food Additives by Reproductive and Developmental Toxicity Studies. Chapter 2; In: *Food Additive*; Yehia El-Samragy (Ed.); IntechOpen.com; **2012**; p. 20; https://doi.org/10.5772/30787; accessed on November 4, 2019.

59. Güngörmüş, C.; Kılıç, A.; Akay, M.T.; Kolankaya, D. (2010). The effects of maternal exposure to food additive E341 (Tricalcium Phosphate) on fetal development of rats. *Environmental Toxicology and Pharmacology*, **2010**, *29*, 111–116.

60. Gurr, S.J.; Rushton, P.J. Engineering plants with increased disease resistance: what are we going to express? *Trends in Biotechnology*, **2005**, *23*, 275–282.

61. Hammes, W.P.; Bantleon, A. Lactic acid bacteria in meat fermentation. *FEMS Microbiology Letters*, **1990**, *87* (1–2), 165–174.

62. Hefferon, K. Nutritionally enhanced food crops: progress and perspectives. *International Journal of Molecular Sciences*, **2015**, *16*, 3895–3914.

63. Horrigan, L.; Lawrence, R.; Walker, P. How Sustainable Agriculture can address the environment and human health harms of industrial agriculture. *Environmental Health Perspectives*, **2002**, 110 (5), 445–450.

64. Humphries, P.; Pretorius, E.; Naude, H. Direct and Indirect Cellular Effects of Aspartame on the Brain. *European Journal of Clinical Nutrition*, **2008**, *62*, 451–462.

65. Inai, K. Hepatocellular tumorigenicity of butylated hydroxytoluene administered orally to B6C3F1 mice. *Japanese Journal of Cancer Research*, **1988**, *79* (1), 49–58; DOI: 10.1111/j.1349-7006.1988.tb00010.x

66. Jay, James M. *Modern Food Microbiology*. 5th edition; New York: Chapman and Hall; **1995**; p. 745.

67. Jone, S.; Parry, S.M.; O'Brien, S.J.; Palmer, S.R. Operational practices associated with foodborne disease outbreaks in the catering industry in England and Wales. *Journal of Food Protection*, **2008**, *71* (8), 1659–1665.

68. Kennedy, J. Segmentation of US consumers based on food safety attitudes. *British Food Journal*, **2008**, *110* (7), 691–705.

69. Kennedy, J. Food Safety Knowledge of consumers and the microbiological and temperature status of their refrigerators. *Journal of Food Protection*, **2005**, *68* (7), 1421–1430.

70. Key, S. Genetically modified plants and human health. *The Journal of the Royal Society of Medicine*, **2008**, *101*, 290–298. DOI 10.1258/jrsm.2008.070372

71. Kishi, M. Relationship of pesticide spraying to signs and symptoms in Indonesian Farmers. *Scandinavian Journal of Work and Environmental Health*, **1995**, *21* (2), 124–133.

72. Koechlin, F. *Genetic Engineering versus Organic Farming*. Okozentrum Imsbach, Tholey-Theley, Germany: IFOAM (International Federation of Organic Agricultural Movements); **2002**; p. 20; https://www.stopogm.net/old/sites/stopogm.net/files/repo/ge_ifoam_2.pdf; accessed on November 4, 2019.

73. Lotter, D.W. Organic Agriculture. *Journal of Sustainable Agriculture*, **2003**, *21* (4), 59–128.

74. MacRae, R. agricultural science and sustainable agriculture: review of the existing scientific barriers to sustainable food production and potential solutions. *Biological Agriculture and Horticulture*, **1989**, *6* (3), 173–219.

75. Mader, P.; Fliessbach, A. Soil fertility and biodiversity in organic farming. *Science*, **2002**, *296*, 1694–1697.

76. Mahmood, Q.; Bilal, M. Jan S, (2014) Herbicides, pesticides and plant tolerance: an overview. In: *Emerging Technologies and Management of Crop Stress Tolerance*; New York: Academic Press; **2014**; pp. 423–448.

77. Mamidi, V.R.; Ghanshyam, C.; Patel, M. Electrostatic hand pressure knapsack spray system with enhanced performance for small scale farms. *Journal of Electrostatics*, **2013**, *71* (4), 785–790.

78. Marreiros, C. Conceptual framework of consumer food choice behavior. CEFAGE-UE Working Paper 2009/06; **2009**; 1–25; http://www.cefage.uevora.pt/en/content/download/1715/22411/version/1/file/2009_06.pdf; accessed on November 4, 2019.

79. Martin, N.H.; Trmcic, A.; Hsieh, T.; Boor, K.J. The evolving role of coliforms as indicators of unhygienic processing conditions in dairy foods. *Frontiers in Microbiology*, **2016**, *7*, article ID: 1549; p. 8; doi: 10.3389/fmicb.2016.01549

80. Miller, H.I. Substantial equivalence: its uses and abuses. *Nature Biotechnology*, **1999**, *17*, 1042–1043.

81. Monney, I.; Agyei, D.; Ewoenam, B.S. Food hygiene and Safety Practices among Street Food Vendors: An Assessment of Compliance, Institutional and Legislative Framework in Ghana. *Food and Public Health*, **2014**, *4* (6), 306–315; DOI: 10.5923/j.fph.20140406.08

82. Motarjemi, Y.; Kaferstein, F. Food safety, hazard analysis and critical control point and the increase in foodborne diseases: a paradox? *Food Control*, **1999**, *10*, 325–333.

83. Mushegian, A.; Shepherd, R. Genetic elements of plant viruses as tools for genetic engineering. *Microbiological Reviews*, **1995**, *59* (4), 548–578.

84. NFPA/CMI Container Integrity Task Force. Botulism Risk from Post-Processing Contamination of Commercially Canned Foods in Metal Containers. *Journal of Food Protection, Microbiological Assessment Group Report*, **1984**, *47* (10), 801–816; http://jfoodprotection.org/doi/abs/10.4315/0362-028X-47.10.801; accessed on November 4, 2019.

85. Ng, C.A.; von Goetz, N. Global Food System as Transport Pathway for Hazardous Chemicals: The Missing Link between Emissions and Exposure. *Environmental Health Perspectives*, **2017**, *125* (1), 1–17; http://dx.doi.org/10.1289/EHP168.

86. Nychas, G.J.E,.; Skandamis, P.N. Meat spoilage during distribution. *Meat Science*, **2008**, *78* (1–2), 77–89; DOI:10.1016/j.meatsci.2007.06.020

87. Oskarrson, A. Environmental contaminants and food safety. *Oskarsson Acta Veterinaria Scandinavica*, **2003**, 54, S1–S5; doi:10.1186/1751-0147-54-S1-S5

88. Paiva De Sousa, C. The impact of food manufacturing practices on food-borne diseases. *Brazilian Archives of Biology and Technology*, **2008**, *51* (4), 815–823.

89. Pandey, R.M.; Upadhyay, S.K. Food additive. In: *Food Additive*; Yehia El-Samragy (Ed.); Open access chapter; **2012**; p. 30; http://www.intechopen.com/books/food-additive/food-additive; accessed on November 4, 2019.

90. Perez, E.; Raposo, A. Microbiological evaluation of Prepared/Cooked Foods in a HACCP Environment. *Food and Nutrition Sciences*, **2011**, *2*, 549–552.

91. Pesavento, G. Antimicrobial resistance profile of staphylococcus aureus isolated from raw meat: a research for methicillin resistant *Staphylococcus aureus* (MRSA). *Food Control*, **2007**, *18*, 196–200; DOI: 10.1016/j.foodcont.2005.09.013.

92. Pimentel, D. Environmental and economic costs of the application of pesticides primarily in the United States. *Environment, Development and Sustainability*, **2005**, *7* (2), 229–252; DOI: 10.1007/s10668-005-7314-2

93. Popek, S. The Implementation of The Requirements of the ISO-22000 Standard on the Basis of an Integrated Management System of Food Industry Organization: Model Solution. *Studia Oeconomica Posnaniensia* (Economic Studies *Posnaniensia*), **2016**, *4* (10), 70–82.

94. Qaim, M.; Kouser, S. Genetically modified crops and food security. *PLOS One*, **2013**, *8*(6), e-article ID: 64879; p. 8.

95. Radhakrishna, R. Food and nutrition security of the poor: emerging perspectives and policy issues. *Economic & Political Weekly*, **2005**, *40* (18), 1817–1821.

96. Rajakaruna, S.S. Application of recombinant DNA Technology (Genetically Modified Organisms) to the advancement of agriculture, medicine, bioremediation and biotechnology industries. *Journal of Applied Biotechnology and Bioengineering*, **2016**, *1* (3), 13–20.

97. Randell, A. *Codex Alimentarius*: How it began. *Food, Nutrition and Agriculture*, **1995**, *13*, 35–40.

98. Ray, B. *Fundamental Food Microbiology*. Boca Raton, FL: CRC Press; **2004**; p. 663.

99. Redmond, E.C.; Griffith, C.J. Consumer food handling in the home: a review of food safety studies. *Journal of Food Protection*, **2003**, *66*, 130–161.

100. Reij, M.; Schothorst, M. Critical notes on microbiological risk assessment of food. *Brazilian Journal of Microbiology*, **2000**, 31, 1–8.

101. Rohr, A.; Luddecke, K. Food quality and safety: consumer perception and public health concern. *Food Control*, **2005**, *16*, 649–655.

102. Ross, A.P.; Darling, J.N. High energy diets prevent the enhancing effects of emotional arousal on memory. *Behavioral Neuroscience*, **2013**, *127 (*5), 771–779.

103. Rotaru, G.; Sava, N. food quality and safety management systems: a brief analysis of the individual and integrated approaches. *Scientifical Researches—Agroalimentary Processes and Technologies*, **2005**, 11 (1), 229–236.

104. Schauzu, M. The concept of substantial equivalence in safety assessment of foods derived from genetically modified organisms. *Ag Biotech Net*, **2000**, *2*, 44–50.

105. Schroeder, T.; Tonsor, G.T. Consumer food safety risk perceptions and attitudes: impacts on beef consumption across countries. *The B.E. Journal of Economic Analysis & Policy*, **2007**, *7* (1), 65–70; http://www.bepress.com/bejeap/vol7/iss1/art65; accessed on November 4, 2019.

106. Shaker, R.; Osailia, T. Isolation of Enterobacter sakazakii and Other Enterobacter Sp. from Food and Food Production Environments. *Food Control*, **2007**, *18* (10), 1241–1245; DOI : 10.1016/j.foodcont.2006.07.020

107. Silbergeld, E.K.; Graham, J. Industrial food animal production, antimicrobial resistance and human health. *Annual Review of Public Health*, **2008**, *29*, 151–169.

108. Smith, K.R. Human Health: Impacts, Adaptation and Co-Benefits, Climate Change 2014: Impacts, Adaptation and Vulnerability, Part A: Global and Sectoral Aspects. *Contribution of Working Group II to the Fifth Assessment Report of the Intergovernmental Panel on Climate Change*; London, UK: Cambridge University Press; **2014**; pp. 709–754.

109. Sofia, P.K.; Prasad, R. Organic farming-tradition reinvented. *Indian Journal of Traditional Knowledge*, **2006**, *5* (1), 139–142.

110. Stockdale, E.A. Agronomic and environmental implications of organic farming systems. *Advances in Agronomy*, **2001**, *70*, 261–327.

111. Sumaedi, S. The effectiveness of ISO-9001 implementation in food manufacturing companies: a proposed measurement instrument. *Procedia Food Science*, **2015**, *3*, 436–444; doi: 10.1016/j.profoo.2015.01.048

112. Syne, SM.; Ramsubhag, A. microbiological hazard analysis of ready-to-eat meats processed at a food plant in Trinidad, West Indies. *Infection Ecology and Epidemiology*, **2013**, 3, e-article ID: 20450, p. 8; http://dx.doi.org/10.3402/iee.v3i0.20450; accessed on November 4, 2019.

113. Tawfek, N.S.; Amin, H.M. Adverse effects of some food additives in adult male albino rats. *Current Science International*, **2015**, *4* (4), 525–537.

114. Tuormaa, T.E. The adverse effects of food additives on health: review of the literature with special emphasis on childhood hyperactivity. *Journal of Orthomolecular Medicine*, **1994**, *9* (4), 225–243.

115. Vabo, M. The relationship between food preferences and food choice: a theoretical discussion. *International Journal of Business and Social Science*, **2014**, *5* (7), 145–157.

116. Valero, A. Studying the growth boundary and subsequent time to growth of pathogenic *Escherichia Coli* serotypes by turbidity measurements. *Food Microbiology*, **2010**, *27* (6), 819–828; DOI:10.1016/j.fm.2010.04.016

117. Valero, A. Risk factors influencing microbial contamination in food service centers, Significance, prevention and control of food related diseases. InTech Open; **2016**; open access chapter; https://www.intechopen.com/books/significance-prevention-and-control-of-food-related-diseases/risk-factors-influencing-microbial-contamination-in-food-service-centers; accessed on November 4, 2019;

118. Vally, H.; Misso N.L. Clinical effects of sulphite additives. *Clinical & Experimental Allergy*, **2009**, *39* (11), 1643–1651; doi: 10.1111/j.1365-2222.2009.03362.x

119. WHO. *Principles for the Safety Assessment of Food Additives and Contaminants in Food.* Published under the Joint Sponsorship of the United Nations Environment Programme, the International Labor Organization, and the World Health Organization in collaboration with the Food and Agriculture Organization of the United Nations; **1987**; p. 176; https://apps.who.int/iris/handle/10665/37578; accessed on November 4, 2019.

120. WHO. *Evaluation of Certain Food Additives: Some Food Colors, Thickening Agents, Smoke Condensates, and Certain Other Substances.* 19th Report of the Joint FAO/WHO Expert Committee on Food Additives 576; **1975**; https://apps.who.int/iris/handle/10665/37578; accessed on November 4, 2019.

121. Winickoff, D. Science and power in global food regulation: the rise of the *Codex Alimentarius*. *Science, Technology, & Human Values*, **2009**, *35* (3), 356–381; online; DOI: 10.1177/0162243909334242

122. Zhang, M. Agricultural pesticide use and food safety: California's Model. *Journal of Integrative Agriculture*, **2015**, *14* (11), 2340–2357.

# PART II
# Design and Utilization of Healthy Foods

# CHAPTER 7

# GUT MICROBIOTA—SPECIFIC FOOD DESIGN

APARNA V. SUDHAKARAN* and HIMANSHI SOLANKI

## ABSTRACT

The gut microbiota contributes to host health by performing roles in host nutrition, metabolism, immune modulation, pathogen colonization resistance, intestinal epithelial development, and even energy homeostasis. Though the overall health situation of the host and the contribution of intestinal microbiota have been a popular area of research, yet there are numerous gaps to be filled and the exact mechanisms are yet to be found out. This chapter intends to provide an overview of the influence of diet on gut microbiota and interventions on the modulation of gut microbiota.

## 7.1 INTRODUCTION

The humans have coevolved with microbes to form a symbiotic yet complex relationship and are the most studied human-associated ecosystems. The numerous microorganisms that colonize our gut have developed a harmonious ecosystem and have a prominent part in sustaining the homeostatic equilibrium of our body. The entire microbial taxa (bacteria, fungi, archaea, protozoa, fungi) associated with human beings are known as human microbiota, whereas human gut microbiome means the residing microbes and associated genes in the gut [61]. When we compare the genome of humans, it is 99.9% identical but in the case of the gut microbiome, it varies up to 80%–90% in each individual [70]. The dynamic gut microbiome can interact even with our mind and changes constantly according to our physical and mental health status. The human provides a stable habitat for the microbes

*Corresponding author. E-mail: aparna@kvasu.ac.in.

and in turn, microbes contribute to the growth and development by supplying essential nutrients.

Today, the gut microbiota is considered as an essential organ in our body. The gut microbiota contributes to host health by performing roles in host nutrition, metabolism, immune modulation, pathogen colonization resistance, intestinal epithelial development, and even energy homeostasis [15, 71]. The change in the core microbiota by various factors leads to an imbalance in our gut, also known as dysbiosis. Several upcoming kinds of research throw light to the connection between dysbiosis and various disease conditions such as diabetes, heart diseases, autism, asthma, cancer, inflammatory bowel diseases, and kidney diseases [15]. Though the overall health situation of the host and the contribution of intestinal microbiota has been a popular research area, there are numerous gaps to be filled and the complete mechanisms are yet to be elucidated.

The chapter aims to provide information of various gut microbiodata, evelation, relation with diet, nutrient, and overall health benefits.

## 7.2   EVOLUTION AND ESTABLISHMENT OF THE GUT MICROBIOME

Various components contribute to the establishment of the gut microbiome. Understanding these factors helps to correlate the health conditions with microbial composition. Akin to the inevitability of food for our sustenance, the diet or type of nutrients plays a crucial role in establishing the gut microbiome. Several studies are claiming the presence of microbes even before birth that is in the placenta, and mother's microbiome influencing microbial colonization in infants during pregnancy [1]. The legacy of our gut microbiota goes toward the maternal microflora as well as the mode of birth. The predominance of lactobacilli was reported in vaginal birth, whereas in caesarian mainly the facultative anaerobes like *Clostridium* were prevalent [23]. Diversity in the initial stages are less, and *Actinobacteria* and *Proteobacteria* are the most prevalent phyla during this stage. Initial gut microflora has a key part in developing immunity in the host and the occurrence of some diseases in their later-life [17].

The antibiotic disturbance during the critical period in the initial stages has lasting effects on host metabolism and immunity [38, 78]. The feeding pattern also influences the dominant microbiota; the abundance of *Bifidobacteria* and *Lactobacillus* were reported in breast-fed infants, whereas *Atopobium* and

*Bacteroides* predominate in formula-fed infants [77]. The intestinal micro-biota of infants develops into an adult microbiome within 3 years of birth [32]. Each individual will have a core microbiome with distinct composi-tion, a unique "gut print" similar to our "fingerprint". By 2.5–3 years the gut microbiome becomes relatively stable but is strongly influenced by the diet, lifestyle, illnesses, and antibiotic treatment. The composition of microbiota varies both in the transverse and longitudinal axis and is even influenced by the nutritional gradient along the gut. However, the evolution of stable gut microbiota is still poorly understood. The gut microbiome co-evolves with the host and have a crucial role in health during later stages of life.

The human gut microbiota is composed mainly of a complex ecology of three microbial types namely bacteria (predominant), archaea, and eukarya along with some viruses and phages. It is now well recognized that among bacteria, *Bacteroidetes* and *Firmicutes* are the predominant phyla, while *Actinobacteria*, *Proteobacteria*, *Fusobacteria*, *Verrucomicrobia*, and *Cyanobacteria* are present in relatively lower proportions [34, 55].

## 7.3   FUNCTIONS OF GUT MICROBIOTA

The gut microbiota plays numerous roles in host metabolism and maintaining host immunity and health, elevating its status to that of a forgotten organ [15]. The collaborative rapport between the gut microbiota and intestinal mucosa helps to maintain gut integrity, energy harvest, protection from pathogens, immune function, etc.

### 7.3.1   NUTRIENT METABOLISM

In nutrient metabolism, gut microbiota plays an important role. It produces several enzymes that contribute toward the fermentation, biotransformation of dietary compounds, and digestion. The saccharolytic fermentation by microbiota mainly concentrates in the proximal section of the colon, while proteolytic fermentation occurs in the distal region [28].

### 7.3.2   GUT BARRIER INTEGRITY

The function of gut barrier includes three major protective lines: (1) colo-nization resistance by a biological barrier-resident intestinal microflora against pathogens, (2) immune barrier by gut associated lymph tissue, and (3) the cells in lamina propra. The mechanical barrier consists of the closed epithelial cells of the intestines and the capillary endothelial cells. Special structures called "Tight junctions" connect the cells and limit ions, molecules, and cells moving through paracellular space [3]. The mucus layer in the intestine is a system for shielding the epithelial and luminal luminary cells from direct contact. The bowel cells secrete the mucin glycoprotein that in turn provides the organism with nutrition. Mucosal glycosylation patterns, both on the cell surface and subcellular can also be modulated by the gut microbiota. The structural development of the gut mucosa was influenced by the gut microbiota by inducing the transcription factor angiogenin-3 [36]. The barrier integrity is maintained by the Trefoil factor and the resistin-like molecule secreted by goblet cells [36]. The intestinal barrier is compromised during several diseases leading to an increased level of bacterial translocations, further leading to systemic inflammations.

### 7.3.3   ANTIMICROBIAL PROTECTION

The gut has a homeostatic condition in which the beneficial commensal and pathogens reside. The beneficial resident microbes will compete for nutrition and ecological niche and provides an effective barrier against the invasion of pathogenic agents. The mucus layer in the gut is a protective mechanism, which prevents the direct contact between epithelial cells and luminal microbes. The intestinal goblet cells secrete the mucin glycoprotein that in turn provides the nutrition for the organism. The mucosal glycosylation patterns, both on the cell surface and subcellular, can also be modulated by the gut microbiota. The antimicrobial substances produced by the resident microbes also inhibit the growth of pathogens.

### 7.3.4   IMMUNOMODULATION

Throughout development, maturation, and maintenance of gut immune and wellness, gut microbiota plays an active and crucial role. Intestinal bacteria facilitate the normal development of humoral and cellular immune systems. Initial colonization of the microbial cells will improve the development of the child immune system. It can influence innate as well as adaptive immune systems. The signaling between the microbiota, epithelium cells, and the mucus immune system, along with any disruption, may lead to chronic and physiological inflammation. To maintain good health, the intestinal microbiota communicates through the gut–brain axis to provide signage to the brain.

## 7.4   INTERRELATION BETWEEN DIET AND GUT MICROBIOTA

The distribution profile of microbes and exact composition in the gut is still unexplored. Developments in metagenomic technology have initiated to discover our microbial partners. Chemical, metabolic, and immunologic gradients of the intestine affect the density and composition of the microbiota. The factors influencing gut microbiome include the diet, age, medication, sleep, stress, environmental factors, etc.

A crucial role is played by diet in establishing gut microbiota. The micronutrients and macronutrients in the diet can influence the composition and functional potential of the gut microflora [15]. The dietary factors influencing the microbial composition are the nature of substrate consumed, variations in-transit time, pH, microbial composition in the consumed food, diet-related host secretions, and host gene expression regulations [59].

A considerable difference exists in the composition of microbiota among vegetarians and nonvegetarians. Even the animal and plant protein contribute to the compositional change [53]. The beneficial effect of a plant-based diet has been elaborately reviewed by Tomova et al. [70]. It promotes more diverse and constant and evenly distributed microbial systems [40]. Long-term fruit and vegetable intake increase the alpha diversity of gut microbiota [37]. The fiber-rich plant diet enhances the growth of *Bacteroidetes*-related operational taxonomic units (B*acteroidetes, Prevotella, Roseburia*, etc.), *Ruminococcus, E. rectale,* etc., and reduce *Clostridium* and *Enterococcus* species [45].

Zimmer et al. [81] observed that there is a decreased abundance of *Enterobacteriaceae* in vegetarian diet when compared to the omnivorous diet. The fiber-rich plant-based diet promotes the growth of butyrate synthesizing bacteria, which in turn lowers the colonic pH making it adverse for the growth of *Enterobacteriaceae* [81]. This reinforces the enhanced presence of *Roseburia, Lachnospira, and Prevotella* and the elevated production of SCFA by the consumption of a vegan diet [18]. Changing the intake in the type of fibers, could influence bacterial crossfeed patterns and lead to complex variations in the general structure, composition and function of the gut microbiota [15]. In addition, polyphenols in plant diets are reported to increase *Bifidobacterium and Lactobacillus* [70].

In a study comparing the Italian diet (containing less fiber, and more animal proteins, fat, and starch) with the diet of Burkino Faso, Africa (containing more plant proteins and fiber, and fewer animal proteins, fat, and starch), an increased number of *Firmicutes* instead of *Bacteroidetes* were observed in kids from Burkina Faso [19]. There is a lower abundance of *Bacteroidetes* in the Chinese diet, which is rich in animal products when compared with vegetarian Indian diet [35].

Dietary habits affect the composition of intestinal microbiota instantly. When we compare the three major enterotypes in the gut *Prevotella, Bacteroides,* and *Ruminococcus*, the composition significantly varied according to the dietary pattern. *Prevotella* is found significantly in vegan diet [11, 19, 35]. *Bacteroides* are prevalent in animal protein and saturated fat [37, 75] and *Ruminococcus* is largely found in fruit and vegetable-rich diet [74]. The dietary habits can have quick influence on the composition of the intestinal microflora.

## 7.5  NUTRIENT METABOLISM AND GUT MICROBIOTA

The digestion and absorption of dietary components are greatly influenced by the gut microbiota. There are the fundamental role and mutual interaction between the gut microbes and the dietary components. The major components are carbohydrates, proteins, and lipids, which largely define the composition of the gut microbiota as illustrated in Figure 7.1. The relation is vehard to establish and to draw a picture regarding the individual roles of the dietary components [33].

### 7.5.1  CARBOHYDRATE METABOLISM

The simple carbohydrate is metabolized easily and is instantly assimilated in the small intestine. The intake of simple digestible carbohydrates such as glucose, fructose, etc., in the diet reduces the *Bacteroides* and *Clostridia* in the gastrointestinal tract [64]. The complex carbohydrate moves downwards in the small and large intestines where it is broken down by the resident microorganisms. It is reported that the complex nondigestible carbohydrate is favorable for the abundance of lactic acid bacteria, *Ruminococcus, E. rectale, Roseburia* and can reduce *Clostridium* and *Enterococcus* species [64]. Irrespective of the nature of carbohydrates—digestible or nondigestible, an abundance of *Bifidobacteria* is reported [70].

The carbohydrates are metabolized mainly to short-chain fatty acids (SCFAs) as well as carbon dioxide and hydrogen ($CO_2$ and $H_2$) [10]. The major SCFAs synthesized in the gut include acetate, propionate and butyrate that exist in proportions extending between 3:1:1 and 10:2:1 [57]. SCFA plays a substantial role in maintaining intestinal homeostasis, gene expression, cytokine modulation, chemotaxis, proliferation, etc., in the gut epithelial cells. The insulin secretion was correlated with incretin hormone secretion (glucagon-like peptide-1 (GLP-1)), which in turn can be related to SCFA levels in the intestine [44, 79]. SCFAs are the predominant metabolites formed during carbohydrate fermentation, which have local and systemic health benefits. Some of the microflora associated with the production of SCFAs are illustrated in Table 7.1.

The plant-based diet increases the SCFA production [18]. The carbohydrates which can be fermented by microbiota are known as microbiota accessible carbohydrates. The type of the fiber and cross-feeding between the different bacteria determine the extend of digestion of complex polysaccharides and development of individually based bacterial community [12]. The potential of each bacteria to degrade polysaccharides is determined by the enzymes they possess; some bacteria can degrade several carbohydrates that comes in the generalists category (*Bacteroidetes* phylum including *Bacteroides thetaiotaomicron* and *Bacteroides intestinalis*), whereas some can digest only specific carbohydrates known as specialized category (*Prevotella copri* and *Roseburia intestinalis*) [25].

## 7.5.2  PROTEIN METABOLISM

The proteins are digested to smaller peptides, amino acids, and are converted to metabolic active substances by the gut microbes. The proteins are fermented to SCFAs and branched-chain fatty acids, phenol, indole, ammonia, $H_2$, $CO_2$, and $H_2S$ [46]. The aromatic amino acids (phenylalanine, tyrosine, and tryptophan) are digested to phenolic compounds [58]. The source of proteins, namely, an animal or plant origin influence the gut microbial composition. Animal protein-rich diet decreases the abundance of *Roseburia*, *Eubacterium rectale*, and *Ruminococcus bromii* [16] and increases the population of *Bacteroides* and *Clostridia*. In the case of plant proteins like pea protein, there is a rise in *Bifidobacterium* and *Lactobacillus* and fall in *Bacteroides fragilis* and *Clostridium perfringens* [64].

**TABLE 7.1**    The Health Benefits of Short-Chain Fatty Acids and the Associated Gut Microflora

| Short Chain Fatty Acids | Microorganisms | Health Benefits | Ref. |
|---|---|---|---|
| Butyrate | *Faecalibacterium prausnitzii* | The energy source for human colonocytes. | [66] |
| | *Ruminococcus bromii* | Potential to destroy colon cancer cells. | |
| | | Regulate gene expression by inhibiting histone deacetylase. | |
| | *Eubacterium hallii* | | |
| | *Eubacterium rectale* | Most potently increase GLP-1 | [78] |
| | *Roseburia intestinalis* | Induce mucin synthesis. | [49, 54] |
| | | Improve gut integrity by increasing tight junction assembly. | |
| | *Clostridium symbiosum* | | |
| | | Decrease bacterial transport across the membrane. | |
| | | Suppression of proinflammatory cytokines. | |
| | | Activate intestinal gluconeogenesis (IGN) via a system depending on cyclic adenosine monophosphate (cAMP) favoring glucose and energy balance. | [20] |
| | | Butyrate influence differentiation of naive T cells into Tregs. | [2] |
| | | Suppression of colonic inflammation. | [6, 63] |
| Propionate | *Akkermansia municiphilla* | Enhance Iron absorption. | [8, 54] |
| | | The energy source for epithelial cells. | [20] |
| | *Bacteroides fragilis* | Role in gluconeogenesis. | |
| | *Veillonella parvula* | | |
| | *Bacteroides eggerthii* | Modulate satiety signaling by interaction with G protein-coupled receptor. | |
| | | Inhibition of histone deacetylation, limiting inflammation in the gut. | [21, 24] |
| Acetate | *Bacteroides thetaiotaomicron* | Used in cholesterol metabolism and lipogenesis. | [29, 65] |
| | *Bifidobacterium adolescentis* | Role in central appetite regulation. | |
| | | A significant role in central appetite regulation. | |
| | *Collinsella aerofaciens* | | |
| | | Beneficial in terms of gut barrier maintenance. | |
| | *Bacteroides vulgates* | | |

The plant proteins have a positive correlation on intestinal homeostasis. The animal-based proteins are linked to the development of atherosclerosis. Meat and egg are loaded with L-carnitine and phosphatidylcholine that are converted to trimethylamine by the gut microflora and further to its oxide form (into trimethylamine oxide—TMAO) in the liver [39, 68]. In case of milk proteins (casein and whey rich in branched-chain amino acids (BCAAs): valine, leucine, and isoleucine), it was reported to prolong the age-related changes in the gut flora [79]. It also enhances the healthy *Lactobacillaceae*/*Lactobacillus* and decreases the abundance of *Clostridiaceae*/*Clostridium* in the gut [50].

### 7.5.3   LIPID METABOLISM

A change in the dietary lipid can cause modulation in the gut microbiota composition [56]. The ingested lipids will be digested mainly in the small intestine. A low-fat diet (plant-based) favors the growth of Lactic acid bacteria, *Bifidobacteria* and *Bacteroidetes* [64]. A walnut-enriched diet was reported to increase *Ruminococcaceae* and *Bifidobacteria*, and decrease the *Clostridium* sp. cluster XIVa species [5]. The saturated fat predominant western diet was found to enhance *Bilophila* and *Faecalibacterium*, and reduce *Bacteroidetes, Bacteroides, Prevotella, Lactobacillus,* and *Bifidobacterium* [13, 64].

Coelho et al. [13] also reported that the N-3 polyunsaturated fatty acids have a neutral effect or in turn a beneficial effect as it increases *Bifidobacterium, Adlercreutzia, Lactobacillus, Streptococcus, Desulfovibrio*, and *Verrucomicrobia* (*Akkermansia muciniphila*) in the gut. There are many areas to be explored like the effect of lipids in transforming the microbiota in the large intestine, the effect of fatty acid composition in the diet, n-6/n-3 polyunsaturated fatty acid ratio and its impact in humans, etc. More in-depth research can throw light on how lipids can have an impact on gut microbiota.

### 7.5.4   BILE ACID METABOLISM

Bile acids in the small intestine largely influence the digestion and absorption of dietary lipids. Chemically, the synthesis of primary bile acids takes place in the liver and secondary bile acids take place in the large intestine. Majority of primary bile acids (cholic acid and chenodeoxychlic acid) will be absorbed from Ileum for recycling in the liver. The remaining bile acids (1%–5%) reaching the colon will be modulated by the gut microbiota. The gut microflora regulates the bile acid synthesis as well as the conjugation of secondary bile acids (biotransformation). The secondary bile acids like deoxycholic acid have greater detergent properties thereby controlling the bacterial populations. The gut microbes have bile salt hydrolase (BSH) enzymes, which mediates the biotransformation of bile by hydrolyzing the glycol and tauro conjugates. Some of the genera reported to produce BSH are the *Bacteroides, Bifidobacterium, Clostridium, Lactobacillus,* and Listeria.

The deconjugation mechanism reduces the antimicrobial potential as well as the emulsification property of the bile. Another reported modification of bile by gut bacteria is the epimerization of hydroxyl groups leading to the formation of Ursodeoxycholic acid. This is a survival strategy by bacteria, thereby decreasing the toxicity of the bile acids. Bile acid can modify gut microbiota by stimulating the growth of bacteria which can utilize bile as a substrate [73]. The integral regulatory role of bile acids can determine the metabolic status and microbial composition of the host [57].

### 7.5.5   VITAMIN SYNTHESIS

Several gut microbes can de novo synthesize the essential vitamins (K, B, etc.), which the host is incapable of producing and is crucial for health maintenance. The presence of biosynthetic pathways for mainly B vitamins is reported in the genome of gut microbes [47]. The bacteria capable of vitamin synthesis include *Bacteroidetes, Fusobacteria,* and *Proteobacteria* ($B_2$ and $B_7$); *Firmicutes* and *Actinobacteria* (B vitamins); *Bifidobacterium* (B vitamins, K); *B. subtilis* and Escherichia *coli* ($B_2$) [18]; and *Lactobacillus* (B vitamins) [41].

### 7.5.6   POLYPHENOLS AND PHYTOCHEMICALS SYNTHESIS

Polyphenols and phytochemicals are generally metabolized in the colon by the intestinal microflora. It converts the primary compounds to easily absorbable and more biologically active forms [60]. The conversion of complex conjugated and polymeric forms of polyphenols into easily absorbable aglycones is performed by intestinal mucosal enzymes and colonic microbiota. Some of the genera involved in polyphenol metabolism include *Bacteroides, Enterococcus, Eubacterium,* etc. and species involved are *Bacteroides distasonis, Bacteroides uniformis, Bacteroides ovatus, Enterococcus casseliflavus, Eubacterium cellulosolvens, Lachnospiraceae* CG19-1, and *Eubacterium ramulus* [9, 48].

In a recent study, it was reported that *Lactobacillus acidophilus* converts the plant glycosides to aglycones, which can be readily used by the host [69]. The specific microbial enzymes like esterase and glucosidase involve in the biotransformation of polyphenols [69]. The tea polyphenols have a positive impact on the abundance of *Bifidobacterium*, *Lactobacillus,* and *Enterococcus* genus like *Akkermansia* spp., *Faecalibacterium* spp., and *Roseburia* spp. [26, 52], whereas negative impact of *Bacteroides*, *Prevotella,* and *Clostridium histolyticum* that can be linked with its prebiotic effect [67]. The association of a consortium of microbes is integral for the entire metabolism of polyphenols in the gut.

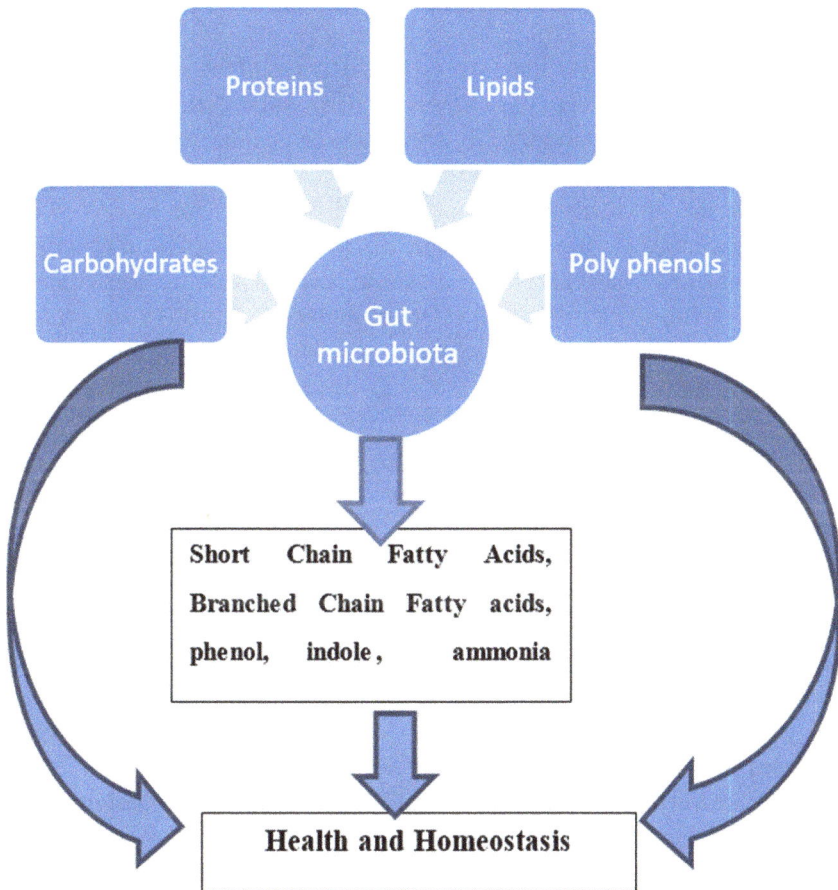

**FIGURE 7.1**  Gut microbiota in nutrient metabolism.

## 7.6  THERAPEUTIC MANIPULATION OF GUT MICROBIOTA

There exists a mutually beneficial relationship between the mucosa and the microflora of the gut. This relation aids the host individual by supporting metabolism and immunity. There is a shift in recent researches from compositional analysis of the gut to the specific role of gut microbiota on various diseases. There are several dietary (prebiotic, probiotic, symbiotic, and postbiotics) and nondietary interventions (microbial transfer therapy) gaining popularity in treating dysbiosis and restoration of healthy gut microflora.

### 7.6.1  DIETARY INTERVENTIONS

The dietary intervention is the most cost-effective and the easiest method to manipulate the gut microbiome. Some of the popular dietary interventions are prebiotic, probiotic, symbiotic, and postbiotics. The basic mechanisms involving dietary interventions are the direct modulation of the gut microbiota or by the production of metabolic end products like SCFAs, which have the potential to regulate the gut microbiota [72]. The diet-induced modifications are transient and the habitual diets have more consequences on gut microbiota. The prolonged effect of dietary changes is still unknown and needs to be addressed [42].

#### 7.6.1.1  PREBIOTIC FOODS

Prebiotics are "substrates that are selectively utilized by host microorganisms, conferring a health benefit to the host" [31]. In simple terms, prebiotics is the food for the beneficial microorganisms in the gut. The prebiotics aids in digestion reduces constipation, resist infections, prevent gastrointestinal diseases, and ameliorate inflammatory bowel disease [30]. The prebiotic supplementation of 1.7 g of galactooligosaccharides (GOS) per day increases the frequency of bowel movement, reduces straining during defecation, and decreases stool consistency when compared with maltodextrin [7].

In a research conducted by Azcarate-Peril et al. [4], *Bifidobacterium, Faecalibacterium,* and *Lactobacillus* increased substantially, when fed with GOS which improves lactose tolerance. It is important to note that prebiotics may not only exert their effects by modifying the abundance or activity of microbes. A novel mechanism based on specific and direct prebiotic interactions using inulin and short-chain fructooligosaccharides demonstrated improved ability to maintain epithelial barrier function and to protect from injury caused by the noninvasive pathogen enterohemorrhagic *E. coli* O157: H7 (EHEC) despite the absence of other microbes [76]. GOS may also inhibit the adherence of *E. coli* to enterocytes [62]. These results suggest that prebiotics may improve gut barrier function, and maybe relevant for specific consumer groups during certain phases of life. A high fiber plant-based diet (onions, garlic, leeks, oatmeal, banana, chicory root, cruciferous vegetables, beans) and whole-grain diet [14] are prebiotic-rich diets, which can control the possibility of conditions such as cardiovascular diseases, Type 2 diabetes, obesity, and cancer.

## 7.6.1.2  PROBIOTICS

Probiotics are "live microorganisms that, when administered in adequate amounts, confer a health benefit on the host" [27]. Recent gut microbiota studies have opened new avenues for personalized healthcare strategies associating the potential use of selected probiotics strains for restoring the gut balance. The basic mechanism by which the probiotics regain the gut homeostasis is by competitive exclusion, improve intestinal barrier functions, production of antimicrobial substances and immune modulation. Probiotics as a concept acquired scientific credibility when Russian scientist E. Metchnikoff proposed the theory of longevity and attributed the long life of Bulgarians to the consumption of traditional fermented dairy products [51]. The fermented foods such as fermented dairy products, vegetables, sauerkraut, kimchi, and wine are a rich source of probiotics. The probiotics can be a single strain or a combination of strains. The most common genera of probiotics are *Lactobacillus*, *Bifidobacterium*, and *Saccharomyces boulardii* (yeast). The combination of prebiotics and probiotics is known as synbiotics.

The knowledge gained in recent years about the ability of gut microbes to influence brain opens new windows of opportunity for probiotics and prebiotics. The recent advancement in probiotics is psychobiotics, which play a functional role in neurological disorders. In this context, they can be defined as "live organisms that, when ingested in adequate amounts, produce a health benefit in patients suffering from psychiatric illness" [22].

### 7.6.1.3 POSTBIOTICS

Postbiotics are the nonviable bacterial products or metabolites produced by the probiotic strains having biological effects on the host. It is an effective alternative method to increase the potential and functionality of each probiotic strain. Moreover, it avoids the risk associated with handling live bacterial cells. It can be developed as a novel therapy for many inflammatory diseases [72].

### 7.6.2 NONDIETARY INTERVENTIONS: FECAL MICROBIOTA TRANSPLANTATION (FMT)/MICROBIOTA TRANSFER THERAPY (MTT)

A person having impaired gut microbiota, mostly due to inflammatory diseases, can be treated by replenishing his/her gut with the microflora of fecal origin collected from a healthy person. This intervention is known as FMT. The history of this technique can be traced back to fourth-century China, where a fecal suspension was fed orally to treat food poisoning and acute diarrhea [80]. FMT involves the administration of distal gut microbiota-containing fecal material from a healthy person (donor) to a patient with an altered gut microbiota that is causing disease. The modulation of the gut microbiota by FMT primarily follows the probiotic principle, but instead of treating the patient with specific strains, a community of microorganisms is used.

A revised technique based on FMT, called MTT, uses colon cleansing along with administration of antibiotics and Standardized Human Gut Microbiota [43]. FMT/MTT is expected to become popular in the future for intestinal disorders and gastrointestinal diseases, but difficulties associated with handling the consortium of microbes are to be addressed.

### 7.7 SUMMARY

Gut microbiota takes part in diverse functions including nutrient metabolism, gut barrier integrity, antimicrobial protection and immunomodulation. The composition of microbiota varies significantly among vegetarians and nonvegetarians, enforcing the influence of diet on gut flora. There is a mutual interaction between the gut microbes and the dietary components, the major ones being carbohydrates, proteins, and lipids, which largely define the composition of gut microbiota. Several dietary and nondietary interventions are possible in treating dysbiosis and in the restoration of healthy gut microflora. Dietary interventions like prebiotics and probiotics are gaining popularity. Still, there are a lot of unexplored areas and therefore immense scope for further research in this subject.

## KEYWORDS

- **dietary intervention**
- **gut microbiota**
- **homeostasis**
- **nutrient metabolism**

## REFERENCES

1. Aagaard, K.; Ma, J.; Antony, K.M.; Ganu, R.; Petrosino, J.; Versalovic, J. The placenta harbors a unique microbiome. *Science Translational Medicine*, 2014, *6* (237), 237ra65.
2. Arpaia, N.; Campbell, C.; Fan, X.; Dikiy, S. Metabolites produced by commensal bacteria promote peripheral regulatory T-cell generation. *Nature*, **2013**, *504* (7480), 451–455.
3. Assimakopoulos, S.F.; Triantos, C.; Maroulis, I ; Gogos, C. The role of the gut barrier function in health and disease. *Gastroenterology Research*, **2018**, *11* (4), 261.
4. Azcarate-Peril, M.A; Ritter, A.J.; Savaiano, D. Impact of short-chain galactooligosaccharides on the gut microbiome of lactose-intolerant individuals. *Proceedings of the National Academy of Sciences*, **2017**, *114* (3), E367–E375.
5. Bamberger, C.; Rossmeier, A.; Lechner, K. Walnut-enriched diet affects gut microbiome in healthy caucasian subjects: a randomized, controlled trial. *Nutrients*, **2018**, *10* (2), 244–252.
6. Baxter, N.T.; Schmidt, A.W.; Venkataraman, A. Dynamics of human gut microbiota and short-chain fatty acids in response to dietary interventions with three fermentable fibers. *MBio*, **2019**, *10* (1), article ID: e02566-18.
7. Beleli C.A.; Antonio M.A.; Dos Santos R.; Pastore G.M.; Lomazi EA. Effect of 4′ galactooligosaccharide on constipation symptoms. *Jornal de Pediatria*. 2015, *91* (6), 567–573.
8. Bougle, D.; Vaghefi-Vaezzadeh, N.; Roland, N. Influence of short-chain fatty acids on iron absorption by proximal colon. *Scandinavian Journal of Gastroenterology*, **2002**, *37* (9), 1008–1011.
9. Braune, A.; Blaut, M. Bacterial species involved in the conversion of dietary flavonoids in the human gut. *Gut Microbes*, **2016**, *7* (3), 216–234.
10. Chassard, C; Lacroix, C. Carbohydrates and the human gut microbiota. *Current Opinion in Clinical Nutrition & Metabolic Care*, **2013**, *16* (4), 453–460.

11. Claesson, M.J.; Jeffery, I.B.; Conde, S.; Power, S.E. Gut microbiota composition correlates with diet wnd health in the elderly. *Nature*, **2012**, *488* (7410), 178–184.
12. Cockburn, D.W.; Koropatkin, N.M. Polysaccharide degradation by the intestinal microbiota and its influence on human health and disease. *Journal of Molecular Biology*, **2016**, *428* (16), 3230–3252.
13. Coelho, O.G.L.; Cândido, F.G. Dietary fat and gut microbiota: mechanisms involved in obesity control. *Critical Reviews in Food Science and Nutrition*, **2019**, *59* (19), 3045–3053.
14. Costabile, A.; Klinder, A.; Fava, F. Whole-grain wheat breakfast cereal has a prebiotic effect on the human gut microbiota: a double-blind, placebo-controlled, crossover study. *British Journal of Nutrition*, **2008**, *99* (1), 110–120.
15. Danneskiold-Samsoe, N.B.; Barros, H.D.D.F.Q. Interplay between food and gut microbiota in health and disease. *Food Research International*, **2019**, *115*, 23–31.
16. David, L.A.; Maurice, C.F.; Carmody, R.N. Diet rapidly and reproducibly alters the human gut microbiome.*Nature*, **2014**, *505* (7484), 559–563.
17. De Aguero, M.G.; Ganal-Vonarburg, S.C.; Fuhrer, T. The maternal microbiota drives early postnatal innate immune development. *Science*, **2016**, *351* (6279), 1296–1302.
18. De Filippis, F.; Pellegrini, N.; Vannini, L.; Jeffery, I.B. High-level adherence to a mediterranean diet beneficially impacts the gut microbiota and associated metabolome. *Gut*, **2016**, *65* (11), 1812–1821.
19. De Filippo, C.; Cavalieri, D.; Di Paola, M. Impact of diet in shaping gut microbiota revealed by a comparative study in children from Europe and Rural Africa. *Proceedings of the National Academy of Sciences*, **2010**, *107* (33), 14691–14696.
20. De Vadder, F.; Kovatcheva-Datchary, P. Microbiota-generated metabolites promote metabolic benefits via gut–brain neural circuits. *Cell*, **2014**, *156* (1–2), 84–96.
21. Den Besten, G.; Bleeker, A.; Gerding, A.; van Eunen, K. Short-chain fatty acids protect against high-fat diet–induced obesity via a pparγ-dependent switch from lipogenesis to fat oxidation. *Diabetes*, **2015**, *64* (7), 2398–2408.
22. Dinan, T.G.; Stanton, C.; Cryan, J.F. Psychobiotics: a novel class of psychotropic. *Biological Psychiatry*, **2013**, *74*(10), 720–726.
23. Dominguez-Bello, M.G.; Costello, E.K. delivery mode shapes the acquisition and structure af the initial microbiota across multiple body habitats in newborns. *Proceedings of the National Academy of Sciences*, **2010**, *107* (26), 11971–11975.
24. El Hage, R.; Hernandez-Sanabria, E. Propionate-producing consortium restores antibiotic-induced dysbiosis in a dynamic *in vitro* model of the human intestinal microbial ecosystem. *Frontiers in Microbiology*, **2019**, *10*, 1206.
25. El Kaoutari, A.; Armougom, F.; Gordon, J.I.; Raoult, D.; Henrissat, B. The abundance and variety of carbohydrate-active enzymes in the human gut microbiota. *Nature Reviews Microbiology*, **2013**, *11* (7), 497–504.
26. Espín, J.C.; Gonzalez-Sarrías, A.; Tomás-Barberan, F.A. The gut microbiota: a key factor in the therapeutic effects of (poly) phenols. *Biochemical pharmacology*, **2017**, *139*, 82–93.
27. FAO/WHO. Joint Working Group Report on Drafting Guidelines for the Evaluation of Probiotics in Food. 2002. London, Ontario, Canada; p. 30.
28. Fava, F.; Rizzetto, L.; Tuohy, K.M. Gut microbiota and health: connecting actors across the metabolic system. *Proceedings of the Nutrition Society*, **2019**, *78* (2), 177–188.

29. Frost, G.; Sleeth, M.L. The short-chain fatty acid acetate reduces appetite via a central homeostatic mechanism. *Nature Communications*, **2014**, *5* (1), 1–11.

30. Gibson, G.R.; Scott, K.P.; Rastall, R.A. Dietary prebiotics: current status and new definition. *Food Sci Technol Bull Funct Foods*, **2010**, *7* (1), 1–19.

31. Gibson, G.R.; Robert, H.; Sanders, M.E. Expert consensus document: the international scientific association for probiotics and prebiotics (ISAPP) consensus statement on the definition and scope of prebiotics. *Nature Reviews Gastroenterology & Hepatology*, **2017**, *14*, 491.

32. Groer, M.W.; Luciano, A.A. Development of the preterm infant gut microbiome: a research priority. *Microbiome*, **2014**, *2* (1), 38–44.

33. Holmes, A.J.; Chew, Y.V.; Colakoglu, F.; Cliff, J.B. Diet-microbiome interactions in health are controlled by intestinal nitrogen source constraints. *Cell Metabolism*, **2017**, *25* (1), 140–151.

34. Human, M. Project Consortium Structure, Function and Diversity of the Healthy Human Microbiome. *Nature*, **2012**, *486*, 207–214.

35. Jain, A.; Li, X.H.; Chen, W.N. Similarities and differences in gut microbiome composition correlate with dietary patterns of indian and chinese adults. *AMB Express*, **2018**, *8* (1), 1–12.

36. Jandhyala, S.M.; Talukdar, R.; Subramanyam, C. Role of the normal gut microbiota. *World Journal of Gastroenterology: WJG*, **2015**, *21* (29), pages 8787.

37. Klimenko, N.S.; Tyakht, A.V. microbiome responses to an uncontrolled short-term diet intervention in the frame of the citizen science project. *Nutrients*, **2018**, *10* (5), 576.

38. Knoop, K.A.; Gustafsson, J.K. Antibiotics promote the sampling of luminal antigens and bacteria via colonic goblet cell associated antigen passages. *Gut Microbes*, **2017**, *8* (4), 400–411.

39. Koeth, R.A.; Wang, Z.; Levison, B.S. Intestinal microbiota metabolism of l-carnitine, a nutrient in red meat, promotes atherosclerosis. *Nature Medicine*, **2013**, *19* (5), 576–588.

40. Lai, K.P.; Ng, A.H.M.; Wan, H.T. dietary exposure to the environmental chemical, PFOS on the diversity of gut microbiota, associated with the development of metabolic syndrome. *Frontiers in Microbiology*, **2018**, *9*, 2552–2560.

41. LeBlanc, J.G.; Milani, C.; De Giori, G.S. Bacteria as vitamin suppliers to their host: a gut microbiota perspective. *Current Opinion in Biotechnology*, **2013**, *24* (2), 160–168.

42. Leeming, E.R.; Johnson, A.J.; Spector, T.D.; Le Roy, C.I. Effect of diet on the gut microbiota: rethinking intervention duration. *Nutrients*, **2019**, *11* (12), 2862.

43. Li, Q.; Han, Y.; Dy, A.B.C.; Hagerman, R.J. The gut microbiota and autism spectrum disorders. *Frontiers in Cellular Neuroscience*, **2017**, *11*, 120.

44. Lin, H.V.; Frassetto, A.; Kowalik, E.J. Butyrate and propionate protect against diet-induced obesity and regulate gut hormones via free fatty acid receptor 3-independent mechanisms. *PloS One*, **2012**, *7* (4), 188–193.

45. Losasso, C.; Eckert, E.M.; Mastrorilli, E. Assessing the influence of vegan, vegetarian and omnivore oriented westernized dietary styles on human gut microbiota: a cross sectional study. *Frontiers in Microbiology*, **2018**, *9*, 317–327.

46. Macfarlane, G.T.; Cummings, J.H.; Allison, C. protein degradation by human intestinal bacteria. *Microbiology*, **1986**, *132* (6), 1647–1656.

47. Magnúsdottir, S.; Ravcheev, D.; de Crécy-Lagard, V.; Thiele, I. Systematic genome assessment of b-vitamin biosynthesis suggests co-operation among gut microbes. *Frontiers in Genetics*, **2015**, *6*, 148–154.

48. Marín, L.; Miguélez, E.M.; Villar, C.J.; Lombó, F. bioavailability of dietary polyphenols and gut microbiota metabolism: antimicrobial properties. *BioMed Research International*, **2015**, *2015*, 40–51.
49. Marino, E.; Richards, J.L.; McLeod, K.H. Gut microbial metabolites limit the frequency of autoimmune T cells and protect against Type 1 diabetes. *Nature Immunology*, **2017**, *18* (5), 552–561.
50. McAllan, L.; Skuse, P.; Cotter, P.D. protein quality and the protein to carbohydrate ratio within a high fat diet influences energy balance and the gut microbiota in C57BL/6J mice. *PloS One*, **2014**, *9* (2), 102–110.
51. Metchnikoff, E. Optimistic Studies. New York: Putman's Sons; **1908**; p. 161–183.
52. Moreno-Indias, I.; Sánchez-Alcoholado, L. Red wine polyphenols modulate fecal microbiota and reduce markers of the metabolic syndrome in obese patients. *Food & Function*, **2016**, *7* (4), 1775–1787.
53. Muegge, B.D.; Kuczynski, J.; Knights, D. diet drives convergence in gut microbiome functions across mammalian phylogeny and within humans. *Science*, **2011**, *332* (6032), 970–974.
54. Peng, L.; Li, Z.R.; Green, R.S.; Holzman, I.R.; Lin, J. butyrate enhances the intestinal barrier by facilitating tight junction assembly via activation of AMP-activated protein kinase in caco-2 cell monolayers. *The Journal of Nutrition*, **2009**, *139* (9), 1619–1625.
55. Qin, J., Li, R.; Raes, J.; Arumugam, M. A Human gut microbial gene catalogue established by metagenomic sequencing. *Nature*, **2010**, *464* (7285), 59–65.
56. Rampelli, S.; Schnorr, S.L.; Consolandi, C. Metagenome sequencing of the Hadza hunter-gatherer gut microbiota. *Current Biology*, **2015**, *25* (13), 1682–1693.
57. Rowland, I.; Gibson, G.; Heinken, A.; Scott, K.; Swann, J.; Thiele, I.; Tuohy, K. Gut Microbiota functions: metabolism of nutrients and other food components. *European Journal of Nutrition*, **2018**, *57* (1), 1–24.
58. Russell, W.R.; Hoyles, L.; Flint, H.J.; Dumas, M.E. Colonic bacterial metabolites and human health. *Current Opinion in Microbiology*, **2013**, *16* (3), 246–254.
59. Salonen, A.; Lahti, L.; Salojärvi, J. Impact of diet and individual variation on intestinal microbiota composition and fermentation products in obese men. *The ISME Journal*, **2014**, *8* (11), 2218–2230.
60. Selma, M.V.; Espin, J.C.; Tomas-Barberan, F.A. Interaction between phenolics and gut microbiota: role in human health. *Journal of Agricultural and Food Chemistry*, **2009**, *57* (15), 6485–6501.
61. Sender, R.; Fuchs, S.; Milo, R. Are we really vastly outnumbered? Revisiting the ratio of bacterial to host cells in humans. *Cell*, **2016**, *164* (3), 337–340.
62. Shoaf, K.; Mulvey, G.L.; Armstrong, G.D.; Hutkins, R.W. Prebiotic galactooligosaccharides reduce adherence of enteropathogenic *Escherichia coli* to tissue culture cells. *Infection and Immunity*, **2006**, *74* (12), 6920–6928.
63. Singh, N.; Gurav, A.; Sivaprakasam, S. Activation of Gpr109a, receptor for niacin and the commensal metabolite butyrate, suppresses colonic inflammation and carcinogenesis. *Immunity*, **2014**, *40* (1), 128–139.
64. Singh, R.K.; Chang, H.W. Influence of diet on the gut microbiome and implications for human health. *Journal of Translational Medicine*, **2017**, *15* (1), 73–84.
65. Song, M.; Chan, A.T. environmental factors, gut microbiota, and colorectal cancer prevention. *Clinical Gastroenterology and Hepatology*, **2019**, *17* (2), 275–289.

66. Steliou, K.; Boosalis, M.S.; Perrine, S.P.; Sangerman, J.; Faller, D.V. Butyrate histone deacetylase inhibitors. *BioResearch open access*, **2012**, *1* (4), 192–198.
67. Sun, H.; Chen, Y.; Cheng, M.; Zhang, X.; Zheng, X.; Zhang, Z. The modulatory effect of polyphenols from green tea, oolong tea and black tea on human intestinal microbiota *in vitro*. *Journal of Food Science and Technology*, **2018**, *55* (1), 399–407.
68. Tang, W.W.; Wang, Z.; Levison, B.S. Intestinal microbial metabolism of phosphatidylcholine and cardiovascular risk. *New England Journal of Medicine*, **2013**, *368* (17), 1575–1584.
69. Theilmann, M.C.; Goh, Y.J.; Nielsen, K.F. *Lactobacillus acidophilus* metabolizes dietary plant glucosides and externalizes their bioactive phytochemicals. *MBio*, **2017**, *8* (6), article ID: e01421-17.
70. Tomova, A.; Bukovsky, I.; Rembert, E.; Yonas, W. the effects of vegetarian and vegan diets on gut microbiota. *Frontiers in Nutrition*, **2019**, *6*, 47–55.
71. Ventura, M.; O'Toole, P.W.; de Vos, W.M.; van Sinderen, D. Selected aspects of the human gut microbiota. *Cellular and Molecular Life Sciences*, **2018**, *75* (1), 81–82.
72. Vieira-Silva, S.; Falony, G.; Darzi, Y. Species–function relationships shape ecological properties of the human gut microbiome. *Nature Microbiology*, **2016**, *1* (8), 1–8.
73. Wahlström, A.; Sayin, S.I.; Marschall, H.U.; Bäckhed, F.; Intestinal crosstalk between bile acids and microbiota and its impact on host metabolism. *Cell Metabolism*, **2016**, *24* (1), 41–50.
74. Whisner, C.M.; Maldonado, J.; Dente, B.; Krajmalnik-Brown, R.; Bruening, M. Diet, Physical activity and screen time but not body mass index are associated with the gut microbiome of a diverse cohort of college students living in university housing: a cross-sectional study. *BMC Microbiology*, **2018**, *18* (1), 210.
75. Wu, G.D.; Chen, J.; Hoffmann, C. Linking long-term dietary patterns with gut microbial enterotypes. *Science*, **2011**, *334* (6052), 105–108.
76. Wu, Y.; Pan, L.; Shang, Q.H.; Ma, X.K.; Long, S.F.; Xu, Y.T.; Piao, X.S. Effects of isomalto-oligosaccharides as potential prebiotics on performance, immune function and gut microbiota in weaned pigs. *Animal Feed Science and Technology*, **2017**, *230*, 126–135.
77. Wu, Z.A.; Wang, H.X. A systematic review of the interaction between gut microbiota and host health from a symbiotic perspective. *SN Comprehensive Clinical Medicine*, **2019**, *1* (3), 224–235.
78. Yadav, H.; Lee, J.H.; Lloyd, J.; Walter, P.; Rane, S.G. Beneficial metabolic effects of a probiotic via butyrate-induced GLP-1 hormone secretion. *Journal of biological chemistry*, **2013**, *288* (35), 25088–25097.
79. Yang, Z.; Huang, S.; Zou, D., Dong, D. Metabolic shifts and structural changes in the gut microbiota upon branched-chain amino acid supplementation in middle-aged mice. *Amino Acids*, **2016**, *48* (12), 2731–2745.
80. Zhang, F.; Luo, W.; Shi, Y.; Fan, Z.; Ji, G. Should we standardize the 1,700-year-old fecal microbiota transplantation? *The American Journal of Gastroenterology*, **2012**, *107* (11), 1755–1761.
81. Zimmer, J.; Lange, B.; Frick, J.S. Vegan or vegetarian diet substantially alters the human colonic faecal microbiota. *European Journal of Clinical Nutrition*, **2012**, *66* (1), 53–60.

# CHAPTER 8

# HEALTH BENEFITS OF *MUSA* SPP SPECIES (BANANAS) IN INFLAMMATORY BOWEL DISEASE

ANA ELISA V. QUAGLIO, LUIZ D. DE ALMEIDA JUNIOR, and LUIZ CLAUDIO DI STASI*

## ABSTRACT

The chemical composition of pulp and peel of banana fruits is rich in polyphenol compounds and resistant starch, supporting numerous protective properties against several chronical diseases, including Crohn's disease and ulcerative colitis, two intestinal inflammatory process that compose the human inflammatory bowel disease. This chapter reported the ability of banana products to modulate the immune response, oxidative stress, and intestinal microbiota, promoting protective effects on the intestinal inflammatory process. Indeed, we also reported that chemical composition of banana based on glycosylated polyphenols and resistant starch are closely related to their health benefits on the gut, which occurs by different mechanisms, particularly increasing epithelial barriers function, modulating intestinal microbiota, incrementing short-chain fatty acids production and upregulating the immune response.

## 8.1 INTRODUCTION

The banana is a very important and popular fruit consumed either fresh or processed several products. Together with rice, wheat, and maize, banana is a food crop and dietary source of nutrients and energy for the people living in humid tropical and subtropical regions [40]. It is acceptable that the term

*Corresponding author. E-mail: luiz.stasi@unesp.br.

"banana" comes from the Arabic word *banan* meaning "fingers" to represent the morphological aspect of banana fruits grouped in clusters. Bananas have been part of human diet for thousands of years and it has been speculated their origin in the New Guinea ~10,000 years ago. After this, banana spreads by Asia and Pacific, and posteriorly by tropical regions in the entire world [56]. It is likely that several banana species were independently domesticated elsewhere in Southeast Asia and Africa, indicating a long history of banana cultivation in these regions [44].

After domestication, it is probable that marketers and travelers introduced bananas in several world regions, mainly in Australia, Indonesia, India, and Malaysia [31]. There are reports about banana use in old registers dated 500 BC, including Sanskrit documents and Indian inscriptions on the walls of several Buddhist temples. In 327 BC, banana (named Moca) was introduced in Europe at the time that troops of Alexander, the Great invaded India [27, 56].

Marketers from Arab world were responsible for the introduction of the banana into Persia, Iraq, countries of the Mediterranean area, and North Africa, where banana was named as Moza, Mouz, or Moz [27]. In the fifteenth century, the cultivation of banana strongly spreader in the West Coast of Africa, simultaneously with its introduction by the Portuguese sailors in the Spanish Islands and by Spaniards into Santo Domingo and Panama. In the Spanish and Portuguese colonies, the requirement for food assisted an increase in the spread of banana over the America. At the end of the eighteenth century, the dissemination of banana cultivation occurs in the Americas, Pacific Islands, and Caribbean [27].

Currently, banana represents an important fruit in the world market with an annual production surrounding 102 million tons of fresh fruit [18], which represents 16.8% of all worlds' fruit production. The enhancement in banana production has been explained by the population growth [63]. The biggest producers of banana are India, which produced 30 million tons and China with 11 million tons in 2017, but banana is also widely produced in Asia, Latin America, and Africa [17, 27]. Other large producer is Brazil with 6.6 million tons [17].

According to FAO [17], banana production in 2017 was around 113 million tons, being Asia responsible for the production of 61 million tons, Americas (30 million tons), Africa (20 million tons), Oceania (2 million tons), and Europe (0.5 million tons). Moreover, the global banana industry generates in exportations approximately USD 10 billion per year [17]. However, 85% of banana production is consumed locally, mainly in great producers as India, China, and Brazil, whereas only 15% is traded in the international market [17].

In the last years, scientific and commercial interest in bananas markedly increase because the rich chemical composition and several pharmacological activities attributed to their pulp fruits and particularly their fruit peel, a banana by-product with potential use as prebiotic and modulator of intestinal microbiota.

This chapter explores chemical and pharmacological data of banana group, focusing on the relationship between chemical composition and pharmacological activities against digestive disorders, mainly inflammatory bowel disease (IBD).

## 8.2   BANANAS (*MUSA* SPP.): CHEMICAL AND PHARMACOLOGICAL ASPECTS

### 8.2.1   BANANA (MUSA SPP.) BOTANICAL TAXONOMY

Banana is a fruit of monocotyledonous botanical group, subtropical, and perennial, from the *Musa* genera (botanical family Musaceae). It has been speculated that name *Musa* was chosen in honor to muses of Greek mythology, but this name has been also related to Antonius Musa, a Roman physician of the first century B.C. [56].

Musaceae is restricted to only two botanical genera: *Musa* and *Ensete*. Linnaeus was the first researcher to assign scientific nomenclature to bananas when he described at the first time the plant species *Musa paradisiaca*. After this, numerous wild species have been described, domesticated, and categorized into genome groups based on their ploidy levels and the genomes which they contain. Simmonds and Shepherd [55] suggested that edible bananas were originated from two wild species, *Musa acuminata* ($2n = 22$) and *Musa balbisiana* ($2n = 22$), resulting in a series of seedless diploid, triploid, and tetraploid bananas having genome A, relative to *M. acuminata*, and genome B, relative to *M. balbisiana* [23]. *M. acuminata* and *M. balbisiana* are species diploids with genomes AA and BB, respectively [39, 56].

Thus, different genomic associations characterize each cultivar depending on chromosomes number, including two chromosomes (AA and AB), three chromosomes (AAA, AAB, and ABB), or four chromosomes (AAAA, AAAB, AABB, and ABBB) [14]. Currently, many botanical taxonomists agree that scientific name *Musa* spp. can be used for all edible bananas because ploidy arrangement characterizes the majority of bananas [14].

The fruits from diploid AA and triploid AAA banana subspecies are reported as sweeter with wide use as dessert, representing the majority of the cultivars with high market value [39, 56]. Bananas derived from *M. balbisiana* and the hybrids between *M. acuminata* and *M. balbisiana* are known as plantains and contain high starch content [56]. The antique and original bananas are fertile diploids plant species, whereas the bananas currently cultivated are clones, mainly triploids, which reproduces by vegetative system [40].

## 8.2.2  CHEMICAL CONSTITUENTS OF BANANAS (MUSA SPP.)

In genus *Musa*, phenol compounds and carotenoids offer health benefits and antioxidant properties. Indeed, pharmacological analysis and phytochemical profile of bananas have been currently highlighted due to their richness in resistant starch, a plant constituent that function as dietary fiber, promoting many benefits in numerous chronic diseases like diabetes, obesity, hypertension, and IBD. In the last years, special attention has been paid to the banana fruit peel, a subproduct of banana that is usually discarded, but can be represent a rich source of bioactive compounds, resistant starch, and dietary fiber. Several nutritional components, including lignin, pectin, sugars, carbohydrates, carotenoids, vitamins, and minerals as well as polyphenols are either found in banana fruit pulp or fruit peel.

### 8.2.2.1  POLYPHENOLIC COMPOUNDS

Banana fruit pulp and fruit peel contain many polyphenolic compounds, including tannins, flavonoids, catechin, epicatechin, gallic acid, and anthocyanins [56]. Some of these compounds, mainly tannins, promote an astringent taste to the banana in unripe state, with higher amounts in the banana fruit peel than banana fruit pulp [34, 45, 56]. The total phenolic acids content in fruit pulp is ~7 mg/100 g of the fresh weight [34]. On the other hand, free phenol compound amounts in banana fruit pulp ranged between 11.8 and 90.4 mg of gallic acid equivalents/100 g of the fresh weight, while in banana fruit peel the phenol content ranging from 4.95 to 47 mg of gallic acid equivalents/100 g of the fresh weight [56, 63].

The main phenol compounds reported include hydroxycinnamic and benzoic acids derivatives and heterosides such as ferulic, caffeic, sinapic, gallic, syringic, cinnamic, vannilic, tannic, chlorogenic, cumaric, and protocatechic acids (Figure 8.1); flavonoids such as rutin, quercetin glycosides, kaempeferol glycosides, isorhamnetin glycosides, and myricetin glycosides; tannins including catechin, epicatechin, gallocatechin (Figure 8.2). A detailed description of chemical composition in banana fruit pulp and banana fruit peel focusing antioxidant properties can be observed in the extensive review recently published [40, 56, 63].

## 8.2.2.2   CAROTENOIDS AND VITAMINS

The mature fruit pulp of banana is rich in several vitamins including carotene (vitamin A), niacin, thiamine, and riboflavin (vitamin B), and ascorbic acid (vitamin C); however, bananas have moderate content of vitamin B6 [58]. The main carotenoids (Figure 8.1) reported in bananas were lutein, isolutein, β-carotene, autoxanthin, neoxanthin, violaxanthin, β-cryptoxanthin, and α-cryptoxanthin [56].

## 8.2.2.3   RESISTANT STARCH

Bananas represent a rich source of resistant starch, which is recognized as a dietary component with several health benefits. Resistant starch contents present in bananas have been reported as limiting factor in the carotenoid's bioavailability [45, 58]. Thus, amounts of resistant starch in banana fruits dramatically change during ripening process [39, 67], potentially influencing their pharmacological activities. Resistant starch is defined "as the sum of starch and products of starch degradation not absorbed in the small intestine of a healthy individual" [35, 46]. Thus, resistant starch, as a part of total starch present in banana, acts similarly to dietary fiber within the gastrointestinal tract. Resistant starch strength against enzymatic digestion in the small intestine has been closely related to numerous positive health benefits [16].

Bananas have resistant starch type 2, which is characterized by native granular starch. The ripening process of banana includes eight stages. At stages I and II, banana fruit is entirely green, rich in starch, astringent, and very hard. From the stage III, the yellow colors of banana fruit peel are gradually increased and consequently occur a reduction of starch, which is broken to form carbohydrates. The starch alteration during bananas ripening involves some enzymes and several pathways. Starch presents in the green banana fruit is converted into several sugars, mainly sucrose, fructose, and glucose. Indeed, in small quantities, starch can be also converted in maltose and rhamnose. The total content of soluble sugar can reach 16% or higher of the fresh fruit weight, that is, indicating a high conversion rate. The average starch content can be reduced from 70% to 80% in the preclimacteric period (before starch breakdown) to <1% when climacteric period finished [5]. Green banana has the highest resistant starch content (between 47% and 57%) when compared to other unprocessed foods [5, 16].

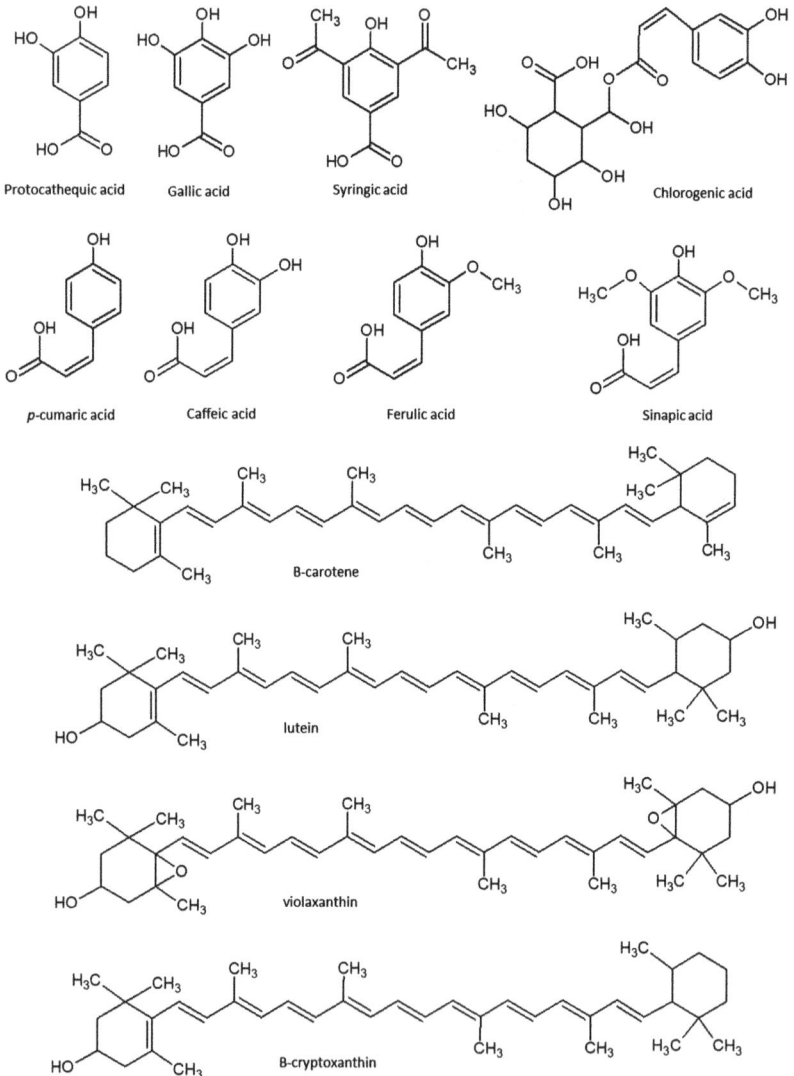

**FIGURE 8.1** Main cynnamic/benzoic acids and carotenoids reported in Bananas (*Musa* spp.) pulp fruit and banana peel.

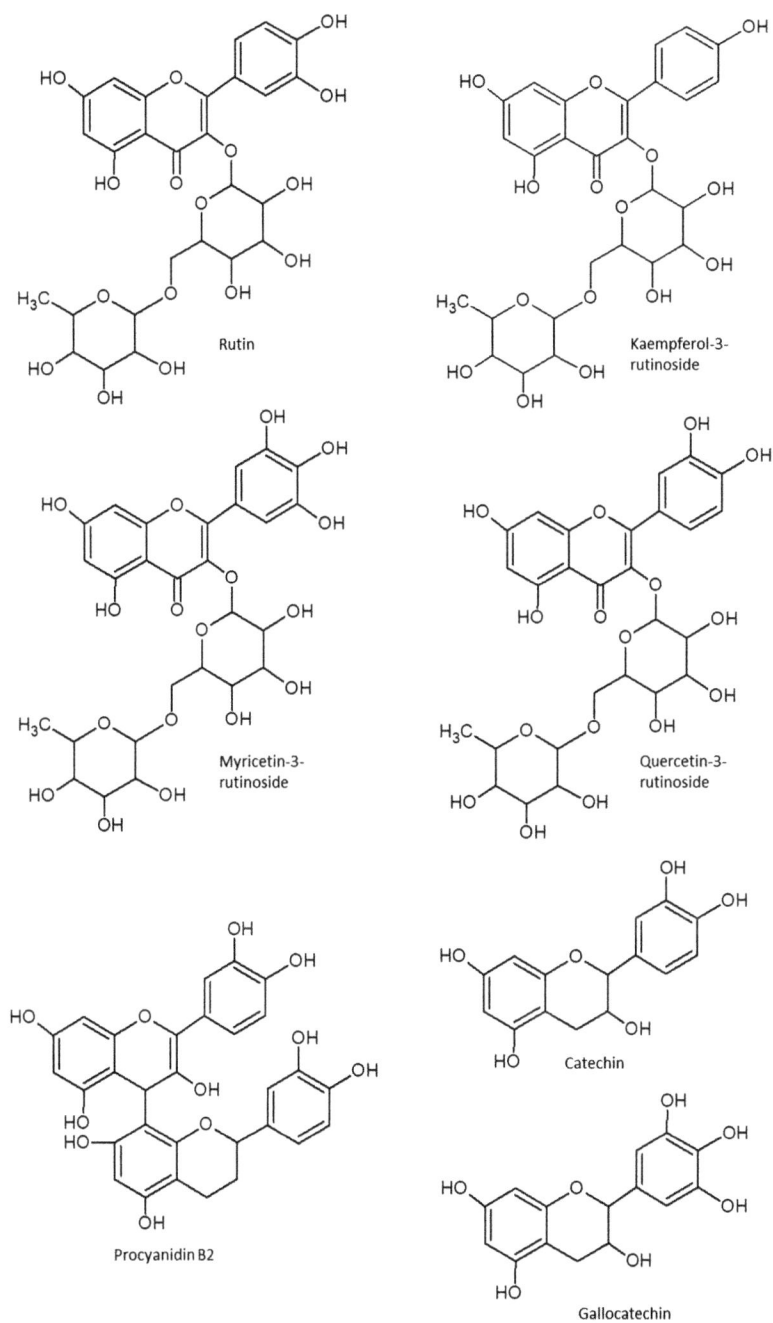

**FIGURE 8.2**   Main flavonoids and tannins reported in Bananas (*Musa* spp.) pulp fruit and banana peel.

## 8.2.2.4  MISCELLANEOUS COMPOUNDS

Banana fruit peel contains higher content of potassium when compared with fruit pulp. In fact, banana plant species are rich sources of potassium when compared with other tropical and subtropical fruits. Banana fruit pulp also contains magnesium, calcium, and phosphorus [45, 58]. Moreover, bananas are poor source of proteins and fats. However, it has been reported a slight increment in protein concentration during changes from unripe to ripe stage, and lipids levels remain almost constant during ripening process [56].

Among different types of lipids, banana fruit peel contains polyunsaturated fatty acids in high amounts, mainly linoleic and linolenic acids [58], which are active compounds useful to treat several chronical disorders. It has been reported that during maturation, the level of polyamines (histamine, serotonin, tryptamine, 2-phenylethylamine, tyramine, dopamine, putrescine, cadaverine, spermine, agmatine, and spermidine) also varies significantly [45].

## 8.2.3  BANANAS (MUSA SPP.): GENERAL BIOLOGICAL ACTIVITIES

The fruit of the ripe banana is a food ready to eat as well as the most available for human consumption. The ripe edible banana functions to promote a good health, due to its great nutritional value associated to its potential therapeutic action [56]. Banana fruit pulp contains many bioactive compounds, like polyphenolic acids and flavonoids with several pharmacological properties, including antioxidant, antitumor, antidiarrheal, antiulcerative, antimicrobial, hypoglycemic, and wound healing activities [2, 4, 7, 22, 49]. Banana fruit pulp also contains resistant starch, a component with lower digestibility, which is very unlike the high glycemic index cereal starches, which can be useful to diabetic people [2].

Consumption of banana protects against vitamin A deficiency since are rich in carotenoids and has been also associated to promote several biological effects, including reduced risk of high blood pressure and stroke associated with cholesterol-lowering effects, protection against ulcers and restoration of normal bowel activity besides protects against neurodegenerative disorders. Banana also contains dopamine, ascorbic acid, and several antioxidants, which help in reducing the oxidative stress and increase the resistance to oxidative alteration of low-density lipoproteins [29]. Moreover, high amounts of resistant starch in bananas have been related to reduce glycemic index, potentially useful to treat diabetes, mainly diabetes type 2 [42].

## 8.3   IBD: GENERAL ASPECTS

IBD includes Crohn's disease (CD) and ulcerative colitis (UC), two chronic diseases of the gut. This chronical disease is a part of a conglomeration of immune-mediated inflammatory diseases that includes psoriasis, psoriatic arthritis, rheumatoid arthritis, and systemic lupus erythematosus [20]. Although IBD etiology is unclear, several factors have been reported to have a key role in its development, including dysregulated immune response, host genotype, oxidative stress, and environmental factors, particularly the composition of intestinal microbiota [33]. Thus, intestinal inflammation results from an exaggerated intestinal immune response to otherwise innocuous stimuli (diet antigens and intestinal microbiota products and metabolites), which persist with the time and it is not conveniently abrogated by the physiological mechanisms that play this role [28]. As consequence, there is an upregulation of the synthesis and release of different mediators including eicosanoids, cytokines and reactive oxygen (ROS), and nitrogen species (Figure 8.3).

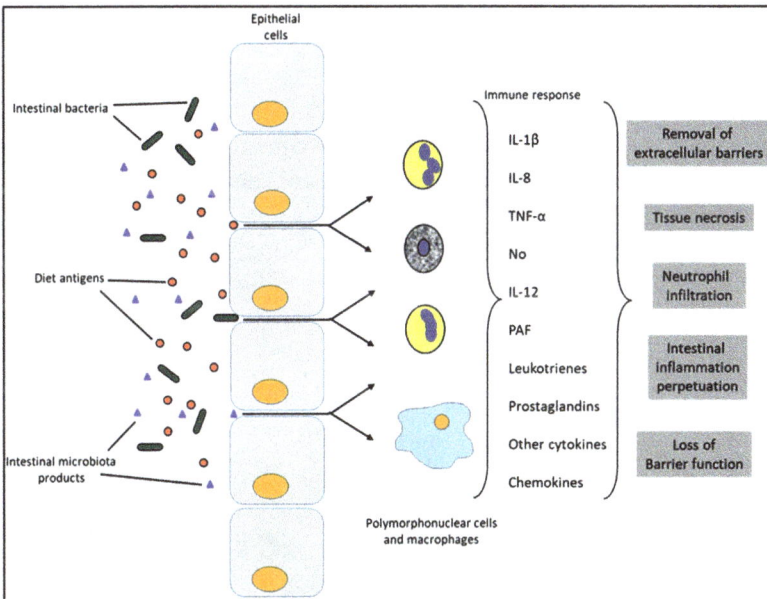

FIGURE 8.3   General aspects of IBD development and perpetuation.

The complex and unclear etiology of IBD is a limiting factor in the discovery and development of new pharmacological treatments and explains the high frequencies of patient's refractory to current available drugs [11]. Moreover, the pharmacological management of IBD, including drugs such as 5-aminosalycic acid derivatives, glucocorticoids, immunomodulatory, and biological therapies produce serious side effects, mainly after long-term use. Thus, current drugs are used to control IBD symptoms or to create a period of deep remission, indicating that there is no IBD pharmacological cure. In addition, dissatisfaction with current IBD therapies has resulted in an increased interest in new treatment approaches, which has been oriented toward IBD etiological factors and new molecular targets [11]. Based on this, we consider important to report the main etiological aspects associated to IBD development in order to identify the potential role of bananas (*Musa* spp.) plant species as complementary therapies to prevent and treat human IBD.

IBD has a complex and imbricated relationship among proinflammatory and anti-inflammatory mediators, which are closely related to innate and adaptive immune response as well as to oxidative stress that occurs in intestinal inflammation (Figure 8.4). Among these mediators, currently, ROS and TNF-α (tumor necrosis factor-α) have been reported as the most important mediators of intestinal inflammation and main target of new drugs. Although the majority of these mediators participates both UC and dendritic cell (DC) etiology, some of them are disease specific and can be used either to better understanding of IBD etiology or to development of new approaches to prevent or treat intestinal inflammation. Moreover, besides of many cytokines, some classical mediators participate in the intestinal inflammatory response, including prostaglandins and nitric oxide.

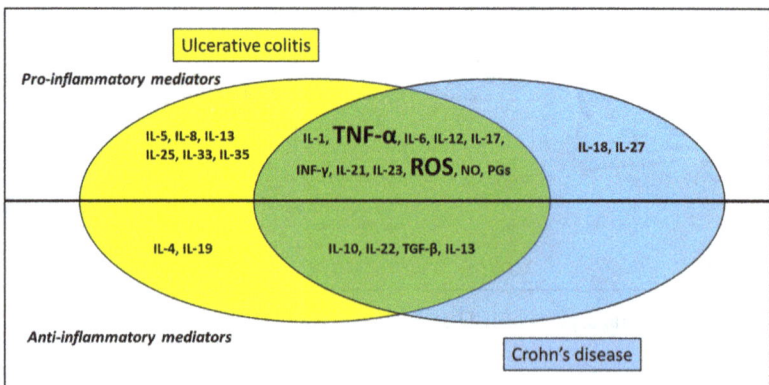

**FIGURE 8.4** The main proinflammatory and anti-inflammatory mediators of inflammatory bowel disease; (Modified and adapted from Müzes et al. [37].)

In the gastrointestinal tract, the innate immune system consists of the several cells including neutrophils, macrophages, DCs, monocytes, natural killer cells, eosinophils, and basophils, and the mucus and epithelial barrier. In the innate immunity process, the recognition of pathogens occurs by an immediate nonspecific response. Generally, activated macrophages lead to the secretion of several proinflammatory and anti--inflammatory cytokines (TNF-α, IL-1β, IL-10, IL-12, IL-18, and IL-23), any chemokines, and ROS. A great number of neutrophils accumulates in inflamed mucosa and promotes crypts architecture damage, leading to the crypt abscess formation, which contributes to the severity of mucosal inflammation [66, 68]. The lymphocytes activation by Th1, Th2, Th17, and Th22 pathways associated to suppression of the activity of Treg cells is one of the main steps in the initiation phase of the adaptive immune response. After T cells activation, the effector T cells enter in the circulation to migrate toward the original site of binding with the antigen [19, 66].

Neutrophils function to eliminate microorganisms namely phagocytosis, degranulation, and ROS production. Excessive activation of macrophage and polymorphonuclear cells infiltration promotes local increase of the cytokines and free radicals production (Figure 8.3). Oxidative stress is considered an important etiologic factor involved in several signals and symptoms of IBD. However, experimental evidences suggest that IBD is associated with an imbalance between increased ROS and decreased antioxidant activity, particularly glutathione and glutathione-related enzymes [6]. This way, antioxidant products can be a therapeutic approach to treat IBD, reducing cytokine and pro-oxidative enzyme concentrations and improving the anti-oxidative cell ability.

The immune system represents one factor in the complex universe of IBD pathogenesis, and it is now widely appreciated that no single component can alone trigger or determine the ultimate fate of IBD. In fact, a combined disruption of all the elements controlling intestinal homeostasis is necessary to the initiation and mediation of this disease. The intestinal microbiota role in developing the host immune innate and adaptive system corroborates the need to understand with more details the human microbiome [24, 61]. There has been increasing evidence that associate intestinal dysbiosis with the origin, manifestation, and development of inflammation of the gut [41, 43, 59].

The gut microbiota can be viewed as a new body organ contributing to the well-being of the host organism. In IBD, an abnormal intestinal micro-biota is clearly associated with some disease phenotypes inducing chronic inflammation [65]. As recently reported, the changes in amounts of the total bacterial within the mucosa as well as reduced bacterial diversity are related to diseases conditions [54]. Although a specific microbial signature has not been identified, several changes in both composition and function of gut microbiota were associated with active IBD [36]. It has been demonstrated that an increase in the biodiversity of the bacterial gut population requires a change in metabolic homeostasis with consequent improvement of its protective effects, while a reduction in bacterial population due to age, illness, or antibiotic therapy, reduces the capacity of the intestinal environment to fight infecting pathogens [32].

In fact, the colonic fermentation of dietary products, particularly dietary fibers and similar compounds with prebiotic properties, allows some of their energy to be salvaged, affects stool transient time, bulking and frequency, influences nutrient bioavailability, and produces short-chain fatty acids (SCFAs) such as acetate, propionate, and butyrate. These gut bacteria metabolites have physiological roles, including epithelial cell proliferation, control of mucosal motility, modulation of immune activity, and endocrine functions. SCFAs act in the prevention and treatment of several chronic diseases, including metabolic syndrome, IBD, and cancer [11, 51]. The beneficial effects of SCFAs are based on several properties because the bacteria metabolites are source of energy for colon cells, regulate the fatty acid synthesis and oxidation, lipolysis, glucose, and cholesterol metabolism, and modulate inflammation by suppression of the proinflammatory mediator's production and enhancement the release of anti-inflammatory cytokine IL-10 [10, 11, 57, 60, 62].

## 8.4   BANANAS (*MUSA* SPP.) AND THEIR POTENTIAL USE IN IBD

Many researchers have suggested banana fruit as an effective product to treat diseases in the gastrointestinal tract. Pannangpetch et al. [38] reported the gastroprotective effect of different banana varieties. They found that extracts of two bananas, *Musa paradisiaca* and *Musa sapientum*, have a potent gastroprotective effect, whereas the extract of *Musa sapientum* had also an ulcer-healing effect. In several countries, banana is consumed as an essential food with nutritional value, but it is also used to treat gastrointestinal tract disorders like diarrhea and gastritis [40]. The juice produced from pseudo-stem is also orally administrated to control diarrhea. The topical use of this juice is also used to wash skin with ulcers and to treat aphtha ulcer in children [40]. The banana fruit peel has also employed as an antacid product against stomach ulcers probably due to presence of leucocyanidin, a flavonoid that act increasing the thickness of the mucous layer of the stomach [26].

The role of several foods in shaping and maintaining of the intestinal microbiota has been widely reported, suggesting that diets with low-fiber amounts have a negative impact on the composition of the intestinal microbiota. Diet with lower amounts of dietary fiber is already a feature of modern diets, which have been related to a progressive loss of intestinal microorganism's diversity [36, 54]. Considering that the nutritional components of diet and their ability to interact with intestinal bacteria community, it seems obvious to consider the direct modulatory potential of a diet rich in fiber on the microbiota composition. On the other hand, components present in the foods have also been linked to their ability to modulate epigenetic mechanisms, increasing the risk of the IBD development and progression. Furthermore, microbiota composition is dynamic and diet-dependent, also influenced by the host age and oscillating according to food intake daily patterns [47].

Several microbiome-based dietary interventions have been studied in IBD, including pre-, pro-, and symbiotics. The use of probiotics, particularly Lactobacilli and Bifidobacteria, has been widely studied. However, new approach of food intervention in the IBD therapy is based on the use of prebiotics, dietary products, which are promptly metabolized by human intestinal bacteria into SCFAs [36, 47, 54]. In fact, a prebiotic product is defined as "a non-digestible food ingredient that beneficially affects the host by selectively stimulating the growth and/or activity of one or a limited number of bacteria in the colon" [21]. This concept claims that several food constituents are resistant to hydrolysis by digestive enzymatic components, passing into the large bowel, where are fermented by the intestinal microbiota [50]. In this context, resistant starch presents in banana (*Musa* spp.) plant species has been considered a prebiotic product because it functions as dietary fiber and a source of SCFAs.

Clinical studies have demonstrated that resistant starch has similar properties to dietary fiber with health benefits in humans [42] and potential use in the prevention of several chronic diseases, including IBD. In fact, the benefits of resistant starch and consequently of bananas are closely related to fermentation of resistant starch by intestinal microbiota with high production of SCFAs, particularly butyrate [1, 42]. Moreover, resistant starch is able to reduce fecal pH, increase fecal mass, and reduce fecal transit time [42].

Banana also represents a rich source of fructo-oligosaccharides (FOS), functional components of foods potentially able to modulate intestinal microbiota. FOS decreases serum cholesterol level, stimulates the growth of beneficial intestinal microflora and improves mineral absorption [30, 52, 63, 64]. Additional studies showed that green dwarf banana fruit pulp and fruit peel flours (*Musa* spp. AAA) were capable to decrease intestinal inflammation and this beneficial effect was related to high production of acetate, propionate, and butyrate [1]. The protective effects of dietary intervention with banana flour were also evidenced by reduction in the colonic damage, inhibition of myeloperoxidase activity, and counteraction of glutathione depletion to take place in inflamed colon, clearly indicating the banana ability to modulate oxidative stress leading to mucosal healing [1, 53]. Indeed, green dwarf banana flour induces colonic mucin production, increasing the epithelial barrier function in the gut [1].

Recent study demonstrated the prebiotic potential of the plantain inflorescence fibers, which promoted the growth of the beneficial *Lactobacillus casei* and *Bifidobacterium bifidum* [3]. This protective effect was evidenced by a lower pH, increased optical density, dry mass and the production of SCFAs. These changes were higher in plantain inflorescence fiber treated group compared with negative and positive (inulin) control [3].

Modulatory properties of plant food on the intestinal microbiota have been reported to other compounds different of the dietary fiber and other polysaccharide products fermentable by gut bacteria. Glycosylated polyphenol compounds, mainly condensed and hydrolysable tannins, anthocyannins and ellagitannins have been also recognized as prebiotic-like products [12, 15], because they modulate intestinal microbiota after metabolism and release of mono- and disaccharides. In fact, prebiotic-like effects of polyphenol compounds have been reported both in vitro assays and in vivo preclinical and clinical trials, in which glycosylated polyphenols-rich foods enhancing the growth of several gut bacteria, such as lactobacilli, bifidobacteria, *Faecalibacterium prausnitzii*, and *Roseburia* spp., with consequent health benefits to the host [12, 15].

The main polyphenol compounds with prebiotic-like effects include tannins, proanthocyanidins, and glycosylated flavonoids [8, 48], chemical constituents reported in banana fruit and banana peel. There are evidences that the interaction between polyphenol compounds and intestinal microbiota resulting in a two-way relationship. Mono- and disaccharides are released after polyphenol deglycosylation by the gut-microbiota mediated hydrolysis products [15], generating phenolic aglycones, which are cleavage and reduced, leading to release of polyphenol metabolites that are often better absorbed than the native phenol compounds, promoting antioxidant properties [15, 25].

Simultaneously, this metabolic process releases mono- and disaccharides, and it is possible to suggest that these sugars can be used as substrate to gut bacteria fermentative process, with consequent production of SCFAs. In fact, fermentative process of glycosylated polyphenols improves antioxidant activity due to an increase in the amounts of phenolic compounds, which is a result of a microbial hydrolysis reaction, whereas saccharides often used in fermentative process [25]. Therefore, polyphenols-rich foods represent an important source of the antioxidant compounds released after fermentative process by gut bacteria to promote their protective effects.

The antioxidant properties of banana were corroborated by many studies. Pereira and Mareschin [40] reported that banana fruit pulp contains several antioxidants, particularly vitamins, carotenoids, and phenolic compounds, which exhibit a wide range of biological effects.

Ara et al. [2] evaluated a methanol extract of *M. balbisiana* flower in diabetic rats and found that banana flower extract increased enzymatic activity of the catalase and superoxide dismutase, associated with a decrease of the malondialdehyde levels [2]. Kumar et al. [29] also described several effects of banana consumption, including reduced risk of high blood pressure and stroke associated with cholesterol-lowering effects, protection against ulcers, and restoration of normal bowel activity. Antioxidant properties of banana plant species were also evidenced by the decrease of the oxidative stress related to enhance of glucose uptake [3].

Based on this data, it is possible to suggest that dietary intervention containing derived banana products is potentially useful to prevent relapse on intestinal inflammation and to increase remission time of symptoms. Although the prebiotic properties in clinical studies are less clear, owing to a lack of scientific data, several studies with different prebiotics, including derived banana products, provide unquestionable evidence for primary and preventive role of these dietary interventions as modulators of the gut microbiota in the intestinal inflammation. Considering the chemical composition and pharmacological activities reported to the banana (*Musa* spp.) plant species, we hypothesize that dietary intervention with banana rich in resistant starch and glycosylated polyphenol compounds are protective products in IBD acting by different mechanisms of action, as described above (Figure 8.5).

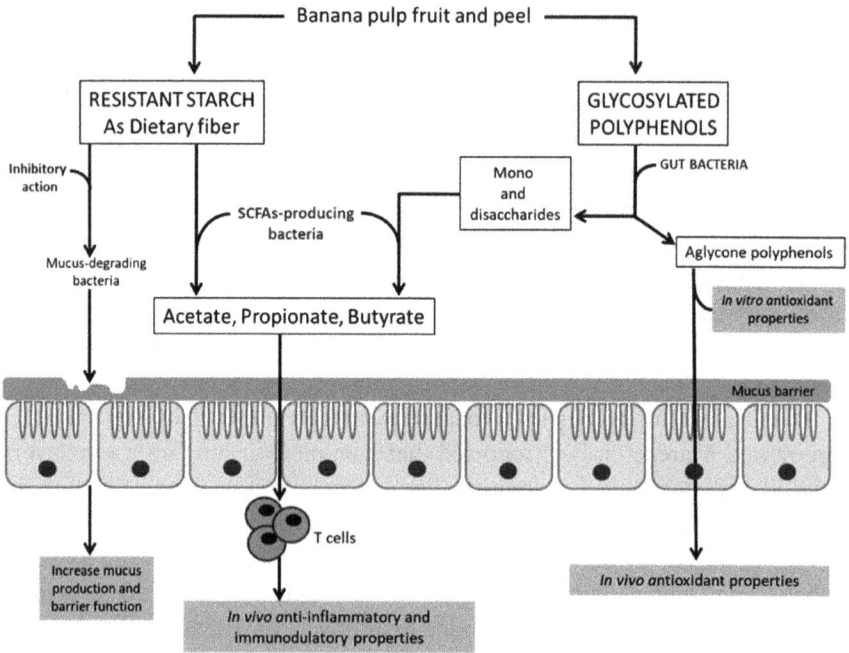

**FIGURE 8.5**  Main potential action site and mechanisms of banana (*Musa* spp.) plant species to control inflammatory bowel disease. (Modified and adapted from Curimbaba et al. [9].)

First, resistant starch present in banana plants acts as a dietary fiber promoting beneficial effects in intestinal inflammation because this product is fermented by bacteria from intestinal microbiota increasing SCFAs production, particularly acetate, propionate, and butyrate, which produce a lot of effects, modulating immune, and anti-inflammatory response. In addition, resistant starch can be act reducing mucus-degrading bacteria, increasing mucus production by this mechanism or acting directly on goblet cells. Second, glycosylated polyphenol compounds present in banana contribute with protective effects in the intestinal inflammation because after their hydrolysis by specific bacteria release glucose and other sugars, which are fermented by intestinal microbiota to increase SCFAs production. Simultaneously, the release of the active aglycone polyphenol molecules, which are promptly absorbed, promote antioxidant properties in different ways, including reduction of mieloperoxidase and counteraction of glutathione depletion to take place in intestinal inflammation.

## 8.5  SUMMARY

New studies in two experimental models of intestinal inflammation, trinitro-benzenesulphonic acid, and dextran sodium sulfate, as well as clinical trial in patients with UC are in development in our laboratories in order to obtain new data on the mechanisms of action and to evaluate beneficial effects of dietary banana intervention in human patients with UC.

## KEYWORDS

- banana
- Crohn's disease
- gut
- inflammatory bowel disease
- intestinal microbiota
- *Musa*
- oxidative stress
- prebiotic
- short-chain fatty acids
- ulcerative colitis

## REFERENCES

1. Almeida-Junior, L.D.; Curimbaba, T.F.S. Dietary intervention with green dwarf banana flour (*Musa* sp. AAA) modulates oxidative stress and colonic SCFAs production in the TNBS model of intestinal inflammation. *Journal of Functional Foods,* **2017**, *38*, 497–504.
2. Ara, F.; Tripathy, A.; Ghosh, D. Possible antidiabetic and antioxidative activity of hydro-methanolic extract of *Musa balbisiana* (Colla) flower in streptozotocin-induced diabetic male albino wistar strain rat: a genomic approach. *Assay and Drug Development Technologies,* **2019**, *17* (2), 68–76.
3. Arun, K.B.; Madhavan, A.; Reshmitha, T.R.; Thomas, S.; Nisha, P. Short chain fatty acids enriched fermentation metabolites of soluble dietary fiber from *Musa paradisiaca* Drives HT29 colon cancer cells to apoptosis. *PLoS One*, **2019**, *14* (5), 1–20.
4. Arun, K.B.; Thomas, S.; Reshmitha, T.R.; Akhil, G.C.; Nisha, P. Dietary Fiber and Phenolic-rich extracts from *Musa paradisiaca* inflorescence ameliorates type 2 diabetes and associated cardiovascular risks. *Journal of Functional Foods,* **2017**, *31*, 198–207.

5. Aurore, G.; Parfait, B.; Fahrasmane, L. Bananas, raw materials for making processed food products. *Trends in Food Science & Technology*, **2009**, *20*, 78–91.

6. Balmus, I.M.; Ciobica, A.; Trifan, A.; Stanciu, C. The implications of oxidative stress and antioxidant therapies in inflammatory bowel disease: clinical aspects and animal models. *Saudi Journal of Gastroenterology*, **2016**, *22* (1), 3–17.

7. Bhaskar, J.J.; S., M.; Chilkunda, N.D.; Salimath, P.V. Banana (*Musa* sp. var. *elakki bale*) Flower and pseudostem: dietary fiber and associated antioxidant capacity. *Journal of Agricultural and Food Chemistry*, **2011**, *60*, 427–432.

8. Cardona, F.; Andrés-Lacueva, C. Benefits of polyphenols on gut microbiota and implications in human health. *The Journal of Nutritional Biochemistry*, **2013**, *24* (8), 1415–1422.

9. Curimbaba, T.F.S.; Almeida-Junior, L.D. Prebiotic, antioxidant and anti-inflammatory properties of the edible amazon fruits. *Food Bioscience*, **2020**, *36*, 100599.

10. Den Besten, G.; Van Eunen, K. The role of short-chain fatty acids in the interplay between diet, gut microbiota, and host energy metabolism. *The Journal of Lipid Research*, **2013**, *54* (9), 2325–2340.

11. Di Stasi, LC.; Costa, C.A.R.A; Witaicenis, A. Products for the treatment of inflammatory bowel disease: a patent review (2013–2014). *Expert Opinion on Therapeutic Patents*, **2015**, *25* (6), 629–642.

12. Dueñas, M.; Muñoz-González, I.; Cueva, C. Survey of modulation of gut microbiota by dietary polyphenols. *BioMed Research International*, **2015**, *2015*, 1–15.

13. Ekesa, B.; Poulaert, M.; Davey, M.W. Bioaccessibility of provitamin a carotenoids in bananas (*Musa* spp.) and derived Dishes in African countries. *Food Chemistry*, **2012**, *133*, 1471–1477.

14. El-Khishin, D.A.; Belatus, E.L.; El-Hamid, A.A.; Radwan, K.H. molecular characterization of banana cultivars (*Musa* spp.) from Egypt using AFLP. *Research Journal of Agriculture and Biological Sciences*, **2009**, *5* (3), 272–279.

15. Espín, J.C.; González-Sarrías, A.; Tomás-Barberán, F.A. The gut microbiota: a key factor in the therapeutic effects of polyphenols. *Biochemical Pharmacology*, 2017, *139*, 82–93.

16. Evans, A. Resistant starch and health, In: *Encyclopedia of Food Grains.* Wrigley, C.W.; Corke, H.; Seetharaman, H.; Faubion, J. (Eds.); Illinois, USA: Academic Press Inc.; **2016**; pp. 230–235.

17. FAO. *Banana Market Review Preliminary Results for 2019.* **2019**; http://www.fao.org/economic/est/estcommodities/bananas/en/; http://www.fao.org/filead min/templates/est/COMM_MARKETS_MONITORING/Bananas/Documents/Banana_Market Review_Prelim_Results_2018.pdf. Accessed on June 17, 2019.

18. Faostat. *FAO Statistical Database. Agricultural data.* **2012**; http://faostat. fao.org/site/339/default.aspxN. Accessed on June 17, 2019.

19. Geremia, A.; Biancheri, P.; Allan, P.; Corazza, G.R.; Di Sabatino, A. Innate and adaptive immunity in inflammatory bowel disease. *Autoimmunity Reviews*, **2014**, *13*(1), 3–10.

20. Ghosh, S.; Pariente, B.; Mould, D.R.; Schreiber, S.; Petersson, J.; Hommes, D. New Tools and approaches for improved management of inflammatory bowel diseases. *Journal of Crohn's and Colitis*, **2014**, *8* (10), 1246–1253.

21. Gibson, G.R.; Roberfroid, M.B. Dietary Modulation of the human colonic microbiota: introducing the concept of prebiotics. *The Journal of Nutrition*, **1995**, *125* (6), 1401–1412.

22. González-Montelongo, R.; Lobo, M.G.; González, M. antioxidant activity in banana peel extracts: testing extraction conditions and related bioactive compounds. *Food Chemistry*, **2010**, *119*, 1030–1039.
23. Häkkinen, M. Reappraisal of sectional taxonomy in *Musa* (Musaceae). *Taxon*, **2013**, *62* (4), 809–813.
24. Honda, K.; Littman, D.R. The microbiota in adaptive immune homeostasis and disease. *Nature*, **2016**, *535*, 75–84.
25. Hur, S.J.; Lee, S.Y.; Kim, Y.C.; Choi, I.; Kim, G.B. Effect of fermentation on the antioxidant activity in plant-based foods. *Food Chemistry*, **2014**, *160*, 346–356.
26. Imam, M.Z.; Akter, S. *Musa paradisiaca* L. and *Musa sapientum* L.: a phytochemical and pharmacological review. *Journal of Applied Pharmaceutical Science*, **2011**, *01* (05), 14–20.
27. Israeli, Y.; Lahav, E. Banana. In: *Encyclopedia of Applied Plant Sciences*, Amsterdam, Netherlands: Elsevier; **2017**, *32017*, pp. 363–381.
28. Katz, J.; Itoh, J.; Fiocchi, C. Pathogenesis of inflammatory bowel disease. *Current Opinion in Gastroenterology*, **1999**, *15*, 291–297.
29. Kumar, K.P.S.; Bhowmik, D.; Duraivel, S.; Umadevi, M. Traditional and medicinal uses of banana. *Journal of Pharmacognosy and Phytochemistry*, **2012**, *1* (3), 51–63.
30. Kurtoğlu, G.; Yildiz, S. Extraction of fructo-oligosaccharide components from banana peels. *Gazi University Journal of Science*, **2011**, *24* (4), 877–882.
31. Lebot, V.; Aradhya, K.M.; Manshardt, R.; Meilleur, B. Genetic relationships among cultivated bananas and plantains from Asia and the Pacific. *Euphytica*, **1993**, *67*, 163–175.B
32. Macfarlane, S.; Macfarlane, G.T. Bacterial diversity in the human gut. *Advances in Applied Microbiology*, **2004**, *54*, 261–289.
33. Maloy, K.J.; Powrie, F. Intestinal homeostasis and its breakdown in inflammatory bowel disease. *Nature*, **2011**, *474* (7351), 298–306.
34. Mattila, P.; Hellström, J.; Törrönen, R. Phenolic acids in berries, fruits, and beverages. *Journal of Agricultural and Food Chemistry*, **2006**, *54*, 7193–7199.
35. Mesquita, C.B.; Leonel, M. Characterization of banana starches obtained from cultivars grown in Brazil. *International Journal of Biological Macromolecules*, 2016, *89*, 632–639.
36. Miyoshi, J.; Chang, E.B. The gut microbiota and inflammatory bowel diseases. *Translational Research*, **2017**, *179*, 38–48.
37. Müzes, G.; Molnár B.; Tulassay Z.: Sipos F. Changes of the cytokine profile in inflammatory bowel diseases. *World Journal of Gastroenterology*, 2012, *18*, 5848–5861.
38. Pannangpetch, P.; Vuttivirojana, A. The anti-ulcerative effect of Thai *Musa* species in rats. *Phytotherapy Research*, **2001**, *15*, 407–410.
39. Pareek, S. Nutritional and biochemical composition of Banana (*Musa* spp.) Cultivars. In: *Nutritional Composition of Fruit Cultivars*; Simmonds, M.; Preedi, V. (Eds.); USA: Academic Press Inc.; **2015**; *Volume 1*; pp. 49–81.
40. Pereira, A.; Maraschin, M. Banana (*Musa* spp) from peel to pulp: ethnopharmacology, source of bioactive compounds and its relevance for human health. *Journal of Ethnopharmacology*, **2015**, *160*, 149–163.
41. Pereira, C.; Grácio, D.; Teixeira, J.P.; Magro, F. Oxidative stress and DNA damage: implications in inflammatory bowel disease. *Inflammatory Bowel Disease*, **2015**, *21* (10), 2403–2417.

42. Pereira, K.D. Resistant starch, the latest generation of energy control and healthy digestion. *Food Science and Technology*, **2007**, *27*(1), 88–92.

43. Pickard, J.M.; Zeng, M.Y.; Caruso, R.; Núñez, G. Gut microbiota: role in pathogen colonization, immune responses and inflammatory disease. *Immunological Reviews,* **2017**, *279* (1), 70–89.

44. Ploetz, R.C.; Kepler, A.K.; Daniells, J.; Nelson, S.C. Banana and plantains – an overview with emphasis on Pacific Island Cultivars. In: *Species Profiles for Pacific Island Agroforestry*. Elevitch, C.R. (Ed.); Hawai, USA: Permanent Agriculture Resources (PAR); **2007**; pp. 1–27.

45. Qamar, S.; Shaikh, A. Therapeutic potentials and compositional changes of valuable compounds from banana— A Review. *Trends in Food Science & Technology*, **2019**, *79*, 1–9.

46. Ramos, D.P.; Leonel, M.; Leonel, S. Resistant starch in green banana flour. *Alimentos e Nutrição Araraquara*, **2009**, *20* (3), 479–483.

47. Rapozo, D.C.M.; Bernardazzi, C.; Souza, H.S.P. Diet and microbiota in inflammatory bowel disease: the gut in disharmony. *World Journal of Gastroenterology*, **2017**, *23* (12), 2124–2140.

48. Rastmanesh, R. High polyphenol, low probiotic diet for weight loss because of intestinal microbiota interaction. *Chemico-Biological Interaction*, **2011**, *189* (1–2), 1–8.

49. Rebello, L.P.G.; Ramos, A.M. Flour of banana (*Musa* AAA) peel as a source of antioxidant phenolic compounds. *Food Research International*, **2014**, *55*, 397–403.

50. Roberfroid, M. Functional food concept and its application to prebiotics. *Digestive and Liver Disease*, **2002**, *34* (2), 105–110.

51. Roberfroid, M. Fructo-oligosaccharide malabsorption: benefit for gastrointestinal functions. *Current Opinion on Gastroenterology*, **2000**, *16* (2), 173–177.

52. Roberfroid, M.; Gibson, G.R.; Hoyles, L.; McCartney, A.L.; Rastall, R.; Rowland, I.; Wolvers, D.; Watzl, B.; Szajewska, H. Prebiotic effects: metabolic and health benefits. *British Journal of Nutrition,* **2010**, *104* (2), 1–63.

53. Scarminio, V.; Fruet, A.C.; Witaicenis, A.; Rall, V.L.M.; Di Stasi, L.C. Dietary intervention with green dwarf banana flour (*Musa* sp AAA) prevents intestinal inflammation in a trinitrobenzenesulfonic acid model of rat colitis. *Nutrition Research*, **2012**, *32*, 202–209.

54. Sheehan, D.; Shanahan, F. The gut microbiota in inflammatory bowel disease. *Gastroenterology Clinics of North America*, **2017**, *46* (1), 143–154.

55. Simmonds, N.W.; Shepherd, K. The taxonomy and origins of the cultivated bananas. *The Journal of the Linnean Society. Botany*, **1955**, *55*, 302–312.

56. Singh, B.; Singh, J.P.; Kaur, A.; Singh, N. bioactive compounds in banana and their associated health benefits—a review. *Food Chemistry*, **2016**, *206*, 1–11.

57. Soldavini, J.; Kaunitz, J.D. Pathobiology and potential therapeutic value of intestinal short-chain fatty acids in gut inflammation and obesity. *Digestive Diseases and Sciences*, **2013**, *58* (10), 2756–2766.

58. Soorianathasundaram, K.; Narayana, C.K.; Paliyath, G. Bananas and plantains. In: *Encyclopedia of Food and Health*, Caballero, B.; Finglas, P.; Toldra, F. (Eds.); Illinois, USA: Academic Press Inc.; **2016**, pp. 320–327.

59. Souza, H.S.P. Etiopathogenesis of inflammatory bowel disease: today and tomorrow. *Current Opinion in Gastroenterology*, **2017**, *33* (4), 222–229.

60. Tang, Y.; Chen, Y.; Jiang, H.; Robbins, G.T.; Nie, D. G-protein-coupled receptor for short-chain fatty acids suppresses colon cancer. *International Journal of Cancer*, **2011**, *128* (4), 847–856.
61. Thaiss, C.A.; Zmora, N.; Levy, M.; Elinav, E. The microbiome and innate immunity. *Nature*, **2016**, *535* (7610), 65–74.
62. Vinolo, M.A.; Rodrigues, H.G.; Hatanaka, E. Suppressive effect of short-chain fatty acids on production of proinflammatory mediators by neutrophils. *The Journal of Nutritional Biochemistry*, **2011**, *22* (9), 849–855.
63. Vu, H.T; Scarlett, C.J.; Vuong, Q.V. Phenolic compounds within banana peel and their potential uses: a review. *Journal of Functional Foods*, **2018**, *40*, 238–248.
64. Walker, W.A.; Duffy, L.C. Diet and bacterial colonization: role of probiotics and prebiotics. *The Journal of Nutritional Biochemistry*, **1998**, *9*, 668–675.
65. Weingarden, A.R.; Vaughn, B.P. Intestinal Microbiota, fecal microbiota transplantation, and inflammatory bowel disease. *Gut Microbes*, **2017**, *8* (3), 238–252.
66. Xavier, R.J. & Podolsky, D.K. Unravelling the pathogenesis of inflammatory bowel disease. *Nature*, **2007**, *448*, 427–434.
67. Zhang, P.; Whistler, R.L.; BeMiller, J.N.; Hamaker, B.R. Banana Starch: production, physicochemical properties, and digestibility—a review. *Carbohydrate Polymers*, **2005**, 59, 443–458.
68. Zhou, G.X.; Liu, Z. potential roles of neutrophils in regulating intestinal mucosal inflammation of inflammatory bowel disease. *Journal of Digestive Diseases*, **2017**, *18* (9), 495–503.

# CHAPTER 9

# ANTICANCER PROPERTIES OF SILVER NANOPARTICLES FROM ROOT EXTRACT OF TRIGONELLA FOENUM-GRAECUM

RAMASAMY HARIKRISHNAN*, LOURTHU SAMY SHANTHI MARI, GUNAPATHY DEVI, and CHELLAM BALASUNDARAM

## ABSTRACT

The present study reports on the biosynthesis of silver nanoparticles (AgNPs) with the root extract of *Trigonella foenum-graecum* (TFAgNPs) and its anticancer activity against A498 cancerous cells by apoptosis through mass drug administration (MDA). The characteristic reaction observed by the color change from neutral to visible brown at pH 11.0 was due to SPR. The scanning electron microscope (SEM) analysis indicated that the spherical shape with size between 20 and 40 nm. In the UV–Vis spectral study was maximum absorption peaks were noted at 420 and 430 nm, respectively. The particle size distribution (PSD) of the TFAgNPs using dynamic light scattering showed that their average size is 120 nm. The X-ray diffraction (XRD) patterns indicate that TFAgNPs comprise a high-intensity diffraction peak at 38.18° corresponding to that of the crystalline Ag. The Fourier transform infrared spectroscopy (FTIR) spectra study confirmed that many functional groups are associated in TFAgNPs; they could eliminate the cancerous A498 cells better than the normal PBMCs. TFAgNPs exhibited a dose-dependent decline in cell viability with an increasingly significant in MDA and decrease intracellular. The apoptosis significantly increased in FTAgNPs treated cells and resulted in a significant decline in caspase-8 role with conflicting upturns in caspase-3/-7/-9 roles. Further, the western

*Corresponding author. E-mail: rhari123@yahoo.com.

blots revealed an augmented expression of smac/DIABLO, p53, Bax, and PARP-1. These results suggest that FTAgNPs induce cell death with A498 via mt facilitated key apoptotic program. Further detailed exploration is necessary to promising using of TFAgNPs in other cancer cell therapy trials.

## 9.1   INTRODUCTION

Nanotechnology continues to play a significant role in the biotechnology-related industry for the past several years. However, the annual global investment by the government and private sector in this promising sector exceeds several billion dollars [61]. Though the NPs synthesis can be accomplished by chemical, physical, and biological means, the use of NPs critically depends on the particle size, shape, and composition. Since NPs-based gold (Au), silver (Ag) as well as platinum (Pd) is expansively useful in human health; there is a dire necessity to progress eco-friendly NPs synthesis using without any toxic compounds. In this regard, NPs synthesis, biological methods using microorganisms, enzymes, and plant products have been offered a promising alternating environ-friendly *in lieu* of chemical as well as physical procedures [2].

In order to effectively synthesize NPs of desired size and shape, attention should be paid to three important factors, that is, the choice of solvent, reducing agent, and a biocompatible stabilizer [32]. In physicochemical methods, elimination of organic solvents is usually impossible to achieve because of the structure of stabilizers, which are rarely soluble in water; hence the biological methods are favored.

In recent years, attempts to make metallic nanoparticles (MNPs) from noble metals such as Ag, Au as well as Pd have succeeded through unicellular microorganisms like bacteria [39, 51], fungi [1], and plant parts [4, 6]. The abundant availability of biological materials for the synthesis of AgNPs bears tremendous hope for applications in pharmaceutical and biomedical industry especially since they are not using any toxic compounds in the synthesis techniques [45]. Besides it being cheap and eco-friendly not using high energy, temperature, pressure as well as toxic compounds [15]. Further, it was described that AgNPs are lesser or nontoxic to humans but it is most efficient to bacteria, virus as well as other eukaryotes at less concentrations without side effect [23].

The primary important utilization of Ag and AgNPs is in the medicinal field in the production of humid creams to inhibit infection from burns and open injuries [20]. Moreover, numerous salts containing Ag and its byproducts are commercially produced as antimicrobial agents [27]. As active component, Ag has been widely applied in wound dressings and bandages due to its wide-spectrum antibactericidal against Gram-positive or bacteria [56]. AgNPs had been used as potent bactericide [41], antimicotic [43], and anticancer [55] agents.

Recently, plant tissues or fruits have been used in the synthesis of NPs. Extracts from plants usually contain various polyphenols, which form excellent reducing agents and hence synthesis Ag or Au NPs beneficially used of the chosen size. Indeed, it is continuously used as the best methods for treating different diseases associated with cell proliferation or cell death [58].

Renal cell carcinoma (RCC) recorded nearly 3% of adult malignancies and over 90% for renal cancers [10]. After the prostate and bladder cancer, RCC is a third most common urino-genital cancer that produces over 40% mortality [59]. Therefore, the preventive and management of measure of RCC, particularly metastatic RCC, pose a dangerous task as a major health issue. Hence further clear empathetic of RCC pathogenesis is necessary for producing new target therapies or biomarkers to enhance the efficiency of treatment.

*Trigonella foenum-graecum* is the major fenugreek, distributed in various countries like Pakistan, India, Iran, Nepal, Bangladesh, and Egypt. Fenugreek has the most beneficial action on cold, hay fever, catarrh, bronchial asthma, influenza, emphysema, laryngitis, pneumonia, pleurisy, tuberculosis, complaint, sore throat, and sinusitis. Several studies indicate that the active ingredients sourced from this plant can control various cancer cells.

This chapter focuses on the biosynthesis of AgNPs from root extract of *Trigonella foenum-graecum* and discusses the effects of its anticancer properties on A498 cancerous cells by apoptosis through MDA.

## 9.2 MATERIALS AND METHODS

### 9.2.1 BIOSYNTHESIS OF TFAGNPS

Fresh healthy plant roots of *Trigonella foenum-graecum* (L) were collected, thoroughly washed in purified water, air-dried for several days, and pulverized into a fine powder. Twenty grams of this taken in a conical flask was dissolved in 200 mL of distilled sterile water and mixed with 1 mM of silver nitrate ($AgNO_3$); the solution was mixed well for a few minutes and then incubated 30 min in a water bath, and filtered in Whattman (No. 1) paper and then extract was collected using as reducing agent and stabilizer. The color change observed from neutral to brown at pH 11.0 exhibited the formation of AgNPs. After this, solution was centrifugated for 20 min (5000 rpm) to collect the precipitate, which was air dried and powdered for nanocharacterization by using UV–Vis., SEM, dynamic light scattering (DLS), zeta potential, XRD, and FTIR analysis.

### 9.2.2   REDUCTION OF BIOSYNTHESIZED TFAGNPS

Reduction of $AgNO_3$ to $Ag^+$ was proved by color changes (from neutral to brown) at pH 11.0 in aqueous resolution because of the excitation of SPR in AgNPs, which indicated the formation of biosynthesized TFAgNPs.

### 9.2.3   UV–VIS SPECTRUM ANALYSIS

The biosynthesized TFAgNPs remained characterized by UV–Vis spectroscopy, a widely used technique to characterize the AgNPs. The drop of pure $Ag^+$ into $Ag^0$ was confirmed by determining using UV–Vis spectrum by dissolving a small quantity of the sample in sterile distilled water. Reduction of $Ag^+$ ions was analyzed using UV-spectrophotometer (SYSTRONICS) determination of 1 nm ranging from 300 to 1100 nm with a scanning speed 300 nm/min at room temperature (RT). To observe the absorption peaks, indicating the presence of AgNPs due to SPR phenomenon, the reduction of $Ag^+$ was determined by UV–Visible spectrum response at various time periods using at 1 mL sample corresponding blank containing at 1 mL distilled water.

### 9.2.4   SEM

SEM study was done using a SEM machine (Thermo Scientific, Carl Zeiss Sigma model-FESEM). A thin film was prepared using TFAgNPs sample in carbon glazed copper grid using a very little quantity dropping of TFAgNPs sample; the excess sample is expel by blotting paper. The prepared thin-film was put on the SEM grid and allowed for 5 min drying using a mercury lamp.

### 9.2.5  DLS

The biosynthesized TFAgNPs were further discriminated using DLS by a Zeta Potential analyzer (Brookhaven). The TFAgNPs average particle size and polydispersity described relative thickness of the size scattering by DLS.

### 9.2.6  ZETA POTENTIAL

Size as well as zeta potential of the biosynthesized TFAgNPs were measured by Malvern Zetasizer (ZEN 3600, UK), which allowed the analysis of scattering particle size range 2–3 nm.

### 9.2.7  XRD

The examination of biosynthesized TFAgNPs was completed in an X'Pert Pro X-ray diffractometer manufactured by PANalytical, The Netherlands. Drop-coated films sample was prepared to determine the formation of TFAgNPs functioned at 40 kV intensity and 30 mA electric current with CuKα energy in θ–2θ composition. Debye–Scherer's formula was carried out to measure the TFAgNPs size and the two values of the XRD peaks.

Debye–Scherrer's formula:

$$D = [K\lambda] / [\beta \cos q] \tag{9.1}$$

where $K$ is a constant, $\lambda$ is wavelength of the X-ray, $\beta$ is full-girth-half maximum of XRD peak or radians, and $q$ is Bragg's position of the XRD peak.

### 9.2.8  FTIR

Ten milligrams of the powdered sample was taken from the biosynthesized TFAgNPs and was imperiled to FTIR examination in a Perkin Elmer-RX1 spectrophotometer (Paragon 500) in the distributed reluctancy mode at $4\ cm^{-1}$ resolution in KBr pellets. The measurement was carried out by JASCO (FTIR-6200) spectra. FTIR analysis is attempted to ensure the crystalline formation of nanocrystals and determine the adsorbed classes on the surface of crystal and the associated functional groups. The FTIR spectroscopy was analyzed in the wave ranging from 400 to 4000 cm$^{-1}$.

## 9.2.9 ANTIMICROBIAL ACTIVITY

Following microbial cultures were purchased from MTCC, IMTECH, Chandigarh and used in the study:

- *Aeromonas hydrophila* (MTCC 1739),
- *Arthrobacter* sp. (MTCC 2937).
- *Candida albicans* (MTCC 227),
- *Escherichia coli* (MTCC 2939 & MTCC 739),
- *Pseudomonas aeruginosa* (MTCC 1934 & MTCC 2453),
- *Rhodococcus rhodochrous* (MTCC 265),
- *Staphylococcus aureus* (MTCC 96 & MTCC 2940),

New overnight cultures of each pathogen were inoculate (100 μL) and evenly spread on NA plate's surface in different plates. These organisms are commonly isolated as multidrug resistant human pathogens.

Mueller–Hinton Agar (MHA) was prepared and disinfected in a autoclave at 121 °C for 15 min (15 psi pressure) to investigate the antibacterial activity of biosynthesized TFAgNPs. Then sterile MHA (20 mL) was poured aseptically into each sterile petridish and accepted for solidification at RM under sterile conditions. After solidifying, petriplates were spread with MTCC cultures. The wells were bored in each plate by using a sterile borer. Twenty microliters of the sample (containing 5 mg/L) of the biosynthesized TFAgNPs together with standard antibiotic were laden with equal quantity in each well on the plates. Dimethyl sulfoxide (DMSO) and AgNO$_3$ were used and loaded in respective wells for control. The petri plates were then kept at 37 °C and they measure the activity of clearly visible after 24 h. The ZI was determined and the sample of the biosynthesized TFAgNPs was noted as the highest antimicrobial activity.

## 9.2.10 CYTOTOXICITY ASSAY

The cells were then treated with biosynthesized TFAgNPs at 0, 50, 100, 150, 200, 250, 300, 350, 400, 500, and 1000 μg mL$^{-1}$ concentrations for 24 h. The 1% methanol was used negative control for comparison. Following 24 h of cell treatment, 0.5 mg mL$^{-1}$ of MTT dye is included in every well and then kept for 3 h for the formation of formazan crystal products. It was dissolved with 100 μL of DMSO and incubated for 15 min. After the quantity of purple formazan products was analyzed by measuring O.D. at 595 nm using a microplate reader following ELISA assay. It was executed in triplicate plates and calculated the percentage of cell viability. The cell growth was revealed as the percentage of absorbance in cells with biosynthesized TFAgNPs treatment to those in cells with AgNPs treatment (100%).

### 9.2.11 ADENOSINE TRIPHOSPHATE (ATP) ASSAY

About 20,000 cells were allocated with O 96-w microtitre plate in six replicates containing 50 μL ATP CellTitre Glo (Promega, Madison) reagent (50 μL) and kept 30 min in dark RT. After the signal proportional of luminescent in the nuclear or cellular ATP contents were sensed by a microplate reader manufacturing by Modulus™ at Turner Biosystems. Then the obtained data were asserted as ± RLU.

### 9.2.12 GSH ASSAY

For GSH assay, GSH-Glo™ manufacturing by Promega at Madison was used to estimate intracellular GSH levels. Consequently, 10,000 cells were taken in each well of O 96-w microtitre plate culture medium in six replicates and discarded medium then 25 μL of 1X GSH-Glo™ reagent was added according to GSH-Glo™ kit instructions in each well. At range, 0-5M GSH standards were consecutively twofold diluted from a 5 mM standard in deionized water and mixed well. After 30 min in the shaken incubator at RT, each well 100 μL Luciferin detection reagent was added and then incubate RT for 15 min, then luminescence was sensed in a luminometer microplate reader manufacturing by Modulus™ at Turner Biosystems. Based on the obtained results, a standardization curve was prepared and concentrations of sample GSH (μM) were calculated.

### 9.2.13 MDA

The synthesis of AgNPs-mediated ROS generation of MDA levels was determined by TBARS assay. Briefly, the test tubes were added 2% $H_3PO_4$

for 200 μL, 7% $H_3PO_4$ for 400 μL, 400 μL of *tert*-butyl alcohol/BHT solution, and 200 μL of 1M HCL. Each well of six-well plate was added 50,000 cells and incubated in RT then recovered supernatants. Each test tubes of 100 μL cell supernatant was added and all in triplicate. Subsequently, a positive control test tube was prepared by adding 1 μL of MDA reagent and all tubes kept in a hot water bath at 100 °C for 15 min and then cooled to RT. Then each tube was added with 1.5 mL butanol, vortexed for 10 s, and left undisturbed for a few minutes to enable separation into two different phases. From the top, butanol phase layer was taken 800 μL each into 1.5 mL test tubes and centrifuged (840g) for 6 min at 24 °C. From this 100 μL of the supernatant was shifted in six replicates to a 96-well micotitre plate, and the O.D. absorbance was measured at 532/600 nm in a spectrophotometer. The ±O.D. absorbance is divided by the loss coefficient (156 mM$^{-1}$) stated as μM concentrations.

### 9.2.14   CASPASE ASSAY

The activity of caspase (-3/-7,/-8,/-9) was quantified using Caspase-GloW® kit (Promega, Madison, USA) according to the manufacturer's procedure. The Caspase-GloW® reagents (-3/-7,/-8,/-9) were reconstituted and added in each O 96-w microtitre plate as maintained in six replicates (each well 40 μL of reagent/100 μL suspension containing 10,000 cells). It was mixed properly, incubated for 30 min in dark RT, and the luminescent signal in a microplate luminometer (Modulus™, Turner Biosystems) was measured. The obtained caspases activities data were expressed as RLU.

### 9.2.15   APOPTOSIS ANALYSIS

After incubation and washing the cells, about $1 \times 10^6$ cells picked with Annexin V-FITC (invitrogen) and PI (invitrogen) reagents using color binding buffer as per the manufacturer's procedure. The obtaining FITC or PI fluorescent signals were determined at 518 and 620 nm by using Beckman coulter FACS machine manufacturing by Beckman. There were 30,000 events that were observed in each time/analysis using FCS Express V3 software developed by De Novo Software, Canada and Microsoft Excel using for calculation. The percentage (%) apoptosis is the calculation of Annexin V (FITC$^+$/PI$^-$) and Annexin V (FITC$^+$/PI$^+$) cells.

## 9.2.16   MITOCHONDRIAL MEMBRANE POTENTIAL (ΔΨ)

The ΔΨ assay was performed by BD™ MitoScreen kit manufacturing by BD Biosciences. Cationic dye, JC-1 is highly sensible to ΔΨ which gathers in mt-polarized membranes part. A 100 µL working JC-1 solution and 100 µL of cell suspension added in each flow cytometry tube, incubated for 15 min at 37 °C containing with 5% $CO_2$. Then 100 µL JC-1 wash buffer was added in each tube. Around 50,000 events were gated to exclude cellular debris by FACS Calibur flow cytometer (CellQuest PRO v4.02 software/ FlowJo v7.1 software) for mt depolarization and the results were stated as % of total events.

## 9.2.17   COMET ASSAY

DNA fragmentation in the AgNPs treated cells and control cells were used to observe in the comet assay. Briefly, each sample three slides were prepared: (1) 1st layer contains with 400 µL of 1% LMPA at 37 °C; (2) second layer cells contains with 25 µL in each sample along 0.5% LMPA for 175 µL at 37 °C; (3) third layer contains with 200 µL of 1% LMPA at 37 °C. The coverslips were detached in each layer and the slides were exposed to lysis (at 4 °C for 1 h to protect from light) by existence flooded in cells lysis buffer containing with 2.5 M NaCl and 100 mM EDTA, 1% Triton™ X-100, 10 mM Tris pH at 10, and 10% DMSO, then slides calibrated for 20 min in electrophoresis buffer pH at 13 that containing 300 mM NaOH, 1 mM $Na_2$EDTA, and finally electrophoresis (300 mA, 25V, 35 min). After electrophoresis, slides wash away three times for 5 min each wash in 0.4 M Tris-buffer (pH 7.4) then marked at 40 µL EtBr. After washing, coverslips laid on slides and kept at 4 °C overnight and observed by fluorescent microscope manufacturing by Olympus IXSI inverted microscope, images captured, and comet tails of 50 cells using Soft Imaging System (Life Science, analySISW v5). The obtained data remained stated as mean tail length in *micrometer*.

## 9.2.18   WESTERN BLOT ANALYSIS

The Cytobuster™ reagent (Novagen) containing inhibitors such as protease (Roche, 05892791001) and phosphatase (Roche, 04906837001) was used for protein purification. Cytobuster (200 µL) was included in cells and incubated at 4 °C for 10 min. The mixtures were centrifuged at 180g for 10 min at 4 °C and then a crude protein extracts was obtained, quantified and standardized to 1 mg mL$^{-1}$ by bicinchoninic assay. An aliquot of 25 μL of each sample was 7.5% electrophoresis and transmitted to nitrocellulose membranes. Then blocking the membranes treated for 1 h with 3% BSA in TBS (20 mM Tris–HCl at pH 7.4, 500 mM NaCl, and 0.01% TBST) and then kept overnight at 4 °C with primary Ab in 1% BSA in TBST. After the membranes were washed three times for 15 min each with 10 mL TBST and after incubated for 1 h in RT with secondary Ab. Again the membranes were washed three times for 15 min each with TBST and then detected immuno-activity using KPL system (UViTech Alliance 2.7). The protein spots were evaluated using UViBand Image software and the obtained data were stated as mean RBI.

### 9.2.19   MEASUREMENT OF ROS GENERATION

The ROS generation determined from intracellular levels by DCFH-DA method. The DCFH-DA is a lipophilic cell-permeable compound; it was de-acetylated to DCF form through cellular esterases in the cytoplasm. The DCF was oxidized by some radicals (peroxyl, hydroxyl, nitrate, carbonate, alkoxyl) measured to a fluorescent marked molecule in 530 nm excitation or 485 nm emission. If the DCF is not oxidized by $H_2O_2$ per se nor $O_2^-$; reflects lysosomal and $\Delta\Psi$ permeabilisation (which implicates to discharge of redox-reactive ions as well as cytochrome c and catalyzed DCF oxidation) and accumulates DCF in cytosol is incapable to enter mt. Black 96-well microtitre plates with transparent bottom were coated with A498 cells and incubated for 24 h with different concentration of TFAgNPs (5, 10, 20 μg m$^{-1}$). Then the cells were cleaned using HBSS and laden with HBSS containing 20 μM DCFHDA incubated for 30 min (37 °C). Then, the cells washing by HBSS and measured every 5 min for 30 min interval at 37 °C to identify fluorescence 485 nm excitation and 535 nm emission measured in a plate reader manufacturing by Tecan Infinite F200. A 15 μM TBP was used for positive control and the ROS rise determination as mean slope/min compared with unexposed control cells as expressed mean ± S.D. of four independent experiments.

### 9.2.20   STATISTICAL ANALYSIS

All the data were calculated by using Biostat software (AnalystSoft Inc., Canada). The statistical significance between groups of the differences determined one-way and two-way ANOVA model with post hoc comparisons of the reaction of treatment by the viability of the cells ($P < 0.05$).

## 9.3 RESULTS

### 9.3.1 VISIBLE REDUCTION OF SILVER IONS

The biosynthesized TFAgNPs was proven through the color variation pH 11.0 (from neutral to brown, Figure 9.1). The biosynthesized TFAgNPs in different pH before adding 1 mM AgNO$_3$ is shown by color change from light yellow solution to brown at pH 11.0 (Figure 9.1A), whereas the TFAgNPs in different pH after adding 1 mM AgNO$_3$ is shown by color change from neutral to brown at pH 11.0 (Figure 9.1B).

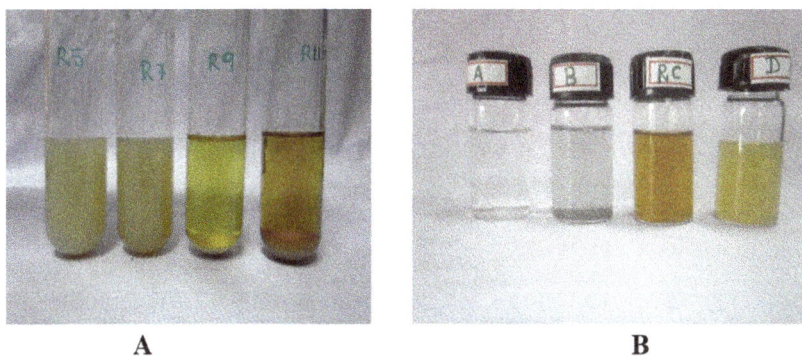

**FIGURE 9.1** Visible reduction of silver ions of biosynthesized TFAgNPs: (A) TFAgNPs in different pH before adding 1 mM AgNO$_3$ shown color change from light yellow solution to brown color at pH 11.0. (B) TFAgNPs in different pH after adding 1 mM AgNO$_3$ shown color change from colorless solution to brown color at pH 11.0.

### 9.3.2 UV–VIS SPECTRUM ANALYSIS

UV–Visible spectroscopic examination was carried out to confirm the synthesis and study the size as well as the shape of NPs in the liquid solution. To verify the biosynthesized TFAgNPs, the test samples were monitored for their absorbance between 300 and 650 nm, respectively, by UV–Visible spectrophotometer. The developmental reaction among metal ions and

herbal extracts were distinguished by UV–Visible spectrum of the biosynthesized TFAgNPs in a liquid solution at different wavelengths (Figure
9.2). The maximum absorbance was observed at 430 nm thus validating
the biosynthesis of TFAgNPs. The reduction of $Ag^+$ and the development of
constant NPs ensued quickly (within an hour) of response; thus producing
it one rapid bioreduction procedures to provide Ag nanostructures described
until. The surface plasmon band in biosynthesized AgNPs solution in case of
biological method remains closer to 430 nm, while it is close to 450 nm in
case of chemically synthesized AgNPs. Plasmon absorption band at 430 nm
indicates the existence of spherical or roughly spherical of TFAgNPs.

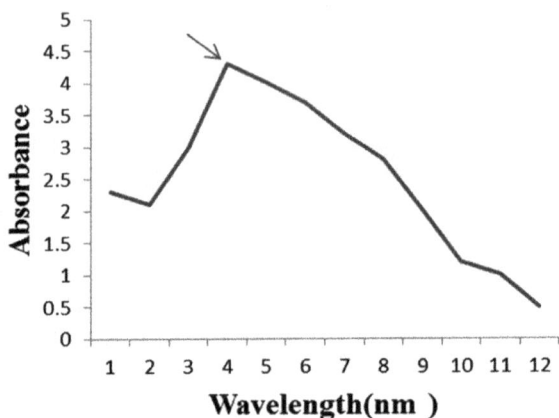

**FIGURE 9.2**    UV-spectrum of biosynthesized TFAgNPs.

### 9.3.3   SEM ANALYSIS

The size, shape, and morphological structure of biosynthesized TFAgNPs
was studied using SEM analysis, which showed that TFAgNPs are spherical
with size ranging between 70 and 90 nm (Figure 9.3).

The particle size average is 82 nm. The size of TFAgNPs using plant
extract is smaller than the chemically synthesized AgNPs, indicating its great
importance in applications (Figure 9.3A and B).

### 9.3.4   DLS ANALYSIS

The particle size distribution (PSD) of the biosynthesized TFAgNPs by
DLS showed that the colloidal solution comprises particles of various size;

some were in average size between 5 and 120 nm. The average size of the nanoparticles is 81.3 nm (Figure 9.4).

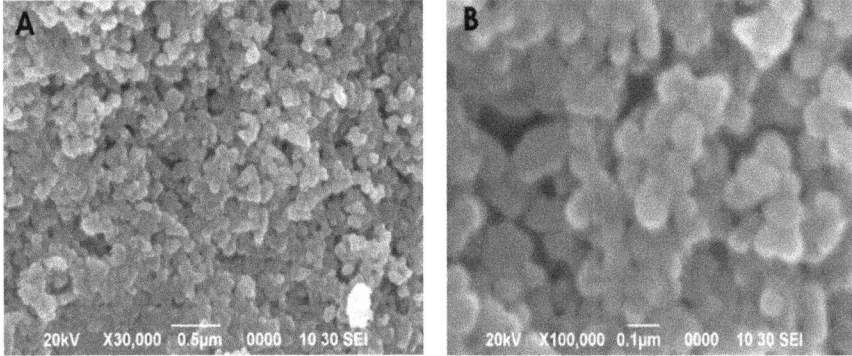

**FIGURE 9.3**    The size and morphological structure of synthesis AgNPs using SEM analysis: (A) low magnification, (B) high magnification.

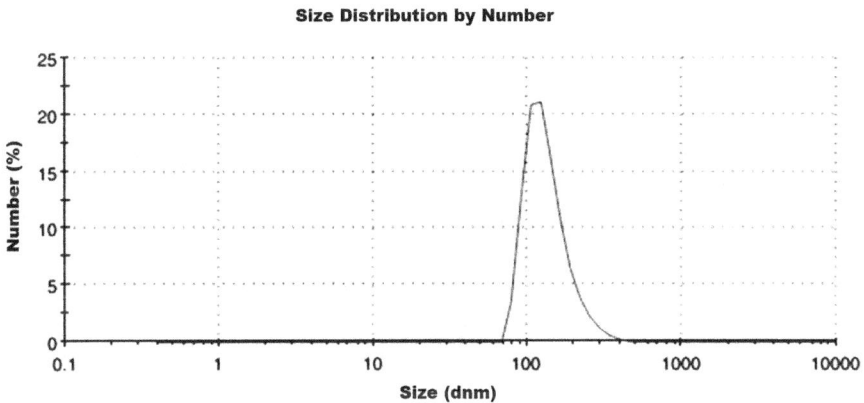

**FIGURE 9.4**    The particle size distributions (PSD) of biosynthesized TFAgNPs by dynamic light scattering (DLS).

## 9.3.5   ZETA POTENTIAL

The nanostructure of biosynthesized TFAgNPs by DLS was advance confirmation by the distinguishing peaks obtained from Zeta sizer image. Further, it designated that the average of NPs distance range is 581 d.nm conforming average zeta potential (−35.3 mV) as suggested highest constancy of AgNPs and indicates good capping of NPs by negatively charged groups. A very high potential negative value might be due to the capping of polyphenolic elements existing in the extract. This study also confirmed the stability of the biosynthesized AgNPs (Figure 9.5).

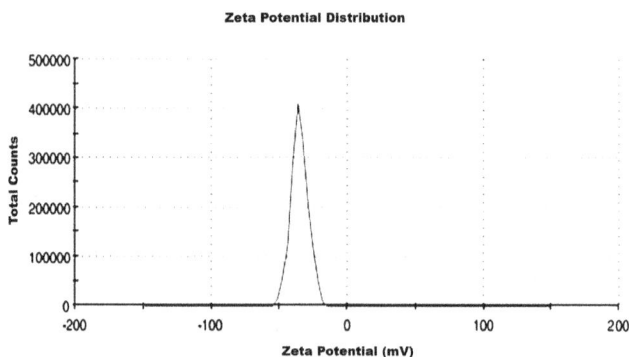

**FIGURE 9.5**   The zeta potential of biosynthesized TFAgNPs by dynamic light scattering (DLS).

### 9.3.6   XRD ANALYSIS

The biosynthesized TFAgNPs nature is crystalline, and the diffraction peaks correspond as hexagonal zincite part of AgNPs. The diffraction configuration and interplanar arrangement are very closely related to standard Ag diffraction configuration. The peaks at $2\theta = 28.71°$, $31.65°$, $47.45°$, $55.63°$, $58.12°$, and $78.87°$ were dispersed to the (111), (100), (200), (311), (110), and (311) reflection lines of AgNPs, respectively. These contracts with the component cell of the FCC structure (JCPDS File No. 04-0783). No other impurities characteristic peaks were sensed, this proposes obtained high-quality AgNPs. In addition, the peak existed extended, indicating that size of NPs looked very small affording to Equation (9.1). The crystallite average size was determined 25 nm by the DS calculation. It is confirmed that the NPs were composed of pure crystalline Ag (Figure 9.6).

### 9.3.7   FTIR ANALYSIS

The FTIR study discovered for carbonyl amino acid residues group as well as proteins is facilitating a strong bind to the metal, which indicates that the proteins might be possible from the MNPs (i.e., AgNPs capping) that could avert accumulation and thus steady the medium. It proposed that the biomolecules might feasibly accomplish twin role in the development and stabilization of AgNPs in a liquid medium. The obtained effects suggest that sugars, proteins, amino acid existing in the extracts, which play a key role in the drop of Ag$^+$. The FTIR measurement was agreed to categorize the potential molecules involved during the biological reduction reactions of biosynthesized TFAgNPs before and after adding 1 mM AgNO$_3$. The spectrum of TFAgNPs was found ranging between 400 and 4000 cm$^{-1}$ and observed different bands at 3907.08 cm$^{-1}$, 3870.0 cm$^{-1}$, 3357.10 cm$^{-1}$, 2925.81 cm$^{-1}$, 2371.55 cm$^{-1}$, 2148.58 cm$^{-1}$, 1653.61 cm$^{-1}$, 1427.02 cm$^{-1}$, 1252.04 cm$^{-1}$, 1055.53 cm$^{-1}$, 634.67 cm$^{-1}$, and 539.08 cm$^{-1}$; thus related with amide, thiocynate (–SCN), carbonate ion, organic phosphates (P=O), aliphatic iodo compounds, thio ethers (CH3-S-(C-S), methylene-C–H asym/sym, normal polymeric, and phosphate ion (Figure 9.7).

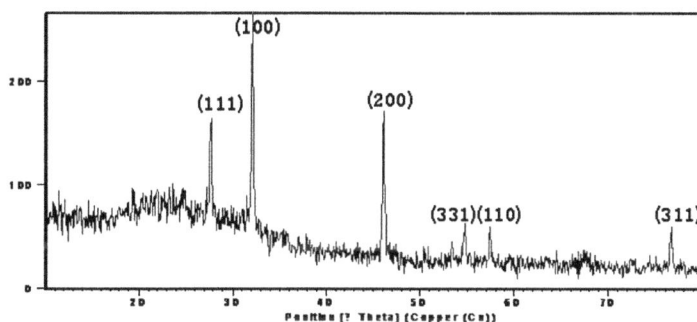

FIGURE 9.6   The XRD analysis of biosynthesized TFAgNPs.

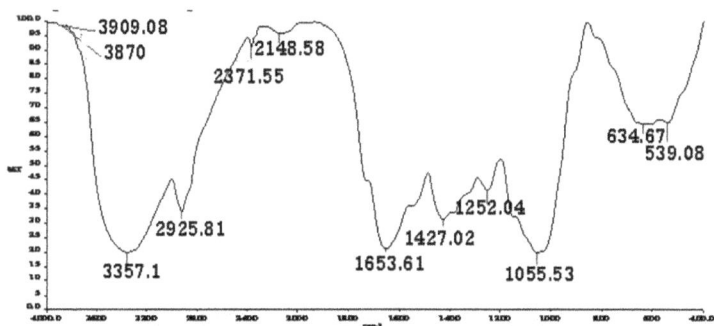

FIGURE 9.7   FTIR measurement of the possible molecules responsible for the reduction of biosynthesized TFAgNPs.

## 9.3.8 ANTIBACTERIAL ACTIVITY

The antibactericidal effect was carried out using biosynthesized TFAgNPs through the formation of ZI. The ZI is the zone area on control agar plate where the growth of tested microorganism is inhibited by an antibiotic commonly employed on the surface agar. If the tested microorganism is susceptible to the antibiotic, it never grows in the presence of the antibiotic. The ZI size is a quantity of the biocompound's efficacy, the large clear inhibition zone around the antibiotic is the highest activity of the compound. The clear zone surrounding the wells in the other plates demonstrated the activity of TFAgNPs (Tables 9.1 and 9.2). The measurement of ZI before adding 1 mM of biosynthesized TFAgNPs at various concentrations against all the tested multidrug resistance human pathogens ranged from 1 to 3 mm. The ZI after adding 1 mM AgNO$_3$ at a concentration of 100 $\mu$g mL$^{-1}$ of the root extract against all the tested human pathogens was between 2 and 5 mm. However, after adding 1 mM AgNO$_3$ at a concentration of 150 $\mu$g mL$^{-1}$ of the root extract was tested against human pathogens with the ZI between 4 and 7 mm indicating high potency.

**TABLE 9.1**  Measurement of Zone of Inhibition of Biosynthesized TFAgNPs Before Adding 1 mM AgNO$_3$ Against Human Pathogens

| Tested Pathogens | Zone of Inhibition (mm) at Different Concentrations | | | |
|---|---|---|---|---|
| | 0 $\mu$g mL$^{-1}$ | 50 $\mu$g mL$^{-1}$ | 100 $\mu$g mL$^{-1}$ | 100 $\mu$g mL$^{-1}$ |
| *Aeromonas hydrophila* (MTCC 1739) | – | – | 1 | 2 |
| *Arthrobacter* sp. (MTCC 2937) | 1 | – | 1 | 2 |
| *Candida albicans* (MTCC 227) | – | 1 | 2 | 2 |
| *Escherichia coli* (MTCC 2939) | 1 | 1 | 1 | 4 |
| *Escherichia coli* (MTCC 739) | – | – | 1 | 2 |
| *Pseudomonas aeruginosa* (MTCC 1934) | – | – | 1 | 2 |
| *Pseudomonas aeruginosa* (MTCC 2453) | – | 1 | 2 | 4 |
| *Rhodococcus rhodochrous* (MTCC 265) | – | – | 1 | 2 |
| *Staphylococcus aureus* (MTCC 2940) | – | – | 2 | 3 |
| *Staphylococcus aureus* (MTCC 96) | – | 2 | 3 | 4 |

TABLE 9.2  Measurement of Zone of Inhibition of Biosynthesized TFAgNPs After Adding 1 Mm AGNO$_3$ Against Human Pathogens

| Tested Pathogen | Zone of Inhibition (mm) in Different Concentration | | | |
| --- | --- | --- | --- | --- |
| | 0 µg mL$^{-1}$ | 50 µg mL$^{-1}$ | 100 µg mL$^{-1}$ | 100 µg mL$^{-1}$ |
| *Aeromonas hydrophila* (MTCC 1739) | 1 | 3 | 5 | 6 |
| *Arthrobacter* sp. (MTCC 2937) | 1 | 4 | 5 | 7 |
| *Candida albicans* (MTCC 227) | 1 | 3 | 5 | 6 |
| *Escherichia coli* (MTCC 2939) | 1 | 3 | 4 | 6 |
| *Escherichia coli* (MTCC 739) | 1 | 3 | 4 | 5 |
| *Pseudomonas aeruginosa* (MTCC 1934) | – | 3 | 4 | 5 |
| *Pseudomonas aeruginosa* (MTCC 2453) | – | 1 | 2 | 4 |
| *Rhodococcus rhodochrous* (MTCC 265) | 1 | 3 | 5 | 7 |
| *Staphylococcus aureus* (MTCC 2940) | – | 3 | 4 | 5 |
| *Staphylococcus aureus* (MTCC 96) | 2 | 4 | 4 | 6 |

The zone of inhibitions of TFAgNPs against different bacterial strains was observed and it indicates that the AgNPs control or arrest the growth. The control plates failed to show any growth progress of bacteria in the lack or the absence of antibacterial agents.

### 9.3.9   CELL MORPHOLOGY AND MTT ASSAY FOR CELL CYTOTOXICITY

The obtained results suggested that biosynthesized TFAgNPs treated A498 cells undertaken cell death; however, the nontreated cells observed very active. Therefore, TFAgNPs did not show distinctive morphological variations on A498 cells (Figure 9.8A and B). Biosynthesized TFAgNPs pointedly reduced the growth of A498 cells at a concentration ranging from 0 to 1000 µg used in this study. The IC$_{50}$ value was found to be 300 µg for A498 cells. A498 cells as well as normal PBMCs were evaluated the toxicity of TFAgNPs by MTT analyze; thus suggested that TFAgNPs dose-dependent cytotoxicity activity against A498 cells with a CC$_{50}$ value was 62.4 µg mL$^{-1}$;

however, the $CC_{50}$ value in the normal PBMCs is 768.2 µg mL$^{-1}$. Thus A498 cells demonstrated extremely better sensitivity ($P < 0.005$) to TFAgNPs as compared to normal PBMCs (Figure 9.9). However, TFAgNPs with a high concentration that is 1000 µg m$^{-1}$ did not display any cytotoxicity effect on A498 cells. Further detailed analyzed of the A498 cells were need to discovered whether the cytotoxicity due to apoptosis.

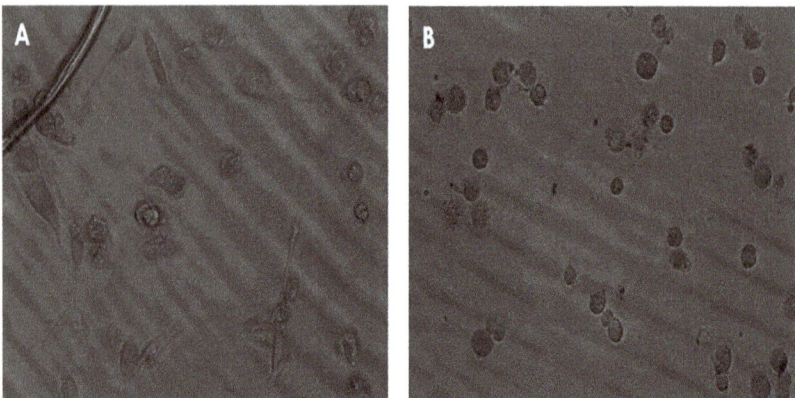

**FIGURE 9.8**  Effect of cell viability (cytotoxicity): before (A) and after (B) treated with biosynthesized TFAgNPs against A498 cells (human kidney carcinoma cell).

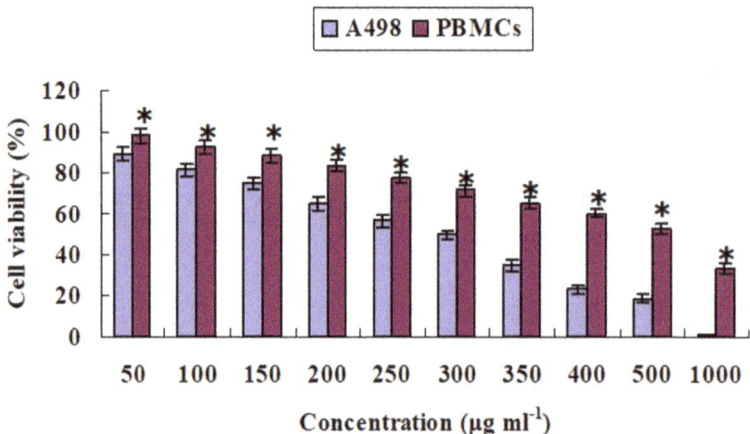

**FIGURE 9.9**  Differential cytotoxic effects of biosynthesized TFAgNPs on PBMCs cells and A498 cancerous. Data from a representative experiment are presented with error bars depicting standard error, $n = 3$. A two-way analysis of variance combined with a model-based means test indicates significant differences in viability between PBMCs cells and A498 ($P < 0.005$).

## 9.3.10   ATP ANALYSIS

The ATP levels were evaluated by luminometric assay. The biosynthesized TFAgNPs treated significantly decreased the levels of ATP with a 2.6-fold (treated $354,000 \pm 13,240$ RLU) compared to the control ($995,000 \pm 25,630$ RLU) (Figure 9.10).

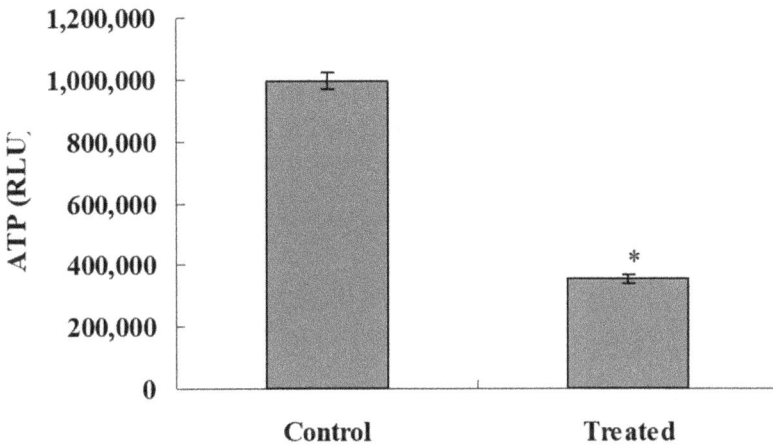

**FIGURE 9.10**   Levels of ATP in A498 Cells: Control and TFAgNPs Treated.

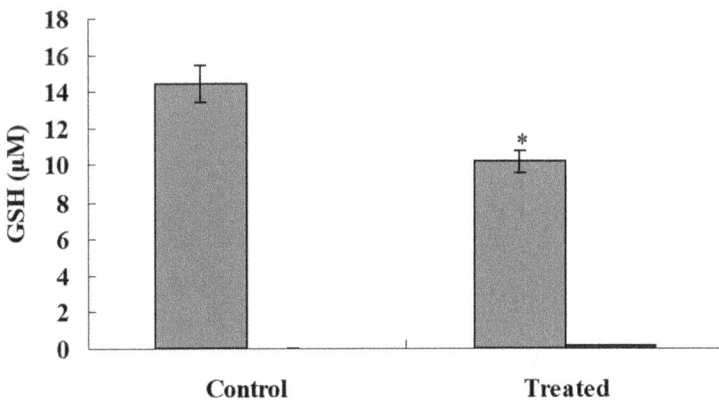

**FIGURE 9.11**   Level of glutathione (GSH) in A498 cells: control and TFAgNPs treated.

### 9.3.11   GLUTATHIONE (GSH) STATUS

The concentrations of GSH were quantified as a marker to determine the capacity of intracellular antioxidant. As shown in Figure 9.11, the concentration of GSH significantly decreased in biosynthesized TFAgNPs treated cells $(10.2 \pm 0.6 \ \mu M)$ compared to untreated cells $(14.5 \pm 1.0 \ \mu M)$.

### 9.3.12   LIPID PEROXIDATION (MDA)

MDA was shown significantly increased in cells reacted with the biosynthesized TFAgNPs $(0.15 \pm 0.008 \ \mu M)$ as related to controls $(0.02 \pm 0.004 \ \mu M)$ as seen in Figure 9.12.

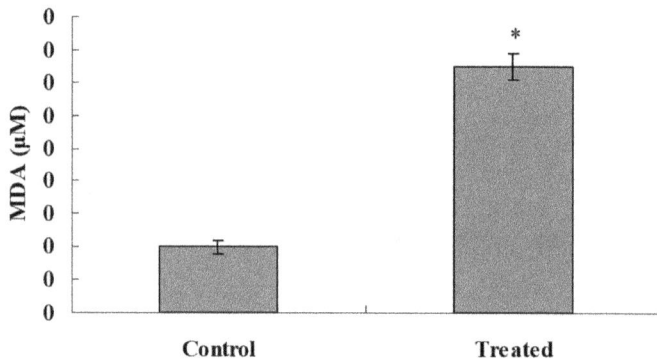

**FIGURE 9.12**   Lipid peroxidation (MDA) level in A498 cells: control and TFAgNPs treated.

### 9.3.13   ANALYSIS OF CASPASES

The biosynthesized TFAgNPs treated cells, caspase-3/-7 $(1.3 \times 10^5 \pm 8.2 \times 10^4)$ and caspase-8 $(4.4 \times 10^5 \pm 2.1 \times 10^4)$ significantly decreased when compared to the control $(8.9 \times 10^5 \pm 3.8 \times 10^2$ and $1.1 \times 10^6 \pm 2.3 \times 10^4)$. However, the cells were treated with biosynthesized TFAgNPs, caspase-9 $(1.2 \times 10^6 \pm 3.2 \times 10^4)$ significantly increased compared to the control $(9.1 \times 10^5 \pm 3.1 \times 10^4)$ as shown in Table 9.3.

**TABLE 9.3** Caspases Activity in Control and Biosynthesized TFAgNPs Treated Cells

| Caspases | Control (Mean ± SEM RLU) | Treated (Mean ± SEM RLU) |
|---|---|---|
| Caspase-3/-7 | $8.9 \times 10^5 \pm 3.8 \times 10^2$ | $1.3 \times 10^5 \pm 8.2 \times 10^4$* |
| Caspase-8 | $1.1 \times 10^6 \pm 2.3 \times 10^4$ | $4.4 \times 10^5 \pm 2.1 \times 10^4$* |
| Caspase-9 | $9.1 \times 10^5 \pm 3.1 \times 10^4$ | $1.2 \times 10^6 \pm 3.2 \times 10^4$* |

RLU: relative light units.

*Symbol indicates values are significantly different at ($p < 0.005$).

### 9.3.14 APOPTOSIS ANALYSIS BY FLOW CYTOMETERY

To confirm the apoptotic action further FACS examination. Apoptosis is inherently modified disassembly within the cell. Disassembly produces the modification of phospholipid content on the outer leaflet of cytoplasmic membrane and translocate or phagocytic cell recognition of phosphatidyl-serine on inner to the outer surface of the cell. It is a positive examination for apoptosis of TFAgNPs treated A498 cells (Figure 9.13A and B). To study whether TFAgNPs marks the oxidative role of the cell, we measured ROS in various time points by quantifying the fluorescent indication of DCF by FACS. Cells interacted with TFAgNPs were showed dose and time period and indicates ROS accumulation in cell lines (Figure 9.14).

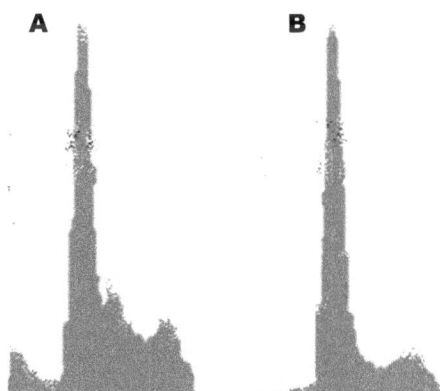

**FIGURE 9.13** FACS analysis for apoptosis induction of A498 cells (treated with biosynthesized TFAgNPs and then stained with Annexin V-PI to apoptotic cells): (A) control cells; (B) TFAgNPs treated cells.

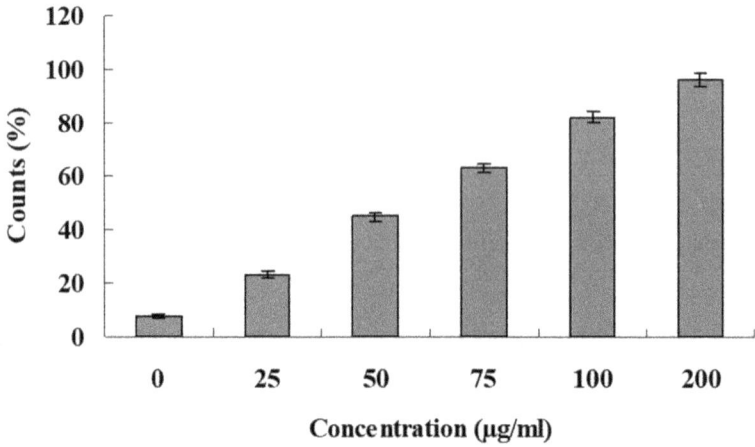

**FIGURE 9.14**   Apoptosis (%) by flow cytometery in A498 cells: control and TFAgNPs treated.

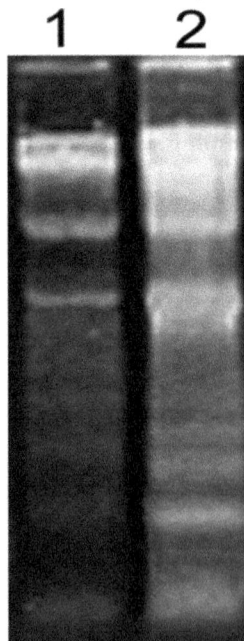

**FIGURE 9.15**   DNA fragmentation analysis was collected cellular DNA extraction after biosynthesized TFAgNPs treatment of A498 cells: Lane 1: Untreated cell (control), Lane 2: TFAgNPs treated.

## 9.3.15   DNA FRAGMENTATION ANALYSIS

The DNA pattern of the cells reacted with biosynthesized TFAgNPs combining with untreated control cells was evaluated. TFAgNPs treated cells start the apoptosis process, as evidenced by DNA fragmenting (Figure 9.15).

## 9.3.16   MITOCHONDRIAL MEMBRANE POTENTIAL (ΔΨ)

The initial intracellular actions happened in apoptosis owing to distraction of the $\Delta\Psi$, which show that biosynthesized TFAgNPs treatment results in loss of $\Delta\Psi$ in A498 cells. The obtained data demonstrated that TFAgNPs results may be due to dose-dependent loss of $\Delta\psi$m (Figure 9.16).

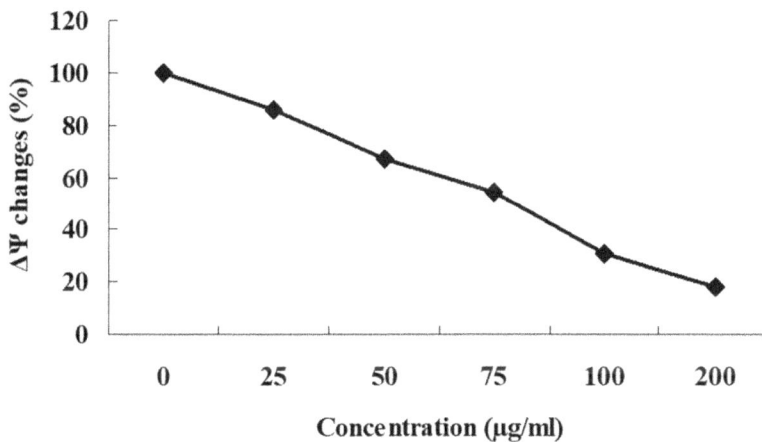

FIGURE 9.16   Quantification of mitochondrial membrane potential ($\Delta\Psi$) in biosynthesized TFAgNPs treated A498 cells.

## 9.3.17   APOPTOTIC PROTEINS INTERACTION

The certain apoptotic proteins expression was confirmed of flow cytometric intracellular marked with smac/DIABLO using western blot technique. The p53 protein manifestation is obtained to be significant when treated with high concentration of biosynthesized TFAgNP (1.12 ± 0.019RBI vs.

control: $0.86 \pm 0.048$RBI, 95% CI = $-0.41$ to $-0.00036$; $p = 0.0494$). On the other hand, a significant increase of PARP-1 after treatment with TFAgNP ($3.63 \pm 0.074$RBI vs. control: $3.32 \pm 0.0046$RBI, 95% CI = $-0.68$ to $-0.061$; $p = 0.0356$) was noted. The estimation of Bax protein is observed at greater levels in cells after treatment with TFAgNP ($3.6 \pm 0.14$RBI) as related to control untreated cells ($2.3 \pm 0.051$RBI, 95% CI = $-1.84$ to $-0.82$; $p = 0.0088$) although there was a highly significant difference in the smac/DIABLO expression among experimental and control cells. Therefore, TFAgNPs exposed cells existing a 4.4-fold high band strength ($1.26 \pm 0.046$RBI vs. control: $0.27 \pm 0.012$RBI, 95% CI = $-0.96$ to $-0.62$; $p = 0.0036$) as shown in Figure 9.17.

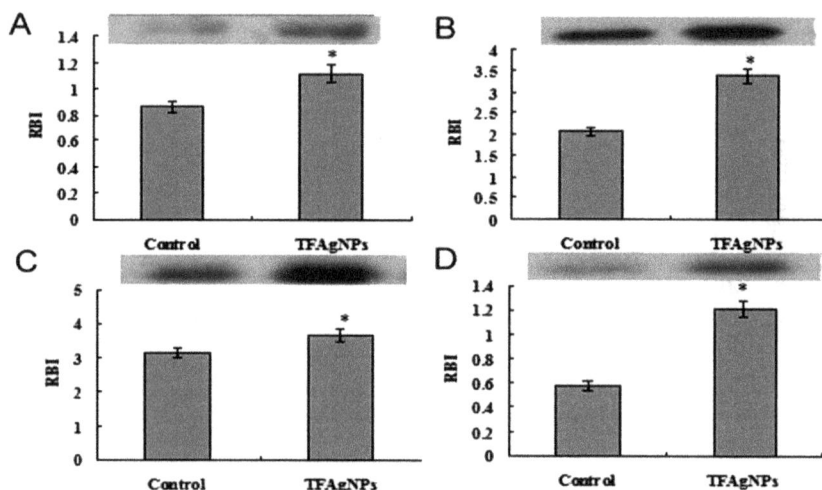

**FIGURE 9.17**   Expression of apoptotic related proteins in biosynthesized TFAgNPs treated and untreated cells: (A) p53, (B) PARP-1, (C) Bax, and (D) smac/DIABLO. Note: Protein bands were standardized against β-actin.

### 9.3.18   MEASUREMENT OF ROS PRODUCTION

The $H_2$DCF-DA experiment is used to evaluate on the effect of AgNPs and $Ag^+$ in the cellular ROS generation (Figure 9.18). After 24 h treatment, at 5, 10, and 20 μg mL$^{-1}$ concentrations TFAgNPs induced significant ROS. After cells were exposed with biosynthesized TFAgNPs (10 mM) for 1 h earlier

AgNPs treatment, the ROS production levels were significantly declining. The $Ag^+$ doses between 5 and 20 μg mL$^{-1}$ similarly increase significant ROS, which decline by pretreatment with AgNPs. Commonly, the AgNPs enhanced higher ROS production than $Ag^+$ as suggested that ROS may be caused by TFAgNPs, are not exclusively owing to the possible release of $Ag^+$.

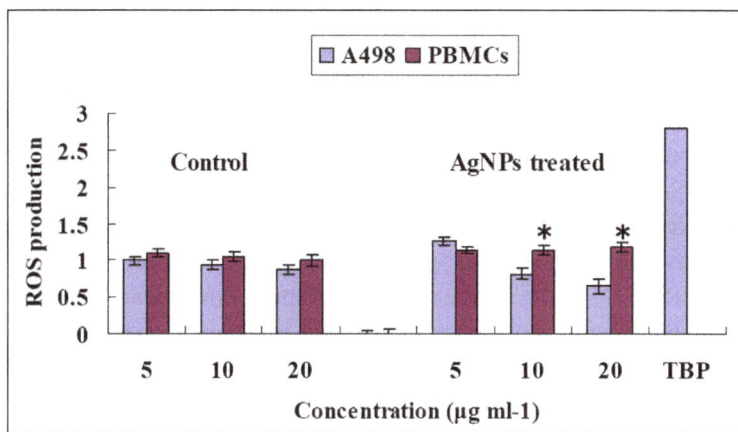

**FIGURE 9.18**    ROS levels in A498 cells after exposure to TFAgNPs. Cells were incubated with AgNPs (5, 10, and 20 μg mL$^{-1}$) for 24 h and then with 20 μM DCF-DA probe for 40 min. Readings (Ex485 nm/Em535 nm) were performed every 5 min over 30 min. *Tert*-butyl hydroperoxide (TBP, 15 μM) was used as a positive control. ROS increase was calculated as the mean slope per min and was normalized to the unexposed control. Results are presented as mean ± standard deviation of four replications.

## 9.4  DISCUSSIONS

Recently, nanoparticles of metals, specifically of gold and silver have drawn significant consideration owing to their immense possible in biomedical fields. In biological methods, adsorption is usually chosen for the exclusion of heavy metal ions owing to its high effectiveness, easy treatment, accessibility of various adsorbents, and cost efficacy. Further green synthesis of NPs is eco-friendly, can be easily synthesize or producted in large quantity; further there was no necessity of high pressure or energy or temperature or toxic chemicals as in the case of chemical as well as physical approaches. Metal NPs such as Au, Ag, Zn, and Pt are widely or directly used in contact with the human body, for example, in the form of shampoos/soaps/detergent/ shoes/cosmetic products/toothpaste, etc., in the medical as well as in pharmaceutical field. All are well-known activities of $Ag^+$ and Ag-based products mostly significant property is that they can kill the microbes effectively [9]. NPs accumulate at particular locations like vesicles and mitochondria from where they exert toxic responses. Particles with minute size contain a larger surface area and thus would involve in the generation of a substantial amount of ROS, which play a major role in NPs toxicity [40].

When a plant extract is mixed in liquid solution of the $Ag^+$ complex, its color modified from colorless to yellow brownish due to decrease of $Ag^+$ demonstrating the AgNPs formation [28]. This study likewise the color change from neutral to brown showed the biosynthesized TFAgNPs from the root extract as suggested in previous study [48]. In this study, the color change appears after the accomplishment of the reaction; it is distinguished that TFAgNPs display yellowish brown color established on their particle size [46]. Noble MPs especially Ag and Au provide a strong immersion band in the observable region afford specific color in the solution.

The SPR of TFAgNPs created a peak spotlighted near 413 nm. UV–Visible absorbance of response combination is obtained from 0 to 8 min. It was detected that the peak absorbance spotlighted near 413 nm representing the reduction of $AgNO_3$ into AgNPs; further it was also represented that the bioreduction of $Ag^+$ into NPs underway at the initiate of response which was accomplished at almost 8 min demonstrating rapid biosynthesized TFAgNPs. With the AgNPs the excitation of surface plasmon sensations color change is manifested yellow brown color [3]; a clearly visible immersion band at 260 nm is qualified to the electronic excitation in tryptophan or tyrosine proteins residues [12]. This indicates the release of extra-cellular proteins in the colloquial resolution and thew promising contribution in the bioreduction progression [13].

UV–Visible spectrum graph of the colloid resolution of biosynthesized TFAgNPs were documented as a functional role of period through exhausting a quartz-cuvette with $AgNO_3$ as the reference. The roots are selected for TFAgNPs since there is a place of photosynthesis and obtainability of higher $H^+$ ions facilitate the reduction of $AgNO_3$ into AgNPs. The molecular basis of biosynthesis Ag crystals might be since the organic matrix contains Ag fixing proteins that afford amino acid moieties and the sites assist for nucleation [49]. The strong SPR band positioned at 430 nm was observed in the biosynthesized TFAgNPs. The site of SPR band in UV–Visible spectrum is specific to shape or size of the particle, and their interface with the medium, native refractive index and the degree of charge transmission among medium and the NPs; numerous reports have proven that the quality of AgNPs peak looks around this district [64].

The morphology of biosynthesized TFAgNPs was characterized by SEM. After the accomplishment of the action, the AgNPs hired on carbon-coating copper grid reveal spherical shape. All the SEM pictures confirm that TFAgNPs morphology is closely spherical in nature, which is in respectable covenant with the SPR band shape in the UV–Vis spectrum. The size of the TFAgNPs was around 50–100 nm. The SEM image of TFAgNPs from the extract is accumulated on the surface owing to the interfaces (hydrogen binding and electricitie exchanges among the bio-organic capping molecules available on the AgNPs [34].

The PSD of TFAgNPs is in various sizes between 5 and 90 nm and the average size was 82 nm. The DLS characterization of the NPs size was colloidal scatterings, which consume the illumination of the particles suspension or molecules undertaking Brownian signal in the laser beam. Time-dependent variations in the strength of dispersed light are examined by autocorrelator, which conclude the autocorrelation reaction of the signal [26]. The measured size with DLS is marginally high as related to the particle size obtained in SEM images since DLS technique determine the hydrodynamic radius [18].

The TFAgNPs is crystalline nature and confirmed in XRD pattern with the diffraction peaks at $2\theta$ values peaks at $2\theta = 28.71°$, $31.65°$, $47.45°$, $55.63°$, $58.12°$, and $78.87°$ allocated to the (111), (100), (200), (311), (110), and (311) reflection lines of AgNPs. It was in contract with FCC structure (JCPDS File No. 04-0783). The standard size of the particle measured in XRD configurations is 28.7 nm, which is in contrast with the size of the particle given in SEM studies. The well determined and strong XRD profile clearly shows that the TFAgNPs produced by $Ag^+$ reduction as crystalline structure as suggested in previous studies [11].

FTIR study was accomplished to detect the potential biomolecules liable for $Ag^+$ reduction and reducing capping of biosynthesized TFAgNPs. FTIR measurement was utilize to examine the chemical configuration on the surface of AgNPs and the native molecular atmosphere/environment of the capping materials on the NPs. The FTIR spectrum suggested that several functional groups (tannins, steroids, triterpenoids, saponins, glycerides, flavonoids, phenols, glycosides) in the root extract at the different site between 400 and 4000 $cm^{-1}$ is mainly liable for the perceived reduction or capping in TFAgNPs.

TFAgNPs showed peaks at 1653.61 $cm^{-1}$ and the bonds due to O–H extending of phenol constituent [47]; whereas the remaining peaks acquired in TFAgNPs sample are 3870.00 and 3907.08 $cm^{-1}$ due to O=H extending of

–OH groups [5]. The stretch at 2925.817 cm$^{-1}$ was identified and it signifies –C–H stretching [57]. The intense peak of 539.08 cm$^{-1}$ shows C–Br group of alkyl halides, whereas the peak at 2925.81 cm$^{-1}$ suggest the occurrence of N–H bend, which demonstrating as secondary amine groups present in the protein. Likewise, 1651 cm$^{-1}$ band resemble to the primary amine groups such as N–H bending or carbonyl extending sensations of protein have been detected [50].

FTIR spectra in this study indicate absorbance bands at 1653.61 cm$^{-1}$ are identified, which correspond to the presence of alkenes [33]. The FTIR peaks of alkanes at 2371.55 cm$^{-1}$ are identified, which are due to carbonyl stretch sensations in the amide relationship of the proteins [44]. A heavy strong absorption peak at 3357.10 cm$^{-1}$ denotes O–H extending vibration which is representative of the occurrence of primary N–H amines [54] and another band at 1055.53 cm$^{-1}$ influence to contribute on –C–O– groups of the polyols (terpenoids, flavones, polysaccharides) existing in the biomass [17]. Another important band at 2148 cm$^{-1}$ is identified that resemble to C=C stretch vibration as suggested alkynes group [31] and 634.67 peak allocated of C–Cl stretching as suggested alkyl halides group [38]. Hence, the FTIR measurement suggested that the amino acid residues of carbonyl group or proteins peptides show a very strong metal-binding competency. Perhaps, the proteins may be coated in NPs and acted as capping agents to the formation AgNPs to prevent the accumulation of the NPs; thus, the NPs are stabilized. This proposes that the biomolecules might perhaps accomplish twin roles in the development and steadiness of TFAgNPs in liquid medium. The TFAgNPs may interface with the proteins in the bacterial membrane and bacterial DNA as they retain sulfur or phosphorus composites and the Ag has a greater attraction to react with these combinations [14]. The amino acid residue of the carbonyl group devours a sturdy binding capacity to metal ions as suggested in the development on the layer of TFAgNPs surface and thus enacting as a steadying promoter to avoid accumulation in liquid medium.

The bactericidal and antiviral roles were extensively investigated in Ag, Ag$^{+}$, and Ag compounds [42]. The zone of inhibition in the study of TFAgNPs after adding 1 mM AgNO$_3$ at 100 µg mL$^{-1}$ concentration against all the tested multi drug resistance human pathogens ranged between 2 and 5 mm. However, the concentration at 150 µg mL$^{-1}$ against all the tested human pathogens a high potency of ZI was observed between 4 and 7 mm. The ZI increased with increasing TFAgNPs concentration as the AgNPs bind to the bacterial cell cytoplasmic membrane causing lysis. Among bactericidal effect of biosynthesized TFAgNPs conformed by a twin roles of mechanism of antibacterial action that is the bacterial activity of $Ag^+$ and mt membrane-disruption activity of the polymer subunits [21].

The key function of AgNPs was obvious act as antibacterial activity either by fastening or entering to the bacterial cell wall and modifying cellular signals [53]. Electrostatic attraction of biosynthesized TFAgNPs can disturb the membrane of bacterial cell wall surface, which structural changes occur owing to cell expiration. Another possibility of AgNPs can attached on the bacterial cell wall surface and interrupts its functional roles such as absorptivity and exhalation [35] followed by metabolic dysfunction pathways including, $Ag^+$ networking favorably in the nucleic acids. The common antibacterial mechanism or activity of AgNPs was suggested by several research workers, but the comprehensive antibacterial mechanism remains to be elucidated.

The biosynthesized TFAgNPs did not exhibit distinct morphological changes on A498 cells. The $IC_{50}$ value obtained was 300 μg for A498 cells. The TFAgNPs cytotoxicity obtained dose-dependent manner to A498 cells with a $CC_{50}$ at 62.4 μg mL$^{-1}$; however, the $CC_{50}$ degree to normal PBMCs obtained at 768.2 μg mL$^{-1}$. In this study, A498 cells demonstrated strikingly more compassion to TFAgNPs toxicity when compared to normal PBMCs ($P < 0.005$). Further, this study likewise investigated the toxicity role in normal human PBMCs as well as A498 cells to TFAgNPs, since the cellular function is aggressive and the eventual phenotype is disturbed by an innumerable of conflicting or touching signals existing in the microenvironment.

The results revealed that the therapeutic index of A498 cells was highly vulnerable to TFAgNPs-mediated toxicity when compared to normal PBMCs. It could be very essential in the clinical study, which is an extreme task facing chemotherapy incompetence of anticancer drugs to successfully discriminate among normal and transformed tissue [16]. Even though several frequently used chemotherapeutic-drugs goal rapidly trigger cell divisions, which may affect from a quite less therapeutic index [37].

TFAgNPs treated A498 cells had underway the process of apoptosis, which is confirmed by DNA destroying where the DNA profiles control or untreated cell DNA is not affected in the present study. It is confirmed that the fixing of the NPs into the bacteria cells may be based on the available surface area for interactional; hence a very small NPs devising a greater surface area that provides more possibility for interface providing highest bactericidal activity than that of big size NPs. Thus it is proposed that the opportunity that the AgNPs may likewise enter bacteria and fungi cells inside may cause impairment by relating between electron phosphorous and sulfur comprising of DNA [37].

Biosynthesized TFAgNPs may toxic to multiple-drug-resistant pathogens. It was demonstrated that they contain a remarkable potential in the biomedical studies and enhance the beneficial effects and fortify the medical properties of herbals. This may be the reason for the higher efficiency of the AgNPs than the silver ions. AgNPs potency may be due to bacterial cell wall denaturation, sugars leaking in the cell wall that may be prime to the hindering of respiration, outer membrane disruption, and intracellular ATP depletion in the bacterial cell [60].

The apoptotic activity was confirmed, labeled with annexin V and FITC can find apoptotic cells present in the population. It was also a congruent experiment of apoptosis when TFAgNPs activated to A498 cells. The MDA was augmented by 126% and 113% when A498 cells were treated with TFAgNPs at 50 and 25 μg m$^{-1}$. The ultrasonic radioactivity affected MDA in the bacterial liposomal membrane. Three reactive products were produced in the ultrasound-treated bacterial liposomal membrane, namely, lipid hydroperoxides, MDA-conjugated dienes, and malondialdehydes [22]. These products were produced in various stages of an MDA chain activity facilitated through free radicals. Our previous experiment confirmed that MDA may be introverted by free-radical scavengers [24]. The ultrasound-initiated MDA performs a result from the chain reaction associated with O$_2$ and intermediated through free radicals. AgNPs enhanced ultrasound-induced MDA.

The apoptosis signal transduction implicates a cascade of originator and killer caspases [8] and the killer caspases-3/-7 cleave particular important substrates to modification accompanying with apoptosis and eventually cell death [25]. The originator caspses-8 or -9 were liable in the stimulation of killer caspases. The present study biosynthesized TFAgNPs considerably upregulated of caspases-3/-7 and -9 the activities and it increased the DNA fragmentation in this study an finale stage representative of apoptosis.

In reaction to this DNA impairment, the PARP-1 catalyzes nuclear enzyme transmission of NAD$^+$ to a particular set of nuclear substrates [52]. At the time of apoptosis, PARP-1 nuclear enzyme is broken or cleaved, by killer caspases-3/-7, to a DNA fixing domain and an 89 kDa part holding catalytic action. TFAgNPs was liable for the broken or cleaved of PARP-1 nuclear enzyme as demonstrated by the considerably augmented of DNA fragment expression when compared with control or untreated cells in this experiment.

The mt performed a significant role of apoptosis via apoptotic intrinsic program. A preliminary stage for stimulating the apoptotic intrinsic pathway is the depolarization of membrane in mt significant the development of mt PT pores, which is related with different metabolic significances such as terminated activity of the electron transportation chain with accompanying of ROS production and declined ATP synthesis [62].

The Bax (proapoptotic gene) is a Bcl-2 family, the transformation of the cytosol to the mt outer membrane through apoptosis, where it interrelates with lipids and prompts mt PT pores in this study with an associated decline in ATP concentration. The significant levels of Bax activation in this study increases the level of mt depolarization and declined ATP concentration as suggested that TFAgNPs stimulate nuclear apoptosis in lung cancer cells through the apoptotic intrinsic pathway.

Ag takes a great similarity for thiol (−SH) groups. In the present experiment, the cysteine-rich GSH levels were declined at the same time as considerably increased MDA by TFAgNPs. This antioxidant or oxidant disproportion has formerly been demonstrated as an apoptotic function through AgNPs-related cytotoxicity. Declining ATP level and improving MDA as a consequence of ROS production, which owing to interruptions in respiratory sequence problem in mt. The NPs differently contain in mt and affected oxidative stress as well as potential structural changes in the bacteria [7].

A number of proapoptotic fragments of molecules are discharged from the mt through the apoptosis. The mt in the presence of ATP discharged cytochrome c that linked with Apaf-1 in the cytosol encouraging its oligomerization. The apoptosome is produced from oligomeric-Apaf-1 combination and pro-caspase-9, which enhances the stimulation of caspase-9, and in chance triggers the effector caspases-3 and -7 [8]. The exciting outcome from this study was that though ATP concentration declined post-TFAgNPs interaction, the caspase-9 activity was quiet prominent in this experiment.

The facility of apoptosis is made by IAP as an autogenous suppressor of pro-caspase stimulation that endorsed to the presence of BIR. In specific, BIR3 and a part of contiguous to BIR2 were liable for blocking of caspases-9, -3, and -7. An mt protein such as Smac/DIABLO capable to eliminate the XIAP prohibiting effects [8]. Both smac/DIABLO and caspases-3, -7, -9 were comprised of IAP-binding patterns that binding into the BIR domains in the XIAP. Thus, smac/DIABLO is the ability to stopping by substituting/ replacing and discharging of caspases-3, -7, -9 from the XIAP inhibitory combination [8].

Authors hypothesized that TFAgNPs may be discharging of smac/ DIABLO from the mt, which express in smac/DIABLO by western blotting in the present study and proven that TFAgNPs stimulate its discharge from the mt. The p53 protein facilitates in a variety of antiproliferative developments in reaction to various anxiety or stress stimuli by straight stimulating apoptosis and endorsing the discharge of Bax [36] and encouraging killer caspase action [30].

Furthermore, p53 protein obstructs with mt reliability and functional activity important to the discharge of pro-apoptotic molecules or ROS production [19]. The present study confirms the augmented p53 protein expression after adding of TFAgNPs to cells. The present study results afford strong confirmation that AgNPs prompted apoptosis in A498. A number of study demonstrated that certain nanomaterials have the ability to display impulsive ROS formation established on physical configuration and surface structure; however, others produce ROS formation merely in the occurrence of particular cell systems. The cellular toxicity mechanisms such as higher ROS generation that surpasses the capability of the cellular or nuclear antioxidant protection system affect cells to arrive from formal oxidative stress, that potency impairment the cellular constituents (lipids, proteins, DNA) [29, 63]. The fatty acids oxidation results in the production of LP that stimulates a chain response ensuing in interruption of plasma or organelle membranes structure and consequently cell death.

## 9.5   SUMMARY

The novel biosynthesized TFAgNPs holds a strong proapoptotic perspective; it has been revealed mechanically that TFAgNPs triggers the inherent apoptotic pathway in A498 cells. This study focuses on the prospective for novel drug development in the management of carcinomas. Nevertheless, advance extensive works are required to determine the consistent effects of TFAgNPs in other cancerous cells and also about nontoxicity on long-term basis.

## ACKNOWLEDGMENTS

This is the part of Mrs. Lourthu Samy Shanthi Mary, M.Phil dissertation work entitle "Characterization of Biologically Synthesized Silver Nanoparticles using *Trigonella foenum-graecum*: Its Anticancer Potential and toxicity Effects in Freshwater fish *Labeo rohita*" submitted at Bharathidasan University, Tiruchirapalli, Tamil Nadu, India, 2014.

## KEYWORDS

- **A498 cells**
- **cytotoxicity**
- **FTAgNPs**
- **reactive oxygen species**
- ***Trigonella foenum-graecum***

## REFERENCES

1. Ahmad, A.; Mukherjee, P.; Senapati, S.; Mandal, D.; Khan, M. I.; Kumar, R.; Sastry, M. Extracellular biosynthesis of silver nanoparticles using the fungus *Fusarium oxysporum*. *Colloids and Surfaces B: Biointerfaces,* **2003**, *28*, 313–318.
2. Ahmad, A.; Sastry, M. A. Biological synthesis of triangular gold nanoprisms. *Nature Materials*, **2004**, *3*, 482–88.
3. Ankanna, S.; Prasad, T. N. V. K. V.; Elumalai, E. K.; Savithramma, N. Production of biogenic silver nanoparticles using *Boswellia ovalifoliolata* Stem Bark. *Digest Journal of Nanomaterials and Biostructures*, **2010**, *5*, 369–372.
4. Badri Narayanan, K.; Sakthivel, N. Coriander leaf mediated biosynthesis of gold nanoparticles. *Materials Letters*, **2008**, *62*, 4588–4590.
5. Baker, C.; Pradhan, A.; Pakstis, L.; Pochan, D. J.; Shah, S. I. synthesis and antibacterial properties of silver nanoparticles. *Journal of Nanoscience and Nanotechnology*, **2005**, *5*, 224–249.
6. Begum, N. A.; Mondal, S.; Basu, S.; Laskar, R.A.; Mandal, D. Biogenic synthesis of Au and Ag nanoparticles using aqueous solutions of black tea leaf extracts. *Colloids and Surfaces B: Biointerfaces,* **2009**, *71*, 113–118.
7. Carlson, C.; Hussain, S. M.; Schrand, A. M.; Braydich-Stolle, L. K.; Hess, K. L.; Jones, R. L.; Schlager, J. J. Unique cellular interaction of silver nanoparticles: sizedependent generation of reactive oxygen species. *The Journal of Physical Chemistry B*, **2008**, *112*, 13608–13619.
8. Chai, J.; Du, C.; Wu, J. W.; Kyin, S.; Wang, X.; Shi, Y. Structural and biochemical basis of apoptotic activation by Smac/DIABLO. *Nature*, **2000**, *406*, 855–862.
9. Chopra, I. The Increasing use of silver based products as antimicrobial agents: a useful development or a cause for concern. *Journal of Antimicrobial Chemotherapy*, **2007**, *59*, 587–590.

10. Chow, W. H.; Devesa, S. S.; Warren, J. L.; Fraumeni, J.F. Jr. Rising incidence of renal cell cancer in the United States. *Journal of the American Medical Association*, **1999**, *281*, 1628–1631.

11. Das, J.; Paul Das, M.; Velusamy, P. *Sesbania grandiflora* leaf extract mediated green synthesis of antibacterial silver nanoparticles against selected human pathogens. *Spectrochimica Acta, Part A*, **2013**, *104*, 265–270.

12. Eftink, M. K.; Ghiron, C. A. Fluorescence quenching studies with proteins. *Analytical Biochemistry*, **1981**, *114*, 199–227.

13. Fayaz, A. M.; Balaji, K.; Girilal, M.; Yadav, R.; Kalaichelvan, P. T.; Venketesan, R. Biogenic synthesis of silver nanoparticles and their synergistic effect with antibiotics: a study against gram-positive and gram-negative bacteria. *Nanomedicine: Nanotechnology, Biology and Medicine*, **2010**, *6*, 103–109.

14. Feng, Q. L.; Wu, J.; Chen, G. Q.; Cui, F. Z.; Kim, T. N.; Kim, J. O. A Mechanistic study of the antibacterial effect of silver ions on *Escherichia coli* and *Staphylococcus aureus*. *Journal of Biomedical Materials Research Part A*, **2000**, *52*, 662–668.

15. Goodsell, D. S. Bionanotechnology: lessons from nature. Hoboken, NJ: John Wiley & Sons Inc.; 2004; p. 227.

16. Hellman, S. Improving the therapeutic index in breast cancer treatment: the richard and hinda rosenthal foundation award lecture. *Cancer Research*, **1980**, *40*, 4335–4442.

17. Hong, N.; Chen, J. Biosynthesis of Silver and gold nanoparticles by novel sundried *Cinnamomum canphora* leaf. *Nanotechnology*, **2007**, *18*, 1–11.

18. Huang, N. M.; Lim, H. N.; Radiman, S.; Khiew, P. S.; Chiu, W. S.; Hashin, R.; Chia, C. H. Sucrose ester micellar-mediated synthesis of Ag nanoparticles and their antibacterial properties. *Colloids and Surfaces B: Biointerfaces*, **2010**, *353*, 69–76.

19. Hwang, P. M.; Bunz, F.; Yu, J.; Rago, C.; Chan, T. A.; Murphy, M. P.; Kelso, G. F.; Smith, R. A.; Kinzler, K. W.; Vogelstein, B. Ferredoxin reductase Affects p53-dependent, 5-fluorouracil-induced apoptosis in colorectal cancer cells. *Nature Medicine*, **2001**, *7*, 1111–1117.

20. Ip, M.; Lui, S. L.; Poon, V. K. M.; Lung, I.; Burd, A. Antimicrobial activities of silver dressings: an *In vitro* comparison. *Journal of Medical Microbiology*, **2006**, *55*, 59–63.

21. Jain, D.; Daima, H. K.; Kachhwaha, S.; Kothari, S. L. Synthesis of plant-mediated silver nanoparticles using papaya fruit extract and evaluation of their antimicrobial activities. *Digest Journal of Nanomaterials and Biostructures*, **2009**, *4*, 557–563.

22. Jana, A. K.; Agarwal, S.; Chatterjee, S. N. The induction of lipid peroxidation in liposomal membrane by ultrasound and the role of hydroxyl radicals. *Radiation Research*, **1990**, *124*, 7–14.

23. Jonge, S. H.; Yeo, S. Y.; Yi, S. C. the effect of filler particle size on the antibacterial properties of compounded polymer silver fibers. *Journal of Materials Science*, **2005**, *40*, 5407–5411.

24. Kanagalakshmi, K.; Premanathan, M.; Priyanka, R.; Hemalatha, B.; Vanangamudi, A. Synthesis, anticancer and antioxidant activities of isoflavanone and 2,3-diarylchromanones. *European Journal of Medicinal Chemistry*, **2010**, *45*, 2447–2452.

25. Kasibhatla, S.; Tseng, B. Why target apoptosis in cancer treatment?. *Molecular Cancer Therapeutics*, **2003**, *2*, 573–580.

26. Kaszuba, M.; McKnight, D.; Connah, M. T.; McNeil-Watson, F. K.; Nobbmann, U. Measuring sub nanometre sizes using dynamic light scattering. *Journal of Nanoparticle Research*, **2008**, *10*, 823–829.

27. Krutyakov, Y. A.; Kudrynskiy, A.; Olenin, A. Y.; Lisichkin, G. V. extracellural biosynthesis and antimicrobial activity of silver nanoparticles. *Russian Chemical Reviews*, **2008**, *77*, 233–240.

28. Linga Rao, M.; Savithramma, N. Biological synthesis of silver nanoparticles using *Svensonia hyderobadensis* leaf extract and evaluation of their antimicrobial efficacy. *Journal of Pharmaceutical Sciences and Research*, **2011**, *3*, 1117–1121.

29. Lovric, J.; Cho, S. J.; Winnik, F. M.; Maysinger, D. unmodified cadmium telluride quantum dots induce reactive oxygen species formation leading to multiple organelle damage and cell death. *Chemistry and Biology*, **2005**, *12*, 1227–1234.

30. MacLachlan, T. K.; El-Deiry, W. S. Apoptotic threshold is lowered by p53 transactivation of caspase-6. *Proceedings of the National Academy of Sciences, USA*, **2002**, *99*, 9492–9497.

31. Mahitha, B.; Prasad Raju, B. D.; Madhavi, T.; Durga Mahalakshmi, D. H. N.; John Sushma, N. Evaluation of antibacterial efficacy of phyto fabricated gold nanoparticles using *Bacopa Monniera* plant extract. *Indian Journal of Advances in Chemical Science*, **2013**, *1*, 94–98.

32. Maliszewska, I. Microbial synthesis of metal nanoparticles, rozdział. In: *Metal Nanoparticles Microbiology*; Rai, M. and Duran, N. (Eds.), Springer-Verlag Berlin Heidelberg; **2011**.

33. Manisha, D. R.; Merugu, R.; Vijay Babu, A. R.; Pratap Rudra, M. P. Microwave assisted biogenic synthesis of silver nanoparticles using dried seed extract of *Coriandrum sativum*, characterization and antimicrobial activity. *International Journal of ChemTech Research*, **2014**, *6*, 3957–3961.

34. Mano Priya, M.; Karunai selvia, B. A.; John Paul, J. A. Green synthesis of silver nanoparticles from the leaf extracts of *Euphorbia hirta* and *Nerium indicum*. *Digest Journal of Nanomaterials and Biostructures*, **2011**, *6*, 869–877.

35. Maribel, G.; Guzmán, J. D.; Stephan, G. Synthesis of silver nanoparticles by chemical reduction method and their antibacterial activity. *International Journal of Chemical Engineering*, **2009**, *2*, 104–111.

36. Miyashita, T.; Krajewski, S.; Krajewska, M.; Wang, H. G.; Lin, H. K.; Liebermann, D.A.; Hoffman, B.; Reed, J. C. Tumor suppressor p53 is a regulator of Bcl-2 and Bax gene expression *In vitro* and *In vivo*. *Oncogene*, **1994**, *9*, 1799–805.

37. Morones, J. R.; Elechiguerra, J. L.; Camacho, A.; Holt, K.; Kouri, J. B.; Ramrez, J. T.; Yacaman, M. J. Green fluorescent protein-expressing *Escherichia coli* as a model system for investigating the antimicrobial activities of silver nanoparticles. *Nanotechnology*, **2005**, *16*, 2346–2353.

38. Moteriya, P.; Chanda, S. Low cost and ecofriendly phytosynthesis of silver nanoparticles using *Cassia roxburghii* stem extract and its antimicrobial and antioxidant efficacy. *American Journal of Advanced Drug Delivery*, **2014**, *4*, 557–575.

39. Nair, B.; Pradeep, T. Coalescence of nanoclusters and formation of submicron crystallites assisted by *Lactobacillus* Strains. *Crystal Growth and Design*, **2002**, *2*, 293–298.

40. Nel, A.; Xia, T.; Madler, L.; Li, N. Toxic potential of materials at the nanolevel. *Science*, **2006**, *311*, 622–627.

41. Niraimathi, K. L.; Sudha, V.; Lavanya, R.; Brindha, P. Biosynthesis of silver nanoparticles using *Alternanthera sessilis* (Linn.) extract and their antimicrobial, antioxidant activities. *Colloids and Surfaces B: Biointerfaces*, **2013**, *102*, 288–291.

42. Nithya, R.; Ragunathan, R. Synthesis of silver nanoparticle using *pleurotus sajorcaju* and its antimicrobial study. *Digest Journal of Nanomaterials and Biostructures*, **2009**, *4*, 623–629.
43. Panacek, A.; Kolar, M.; Vecerova, R.; Prucek, R.; Soukupova, J.; Krystof, V.; Hamal, P. antifungal activity of silver nanoparticles against *Candida* sp. *Biomaterials*, **2009**, *30*, 6333–6340.
44. Paramanantham,. M.; Murugesan, A. Green synthesis of silver nanoparticles from *Physalis Angulatta*: Synthesis and antimicrobial activity. *International Journal of Science and Research*, **2014**, *3*, 40–42.
45. Parashar, U. K.; Saxena, P. S.; Srivastava, A. Bioinspired synthesis of silver nanoparticles. *Digest Journal of Nanomaterials and Biostructures*, **2009**, *4*, 159–166.
46. Prabhu, N.; Divya, T. R.; Yamuna, G. Synthesis of silver phyto nanoparticles and their antibacterial efficacy. *Digest Journal of Nanomaterials and Biostructures*, **2009**, *5*, 185–189.
47. Rajathi1, K.; Sridhar, S. Green synthesized silver nanoparticles from the medicinal plant *Wrightia Tinctoria* and its antimicrobial potential. *International Journal of ChemTech Research*, **2013**, *5*, 1707–1713.
48. Renugadevi, K.; Venus Aswini, R. Microwave irradiation assisted synthesis of silver nanoparticle using *Azadirachta indica* leaf extract as a reducing agent and its *in vitro* evaluation of its antibacterial and anticancer Activity. *International Journal of Nanomaterials and Biostructures*, **2012**, *2*, 5–10.
49. Sathyavathi, R.; Balamurali Krishna, M.; Venugopal Rao, S.; Saritha, R.; Narayana Rao, D. Biosynthesis of silver nanoparticles using *Coriandrum sativum* leaf extract and their application in nonlinear optics. *Advanced Science Letters*, **2010**, *3*, 138–143.
50. Sawle, B. D.; Salimath, B.; Deshpande, R.; Bedre, M. D.; Prabhakar, B. K.; Venkataraman, A. Biosynthesis and stabilization of Au and Au–Ag Alloy nanoparticles by fungus *Fusarium semitectum*. *Science and Technology of Advanced Materials*, **2008**, 9, 035012.
51. Shahverdi, A. R.; Minaeian, S.; Shahverdi, H. R.; Jamalifar, H.; Nohi, A. A. Rapid synthesis of silver nanoparticles using culture supernatants of *Enterobacteriaceae*: a novel biological approach. *Process Biochemistry*, **2007**, *42*, 919–923.
52. Shall, S.; de Murcia, G. Poly(ADP-ribose) Polymerase-1: what have we learned from the deficient mouse model?. *Mutation Research*, **2000**, *460*, 1–15.
53. Shrivastava, S.; Bera, T.; Roy, A.; Singh, G.; Ramachandrarao, P.; Dash, D. Characterization of enhanced antibacterial effects of novel silver nanoparticles. *Nanotechnology*, **2007**, *18*, 225–230.
54. Silverstein, R. M.; Bassler, G. C.; Morrill, T. C. *Spectrometric Identification of Organic Compounds*. 4th ed. New York, John Wiley & Sons Inc.; **1981**.
55. Singh, S.; Saikia, J. P.; Buragohain, A. K. A Novel 'Green' synthesis of colloidal silver nanoparticles (SNP) using *Dillenia indica* fruit extract. *Colloids and Surfaces B: Biointerfaces*, **2013**, *102*, 83–85.
56. Sun, Ch.; Qu, R.; Chen, H.; Wang, Ch. Degradation behavior of chitosan chains in the green synthesis of gold nanopartices. *Carbohydrate Research*, **2008**, *343*, 2595–2599.
57. Thenmozhi, R.; Arumugam, K.; Nagasathya, A.; Thajuddin, N.; Paneerselvam, A. studies on mycoremediation of used engine oil contaminated soil samples. *Advances in Applied Science Research*, **2013**, *4*, 110–118.

58. Vaidyanathan, R.; Kalishwaralal, K.; Gopalram, S.; Gurunathan, S. Nanosilver-the burgeoning therapeutic molecule and its green synthesis. *Biotechnology Advances*, **2009**, *27*, 924–937.
59. van Spronsen, D. J.; Mulders, P. F.; De Mulder, P. H. Novel treatments for metastatic renal cell carcinoma. *Critical Reviews in Oncology/Hematology*, **2005**, *55*, 177–191.
60. Vivekanandhan, S.; Misra, M.; Mohanty, A. K. Biological synthesis of silver nanoparticles using *Glycine max* (Soybean) leaf extract: an investigation on different soybean varieties. *Journal of Nanoscience and Nanotechnology*, **2009**, *9*, 6828–6833.
61. Wagner, V.; Dullaart, A.; Bock, A. K.; Zweck, A. The emerging nanomedicine landscape. *Nature Biotechnology*, **2006**, *24*, 1211–1217.
62. Wang, X. The expanding role of mitochondria in apoptosis. *Genes and Development*, **2001**, *15*, 2922–2933.
63. Xia, T.; Kovochich, M.; Brant, J.; Hotze, M.; Sempf, J.; Oberley, T.; Sioutas, C.; Yeh, J. I.; Wiesner, M. R.; Nel, A. E.. Comparison of the abilities of ambient and manufactured nanoparticles to induce cellular toxicity according to an oxidative stress paradigm. *Nano Letters*, **2006**, *6*, 1794–1807.
64. Zahir, A. A.; Rahuman, A. A. Evaluation of different extracts and synthesized silver nanoparticles from leaves of *Euphorbia prostrata* against *Haemaphysalis bispinosa* and *Hippobosca maculata*. *Veterinary Parasitology*, **2012**, *187*, 511–520.

# CHAPTER 10

# ENVISIONING UTILIZATION OF SUPER GRAINS FOR HEALTHCARE

ANKITA KATARIA* and SAVITA SHARMA

## ABSTRACT

Super grains include amaranth, buckwheat, chia, hemp seed, millets, quinoa, and teff, most of which are gluten free. However, these contain certain antinutritional factors, which can be toxic. However, these antinutrients can be reduced/removed using optimum processing treatments. Apart from nutritional richness, the super grains exhibit good functionality, such as water absorption, water solubility, oil absorption, foaming, emulsification, and gelation making them useful in specialty foods. The processed super grains can be used partially or completely in common products like bread, pasta, noodles, cookies, and beverages to provide specialty characteristics.

## 10.1 INTRODUCTION

The human body is a complex system, which has the unique ability to thrive under diverse environments. The prelude to this, are macronutrients and micronutrients, which should be present in the diet in recommended quantities for people of varied age groups. An important characteristic of the sources of these nutrients is low or no allergenicity.

Out of 250,000 edible species of plant, the world is thriving on only 1% with the major dominance of three crops—(wheat, *Triticum aestivum*; rice, *Oryza sativa*; and maize, *Zea mays*). The scientific community is now keen on finding alternative resources due to the spurring of a presumption that at least 14% decline shall occur in the per capita production of grains by 2030 [41]. Moreover, micronutrient deficiency is a serious global concern

*Corresponding author. E-mail: ankitakataria92@gmail.com.

and is often termed as "hidden hunger" since its impacts on health are not acutely visible. According to World Health Organization (WHO), more than two billion people suffer from micronutrient deficiency globally [151]. Also, 1% of the worldwide population is a patient of gluten intolerance, or celiac disease, wherein the micro-villi of the small intestine are damaged consequently leading to anaemia and osteoporosis [195].

The increased awareness of the consumer regarding micronutrient deficiency and gluten sensitivity, quality protein, essential fatty, amino acids, etc., has led to a shift to those grains, which exhibit superior richness in nutritional values. These include amaranth, buckwheat, chia, hemp seed, millets, quinoa, and teff. These are rightfully termed as the super grains as they exhibit both nutritional and technological superiority. Among these, millets are further defined as certain cereal species that are very tiny/small with an average of 1/10 to 1/4 of wheat kernel size [177].

This chapter elaborates the importance of different super grains with respect to their macronutrients and micronutrients and functional properties. The antinutritional factors present in different grains with their effect on human body has been stated. Major highlight includes the processing interventions required to improve the different grains for their nutrition and functionality followed by their utilization in specialty foods.

### 10.1.1 ANCIENT HISTORY

The pre-Columbian diets were nutritionally superior to modern-day diets, which has been proved by modern science. The dietary recommendations of the WHO and Food and Agricultural Organization (FAO) can be met by the main components of those diets. The ancient civilizations preferred the super grains due to their nutritional superiority of the super grains. For instance, chia seeds were present in human diets since 3500 BC and became an important part of diet in 1500-900 BC [123]. Amaranth seeds were consumed during Mesoamerican festivities by roasting, grinding, and mixing with water or honey for dough formation [188].

The Whole Grain Council defines the term "ancient grains" as "grains that are largely genetically unchanged over the last several hundred years." More recently, a detailed definition is "ancient grains is a category covering grains (cereals), pseudo-grains (more properly pseudocereals) and seeds that are "ancient" in the sense that they have remained largely unchanged over hundreds, even thousands of years, unlike, say modern wheat varieties."

These grains were stapled in the diets of earlier civilizations. These have not been touched for genetic improvement and remain largely outside the mainstream of technological development [178]. These crops are underexploited and unexplored and are highly capable to dominate the food industry.

## 10.1.2 CURRENT NECESSITY FOR FOOD SECURITY

The global population is increasing at an alarming rate, which is and will consequently lead to worldwide increase in the demand of food. The current consumer is well aware of regarding the balanced diet and now prefers, although ready to eat, but nutritionally adequate, safe, and balanced food. The interaction of the diet and human body leads to prevention of certain diseases, which the current developed civilization is facing. These include hypertension, type 2 diabetes, malnutrition, and cardiac issues that can be tackled by a nutritionally superior diet [26]. The alarming situation facing the world is visible by the reports stating 12.9 million deaths due to ischemic heart diseases, 1.3 million from diabetes, and 8 million by cancer [108]. The best alternatives for the food industry for combating the chronic diseases are the ancestral seeds such as quinoa, chia, and amaranth, which have superior nutritional and medicinal properties [137, 147].

The demand for nutritious food with the richness of nutraceutical components and good quality proteins is increasing. The impact of globalization and industrialization has led to biased technological usage of certain plant species, which demand high amount of energy and fertilizers along with the monoculture production thereby reducing the agricultural genetic diversity. With an increasing population, the demand for additional water resources is created. The future will surely lack these required resources with increasing industrial and domestic needs. The food requirements cannot be met by the present major crops, which raises an urgent demand for alternative crops [188].

Due to shrinking number of the crops responsible for the current food security, there is a huge risk on the incomes of those dependent on agriculture and food thereby reducing the global economic growth. This has led to research, retrieval, and dissemination of the information by the scientific community regarding the production, processing, and utilization of the underexploited, neglected, and thereby "anciently novel" crops commonly known as the alternative crops. Since these crops contribute to income generation, environment, nutrition, health, and food security [119], these are rightfully termed as super grains.

## 10.2  COMPOSITION

Super grains exhibit nutritional superiority due to richer lipid, protein and mineral content, and quality. It is the composition of these macro- and micro-nutrients that is responsible for these grains to be termed as "super grains." The presence of essential nutrients such as the essential lipids and amino acids in amounts that are similar or close to the daily intake recommendations provides high potential for regular intake of these products by people of all age groups. The variation in the nutrient concentration of any super grain depends upon the certain factors including soil condition, temperature, and light conditions [173].

Every nutrient plays an important role in the normal growth of the human body. Lipids are the energy source that are made up of glycerol and fatty acids. The length of the fatty acid chains as well as amount of the double or triple bonds defines the functionality of the particular lipid. Lipids provide the calories required for functioning of the body as they are the important component of the cell membranes and help in the regulation of various physiological functions. An important parameter is the degree of saturation/unsaturation, which is based upon the presence of more than one bond along the fatty acid chain. Essential fatty acids such as ω-3 and ω-6 are the prime requirement for optimum growth. The concentration of such fatty acids depends upon the ability of the enzymes to introduce double bond at ω-3 and ω-6 positions of the chain. The European Food Safety Agency recommends the optimum ratio of 3:1 to 5:1 for ω-3 and ω-6, which helps in the significant reduction of heart diseases, chronic diseases, and mortality rate as well as boost immunity system [120, 141]. The higher ratios that is more than 10:1 can impose various health risks including cancer, cardiovascular diseases, and inflammation. Biosynthesis of eicosapentaenoic acid (EPA) ($C_{20:5}$, EPA) and 3-class prostaglandins is not possible due to lack of enzymes in the human body therefore these must be supplied in the diet [49]. Thus, the human diet must contain the required concentration of the lipids.

Proteins are the primary components involved in the muscle formation and are the important part of the cell structure. They are made up of amino acids, which are generally categorized into essential and nonessential ones. Protein-rich foods are gaining attention gradually due to the fact that the high protein foods help in the weight reduction and muscle formation. There are certain parameters that defines the quality of the protein such as in vitro protein digestibility (IVPD), protein efficiency ratio (PER), biological value [171], which essentially depend on the protein molecular structure and associated components that consequently affect the enzyme accessibility [190].

Carbohydrates are the primary source of the energy in the human body. They are the important structural component of the cell wall and also involve in the various body functions. Carbohydrates account for the largest component in the composition of various grains. Major carbohydrates include starch, stachyose, sucrose, fructose, and glucose. The concentration of the starch as well as the activities of starch hydrolysis enzymes are very important factors. At present, the trend is shifting to foods with low starch digestibility as lower digestible starches lead to low glycemic response, which is highly beneficial for diabetic patients [42]. Dietary fiber is also a part of carbohydrates. The optimum concentrations (25–30 g/day) of the dietary fiber imparts various health benefits. Some of the beneficial effects include the reduction of coronary heart disease, cancer, diabetes, cholesterol, weight reduction, and improvement in the gut microflora functioning. The ratio of soluble and insoluble dietary fiber defines the functionality of this component which 1:3 (soluble to insoluble fiber) as recommended by The American Dietetic Association [24, 123]. However, higher levels of dietary fiber can also lower the bioaccessibility of proteins and minerals by binding them [12].

Vitamins and minerals also play an important role in normal growth of human body. They must be present in adequate amount in human body as their deficiency can cause various disorders. Therefore, our diet should contain adequate amount of these nutrient as they are involved in controlling the growth hormones and regulators as well as providing protection from oxidative stress. For instance, tocopherols are mainly responsible for vitamin E activity since they react and deactivate the free radicals responsible for oxidation of unsaturated fatty acids [112]. Minerals are the inorganic matter that cannot be synthesized by the human body. Sodium, calcium, potassium, iron, phosphorus, zinc, sulfur, magnesium, and copper are the few examples of mineral. Among these, iron, calcium, and magnesium are well known for being deficient in gluten-free products. In such cases, super grains like amaranth, buckwheat, and quinoa play an important part as they are rich in these minerals and provide a complete diet to the celiac patients [6]. Also, the high calcium content of these grains protects the celiac patients from disorders like osteoporosis and osteopenia [64]. The proper combinations as well as processing techniques need to be considered for adequate intake of minerals and vitamins [48, 187].

## 10.2.1   AMARANTH (AMARANTHUS SPP.)

Amaranth contains lesser carbohydrates than conventional cereals and starch is the chief component at level of 48%–69% (dry matter basis) [188]. It has lower amylose content which ranges from 0.1% to 11% [138] depending upon the variety. The amount of rapidly digestible starch is 30.7%, which gives a high glycemic index (GI) value (87.2) [35] and starch digestibility. Sucrose is the main component in free sugars apart from raffinose, fructose, glucose, maltose, and stachyose [2].

Proteins constitute 13%–18% (dry matter basis) content in the amaranth grains and are superior to those of conventional cereals. Approximately, 65% is present in the embryo and grain hull and only 35% in the starch perisperm compared to 15 and 85% in the respective parts of the conventional cereals [123, 138]. This leads to a balanced amino acid composition of the grain which is rich in lysine (4.6–6.1 g/100 g protein), tryptophan (0.8–1.8 g/100 g), histidine, and sulfur-containing amino acids (4.4%). The amino acid composition of amaranth is comparable to the FAO/WHO recommendation as well as to animal protein composition, which is required to achieve a balanced diet in humans [148, 188]. The PER and biological value of amaranth are 73%–86% and 2.2, which imply high bioavailability of the essential amino acids [188]. Major fraction is albumins (51%) followed by glutelins (24%) and globulins (16%) with least content of prolamins (2%–3%), thus it is considered to be gluten-free [138].

The lipid content in amaranth, majorly present in the embryo, is 6%–9%, which is more than common cereals. Free lipids are the chief components present at levels of 90%–93%, wherein the major components are triglycerides. Phospholipids and glycolipids constitute the fraction of bound lipids at 85% and 2.6%, respectively. Major phospholipids are phosphoinositol, cefalin, and lecithin. Unsaturated fatty acid content is high at levels of 72%–84% [138, 188]. Linoleic acid (LA) is the dominant fatty acid occupying 50% followed by oleic (23.8%), palmitic (20%), stearic (2%–8%), and linolenic (0.3%–2.2%) acids [119].

High dietary fiber content of 8%–20% is present in amaranth mainly constituted by pectic polysaccharides and xyloglucans. Soluble and insoluble dietary occupy 22% and 78%, respectively, with the former consisting arabinose, glucose, galacturonic acid, arabinose rich polysaccharides and xyloglucans and the latter consisting mainly lignin and cellulose with arabinose, glucose, xylose, galactose, and galacturonic acid. Thus, amaranth seeds work as prebiotics and can be used to improve colon heath since such a constitution is similar to legumes, vegetable, and fruits [101].

Amaranth has a high mineral content of 3.6%, where zinc, magnesium, iron, potassium, calcium, and phosphorus are present in superior amounts. The ratio of calcium to phosphorus ranges from 1:1.9 to 2.7, which is near the optimal value of 1:1.5 making it a good source of these minerals in celiac patients [138, 188]. The major vitamins in amaranth are thiamine, riboflavin, niacin, and ascorbic acid. It is also a good source of vitamin E (tocopherols), which is present in amounts of 7.28–27.9 µg/g. The high content of tocopherols protects the amaranth oil from oxidation despite higher unsaturation degree [188].

## 10.2.2 BUCKWHEAT (FAGOPYRUM ESCULENTUM MOENCH)

Common buckwheat contains 68%–70% carbohydrate content wherein starch occupies 54.5%. The amylose content varies from 15.6% to 17.9%, which is considered to be present as amylose-lipid complexes [105, 198]. The GI is 80 compared to that of wheat bread (100) [195]. The soluble carbohydrates comprise of reducing sugars and fagopyritols [181].

The protein content in buckwheat varies from 6.4 to 13.5%. It is suitable for celiac patients since albumins (12.5%) and globulins (64.5%) are the dominant fractions with very low amounts of prolamin (2.9%) and glutelin (8%) [12]. It is a superior source of the essential amino acids like lysine and arginine, which are generally limiting in conventional cereals. Its strong cholesterol-lowering capacity is attributed to low ratios of methionine/ glycine and lysine/arginine [105]. The biological values of buckwheat proteins are high (90.5–93.1%) due to the richness of essential amino acids but its true digestibility is low (78.8%–79.9%) due to presence of dietary fiber and tannins in higher amounts [12].

The lipid content of buckwheat is 2%–4% most of which is present in the embryo. The free lipids are present at half amounts than bound lipids [32]. The risk of lipid deterioration is high in buckwheat since the embryo is mostly present in the bran fractions [12]. Approximately 75%–80% fatty acid composition is unsaturated wherein 40% are polyunsaturated [181]. The unsaturated and saturated fatty acids are mostly concentrated in the embryo and hull. Oleic acid predominates the fatty acid composition but LA and linolenic acids are also present at high levels of 36.8% and 2.7%, respectively [12].

The dietary fiber content is 12.16%, which is mostly present in the hull or the seed coat. The soluble fiber content (20%–30%) is higher than conventional cereals [181]. Approximately, 33.5% of the total carbohydrate content is resistant starch [12, 105].

Buckwheat has a rich mineral composition, wherein calcium, zinc, chromium, magnesium, potassium, iron, and copper are significantly higher. The magnesium content is 3–4× that of wheat and rice. But, zinc, phosphorus, cobalt, and magnesium are present mainly as phytates deposited in protein bodies thus making them inaccessible by the human body. It is a rich source of B vitamins, which are mainly concentrated in the bran. The bioavailability of thiamine is undetermined since it is present in strong adherence with thiamine-binding proteins [12, 181].

### 10.2.3   CHIA (SALVIA HISPANICA L.)

The lipid content of chia seeds ranges from 25% to 40% in which polyunsaturated fatty acids (PUFAs) are present at maximum levels of 80.5% [84]. Chia lipids contain the highest amount of α-linolenic acid ($C_{18:3}$, ω-3, ALA), that is, 68% compared to other vegetable sources [15]. PUFAs can further form long-chain polyenoic acids like docosahexanoic acid and EPA, which are necessary for brain development especially in children [66]. Chia seeds also possess sterols and tocopherols at higher levels with no cholesterol. The optimal ratio of ω-6 to ω-3 fatty acids is 3–5:1, which is generally not achieved in the regular diets where the ratio is 15–20:1. This can be improved by the chia lipids wherein the value is 0.32–0.35 [43].

Total dietary fiber (TDF) content of chia ranges from 23 to 41% wherein the insoluble and soluble fiber occupy 92% and 8%, respectively [54]. Consumption of chia seeds thus fulfils complete daily recommended fiber intake suggested by American Dietetic Association. TDF in chia is 2× and 4–5× compared to bran and, quinoa, soy, amaranth, and almonds, respectively [182]. The mucilage is mainly the soluble fiber, which is constituted mainly by polysaccharide (48%) of molecular weight 0.8–2 MDa with ash (8%), protein (4%), and fat (1%) [136, 186]. Insoluble dietary fiber is mainly constituted by lignin (Klason lignin), cellulose and hemicellulose. The PUFAs in chia are considered to be protected by Klason lignin since it builds a robust and resistant network with certain antioxidants. Lignin also exhibits hypocholesterolemic properties due to its bile acid absorbing ability [186].

Chia seeds contain the highest protein content (15%–24%) among all cereals thus proving essential to prevent malnutrition associated with protein intake [157, 182]. The main storage protein fraction is globulin (52%–54%) trailed by albumins (17.3%–18.6%), glutelins (13.6%) and prolamins (17.9%) [135, 157]. Thus, chia seeds can be consumed by celiac patients since gluten proteins are absent. Glutamic acid is present at highest levels (123 g/kg of chia protein) followed by arginine (80.6 g/kg of chia protein), and aspartic acid (61.3 g/kg of raw protein). It is not rich in lysine and thus not considered as the sole protein source. The protein digestibility (29.01%) of chia seed is low due to high content of dietary fiber [84, 192].

Chia is also rich in vitamins and minerals. The major macroelements are calcium, phosphorus, magnesium and potassium, and microelements are iron, molybdenum, copper, zinc, sodium, manganese, and selenium. It provides 13–354× calcium, 2–12× phosphorus, and 1.6–9× potassium compared to 100 g of conventional cereals like rice, maize, and wheat. In comparison to 100 g milk, chia seed consumption can provide 6× calcium, 11× phosphorus, and 4× potassium apart from zinc, copper and iron [20]. It is a major source of vitamin B especially niacin compared to soybean, maize, and rice. It is also a good source of vitamins A and C [120].

### 10.2.4   HEMP SEED (CANNABIS SATIVA L.)

The hemp seed is composed of 30%–35% oil wherein unsaturated fatty acids occupy 90% of the total content [103, 189]. Monounsaturated and PUFAs constitute 11.25% and 80%–90%, respectively. LA and α-linolenic acid (ALA) occupy 50%–70% and 15%–25%, respectively, and these two fatty acids along with oleic acid constitute 88% of the total [70]. It also contains γ-linolenic acid (GLA, $C_{18:3}$, ω-6) and stearidonic acid (SDA, $C_{18:4}$, ω-3) at levels of 0.51%–4.55% and 0.26%–1.58%, respectively [49, 141]. SDA is a naturally occurring ω-3 fatty acid, which is generally present in fish and plants at low levels. But it is necessary since it readily converts to EPA compared to ALA because, for the rate-limiting step (Δ6-desaturation) in the synthesis of EPA from ALA, SDA is the resultant product [102]. Moreover, the ratio of ω-6 to ω-3 fatty acids is approximately 2.5–3:1, which is optimal for human nutrition [49]. The hemp seed hull may contain cannabinoids (<0.3%) especially cannabidiol that are generally contaminants from the leaves [70].

The protein content of hemp seed is 25%–30% approximately and is dominated by globulin (edestin 67%–75%), and albumin (25%–37%). Edestin is rich in branched, aromatic, hydrophobic, and sulfur-containing amino acids [91, 103], which are generally present in low amounts in conventional grains. The albumin fraction is comparable to protein present in egg white and human blood [33, 91, 111]. Arginine (12% of total protein) and glutamine acid are present at high levels in the hemp seed proteins, wherein the globulin and albumin fractions have a value of 4.37 and 1.74, respectively, for arginine to lysine ratio (a higher ratio means lower risk of cardiovascular diseases) [91, 111, 190]. The essential amino acid composition of hemp seed is similar to casein and soy protein and adequate according to recommendation of FAO/WHO for infants and 2–5-year-old preschool children. The protein digestibility values of dehulled hemp seed (90.8%–97.5%) are similar to that of casein (97.6%) [190]. Czechoslovakian Tubercular Nutrition Study in 1955 stated that tuberculosis can be treated successfully only by consumption of hemp seed (due to edestin) [91].

Hemp seed contains 5.5% minerals and is a good source of calcium, magnesium, phosphorus, potassium, sulfur, iron, and zinc [34, 52]. It is a superior source of vitamin E, compared to other oilseeds, present at levels of 90 mg/100 g with high amounts of γ-tocopherol (85 mg/100 g) and α-tocopherol (5 mg/100 g) [34, 103]. It also contains fair amounts of β-carotene (a vitamin A precursor) and carotenoids (2–5.3 mg/100 g oil) [70].

The carbohydrate content of hemp seed is ~25% [189], which contains nonstarchy polysaccharides rather than starch, most of which reside in the hull [83, 103]. The *Cannabis* species contain certain sugars like monosaccharides, disaccharides, and cyclitols [29]. The primary sugars of the nonstarchy polysaccharides in hemp seed are xylose and glucose apart from uronic acid, arabinose, and galactose with small amounts of raffinose [82]. Sucrose and a glycerol dihexosylderivative are also found to be present [49]. Hemp seeds contain 28% of TDF, which constitutes 92% of the total carbohydrate fraction [34, 82]. Fiber content mainly contains cellulose, hemicellulose, and lignin. No specific literature is available, which elaborates on the carbohydrate and fiber constitution.

## 10.2.5 MILLETS

Like all cereals, carbohydrates are the main components of millets constituting 56.88%–72.97% [90]. Starch (60%–75%) is the chief carbohydrate, followed by nonstarchy polysaccharides (15%–20%) and sugars (2%–3%). The free sugars prominently include sucrose, glucose, and glucose. Amylose and amylopectin are present in the ratio of 1:3–4. Waxy varieties of certain millets like foxtail and proso also exist [177]. The resistant starch content varies from 21.99% to 30.87%. The GI of millets is generally lower than wheat since it ranges from 40.17 for kodo millet to 52.49 proso millet. This is due to high contents of dietary fiber (arabinoxylan), which reduces the digestive enzymatic activity and high content of fat since fat which adsorbs to the starch surface [162].

Proteins in millets constitute of 10%–11% except finger millet, which exhibits a large variation from 4.76% to 11.7% [90]. They are good sources of essential amino acids particularly sulfur-containing amino acids (cysteine and methionine) [180]. Prolamins are the major storage proteins in all millets except fonio in which glutelins are the chief protein fractions. The IVPD of millets varies from 72.01% for finger millet to 75.41% for foxtail millet [162]. It is lower than wheat flour due to presence of fiber, fat, and antinutritional factors like tannins and phytic acid [60].

The lipid content of millets varies from 1% to 5% with pearl, proso, and foxtail millets containing the highest (5%) and kodo and finger millet containing lowest amounts (1%). Since the germ contains higher content of lipids, pearl, and foxtail millets have higher levels due to larger germs. Approximately 88% of the total pearl millet fat is concentrated in the germ, which contains 32% of the lipid content [177]. The lipids contain neutral lipids (85%), phospholipids (12%), and glycolipids (3%). The unsaturated fatty acids constitute 78%–82% with high levels of LA followed by oleic acid. Linolenic acid and erucic acid are also present in trace amounts [7, 81]. Oleic acid is the chief fatty acid in finger millet, which itself contains lower amount of lipids content, thus accounting for the superior shelf stability [177]. Major phospholipids include lysophosphatidylcholine (42%), phosphatidylcholine (24%), lysophosphatidylethanolamine (21%), and traceable amounts of phosphatidylserine, phosphatidic acid, phosphatidylinositol, and phosphatidylglycerol [81].

Nonstarchy polysaccharides in the millets constitute the dietary fiber content mainly comprised of hemicellulose, cellulose, and pectinaceous material with the absence of arabinose and stachyose (which can cause flatulence) as well as lignin and β-glucan [81] thus providing prebiotic properties. The kernel pericarp contains the cellulose and endosperm contains glucoronoarabinoxylans. Insoluble dietary fiber content (up to 97%) is much higher than conventional cereals, which contain substantial quantities of soluble fiber [176].

Millets are good sources of B vitamins particularly thiamine, riboflavin, and niacin but not cyanocobalamin (vitamin $B_{12}$) [177]. These are present more in bran and germ and less in endosperm [176]. Foxtail millet and pearl millet have the highest content of riboflavin (1.65 and 1.48 mg/100 g, respectively) among all millets [90]. The niacin content of millets is 10.88 mg but its extraction level in cold water is very low (only 13%) [81]. β-carotene content (precursor of vitamin A) is low but zeaxanthin and lutein are the primary carotenoids responsible for yellow color of foxtail millet endosperm but provitamin A activity is very low [177]. Among minerals, millets are good sources of phosphorus and magnesium. Moreover, finger millet is a rich source of calcium (294–390 mg/100 g), barnyard, and little millet are of iron, and common and kodo millets are of copper.

## 10.2.6   QUINOA (CHENOPODIUM QUINOA WILLD.)

Quinoa seeds contain up to 51%–70% carbohydrates [109] majority of which is starch [187]. Starch constitutes 58.1%–64.2% dry weight of seed and contains mainly xylose and maltose at high levels (120 and 101 mg/100 g, respectively) and glucose and fructose at low levels (19 and 19.6 mg/100 g, respectively). The GI values of quinoa seeds vary from 35 to 53, which are much less than wheat and rice [109]. This is attributed to the monosaccharide constitution of dietary fiber content (10%), which is close to that of fruits, vegetables, and legumes. The soluble and insoluble fiber content constitute 22% and 78%, respectively. They are mainly composed of glucose, galacturonic acid, and arabinose monomers and galacturonic acid, arabinose, galactose, xylose, and glucose monomers, respectively [101].

Quinoa is a rich source of proteins, which range from 13.8 to 16.5% [126]. Unlike conventional cereals, prolamin content is low (0.5%–0.7%) and albumins and globulins are the major storage proteins present at 35% and 37% levels, respectively [1], thus it is a gluten-free grain. All the essential amino acids (EAAs) are present in balanced amounts and it is especially rich in lysine (2.4–7.8 g/100 g), threonine (2.1–8.9 g/100 g) and methionine (0.3–9.1 g/100 g), which are limiting in conventional cereals [57]. According to FAO/WHO recommendations, quinoa protein can supply over 180% of the daily recommended intake of essential amino acids for adult nutrition

[193]. Quinoa protein digestibility ranges as high as 91.6% for raw seeds and 95.3% for cooked seeds [153].

The lipid content of quinoa seeds ranges from 5% to 9% with an average of 6.1%, which is higher than wheat, rice, and maize [80]. Alternatively an oilseed [126], the major components are triglycerides (50%) and diglycerides (20%) [80]. The unsaturated fatty acids amount to 89.4% mostly constituted by PUFAs (54.2%–58.3%). The optimal ω-6 to ω-3 ratio of 6:1 makes it more preferable than other oils [175]. The major saturated fatty acid occupying 10% of total fatty acid composition is palmitic acid. Unsaturated fatty acid composition is dominated by LA (49.0%–56.4%), oleic acid (19.7%–29.5%), and ALA (8.7%–11.7%) whose levels are comparable to that in soybean lipid composition [64]. Of the total polar lipids, 57% is composed of two phospholipids, phosphatidyl choline and lysophosphatidyl ethanolamine [80].

The nutritional richness of quinoa is also due to the presence of vitamins which are generally in limited quantities in conventional grains. Riboflavin, pyridoxine, and folic acid are present in higher levels than cereals like wheat, rice, maize, rye, barley, and oats but thiamine is lower than barley and oats. Also, it is a superior vitamin E source thus providing protection from damage due to oxidation. The requirements of children and adults can be met by 100 g of quinoa for pyridoxine and folic acid, which also contribute 80 and 40% of the riboflavin daily requirements for children and adults, respectively [1]. Carotenoids especially lutein and zeaxanthins are also present at levels of 1.2–1.8 mg/100 g [175]. The large reported range of ascorbic acid (0–63 mg/100 g) is due to its high oxidation susceptibility [80].

Quinoa's mineral levels of 2.4% are higher than conventional cereals. The micronutrients mainly include magnesium (26–502 mg/100 g), calcium (27.5–148.7 mg/100 g), phosphorus (140–530 mg/100 g), potassium (0.01–1200 mg/100 g), zinc (2.8–4.8 mg/100 g), copper (0.2–5.1 mg/100 g), and iron (1.4–6.8 mg/100 g). Magnesium, potassium, and calcium are adequately available biologically thus providing a balanced diet [187]. The complete daily requirements of magnesium, iron, and copper (adults and infants), phosphorus and zinc (children) can be met by 100 g quinoa seeds. Approximately 40%–60% of zinc and phosphorus requirements and 22% of potassium of 10% needs for calcium can be met by 100 g quinoa [80] and are considered sufficient for bone and teeth development in children [133]. The ratio of calcium to phosphorus is 1:0.7–3.9, which is superior to that of conventional cereals (1:7.8–54.0) [10].

## 10.2.7   TEFF (ERAGROSTIS TEF)

The teff grains contain 80% carbohydrates, wherein starch is the major component present at the level of 73% [201]. The content of amylose varies from 20 to 30% and no waxy teff varieties are present [19]. Resistant starches occupy 40% of the total carbohydrates in teff [58]. The damaged starch content (2.1%–3.5%), in vitro starch digestibility and GI (74) of teff is remarkably less than conventional grains [195]. The lower damaged starch content, high amylose content, high gelatinization temperature (68 °C–80 °C), and amylose-lipid complex formation explains the low enzymatic activity and digestibility [63, 195]. Teff starch can be used as a vehicle for aroma and flavor compounds due to small, uniformly sized, and smooth starch granules [11].

Teff protein content varies from 8.7% to 11%, which is comparable to common cereals but its composition includes glutelins (45%) and albumins (37%) as the chief storage fractions, while prolamins are minor constituents (12%). In certain cases, prolamins are reported as the major storage proteins of teff [19, 160]. But, it does not contain gluten, which is confirmed by the absence of T-cell stimulatory epitopes thus making it a functional ingredient for patients of celiac disease [19]. Although lysine is a limiting amino acid in teff, its concentration (14–40 g/kg protein) in teff is higher than conventional cereals. Other amino acids in abundance are proline, alanine, glutamic acid, aspartic acid, histidine, and methionine and thus, its amino acid composition is considered to be balanced [11]. The IVPD of teff flour is ~72% due to higher contents of albumins and globulins, which exhibit high digestibility [166].

The lipid content of teff is 2%–3%, which is more than rice and wheat but less than sorghum and maize [19]. Unsaturated fatty acid content values to 84%, which is dominated by oleic acid (32%) and LA (24%) [71]. Palmitic acid is the chief saturated fatty acid constituting 15.9% [62]. It also contains higher levels of ALA. The ratio of LA to ALA is 7:1, which is considered to be optimum for infant formula according to the Codex standards [98].

Dietary fiber constitutes 9.8% (dry matter basis) in the teff grain, which is mostly present in bran. Since teff is consumed as whole without removing the bran, the fiber intake is higher compared to other cereals. Teff contains mineral content of 2.8%–3.4%, which is higher than conventional cereals [11]. It is an excellent source of iron due to which teff consumers have high hemoglobin levels. Other minerals in good amounts are calcium, phosphorus, copper, zinc, and magnesium [160]. The major vitamins in teff are vitamin A, niacin, riboflavin, thiamine, and vitamin A. Vitamin C is highly adequate since it completes the recommended dietary allowance [11].

Table 10.1 elaborates on the macro- and micronutrients of the super grains as reported by the United States Department of Agriculture [184].

**TABLE 10.1** Composition of Super Grains per 100 g Reported under USDA 2019 [184]

| Parameter | Amaranth | Buckwheat | Dried Chia Seeds | Hemp seed (hulled) | Millet | Quinoa | Teff |
|---|---|---|---|---|---|---|---|
| Ash (g) | 2.88 | 2.1 | 4.8 | 6.06 | 3.25 | 2.38 | 2.37 |
| Calcium (mg) | 159 | 18 | 631 | 70 | 8 | 47 | 180 |
| Carbohydrates (g) | 65.25 | 71.5 | 42.12 | 8.67 | 72.85 | 64.16 | 73.13 |
| Copper (mg) | 0.525 | 1.1 | 0.924 | 1.6 | 0.75 | 0.59 | 0.81 |
| Energy (Kcal) | 371 | 343 | 486 | 553 | 378 | 368 | 367 |
| Fat (g) | 7.02 | 3.4 | 30.74 | 48.75 | 4.22 | 6.07 | 2.38 |
| Fatty acids, total monounsaturated (g) | 1.685 | 1.04 | 2.309 | 5.4 | 0.773 | 1.613 | 0.589 |
| Fatty acids, total polyunsaturated (g) | 2.778 | 1.039 | 23.665 | 38.1 | 2.134 | 3.292 | 1.071 |
| Fatty acids, total saturated (g) | 1.459 | 0.741 | 3.33 | 4.6 | 0.723 | 0.706 | 0.449 |
| Fiber (g) | 6.7 | 10 | 34.4 | 4 | 8.5 | 7 | 8 |
| Folate (µg) | 82 | 30 | 49 | 110 | 85 | 184 | Not reported |
| Iron (mg) | 7.61 | 2.2 | 7.72 | 7.95 | 3.01 | 4.57 | 7.63 |
| Magnesium (mg) | 248 | 231 | 335 | 700 | 114 | 197 | 184 |
| Manganese (mg) | 3.333 | 1.3 | 2.723 | 7.6 | 1.632 | 2.033 | 9.24 |
| Niacin (mg) | 0.923 | 7.02 | 8.83 | 9.2 | 4.72 | 1.52 | 3.363 |
| Pantothenic acid (mg) | 1.457 | 1.233 | Not reported | Not reported | 0.848 | 0.772 | 0.942 |
| Phosphorus (mg) | 557 | 347 | 860 | 1650 | 285 | 457 | 429 |
| Potassium (mg) | 508 | 460 | 407 | 1200 | 195 | 563 | 427 |
| Protein (g) | 13.56 | 13.25 | 16.54 | 31.56 | 11.02 | 14.12 | 13.3 |

**TABLE 10.1** *(Continued)*

| Parameter | Amaranth | Buckwheat | Dried Chia Seeds | Hemp seed (hulled) | Millet | Quinoa | Teff |
|---|---|---|---|---|---|---|---|
| Riboflavin (mg) | 0.2 | 0.425 | 0.17 | 0.285 | 0.29 | 0.318 | 0.27 |
| Selenium (mg) | 18.7 | 8.3 | 55.2 | Not reported | 2.7 | 8.5 | 4.4 |
| Sodium (mg) | 4 | 1 | 16 | 5 | 5 | 5 | 12 |
| Thiamine (mg) | 0.116 | 0.101 | 0.62 | 1.275 | 0.421 | 0.36 | 0.39 |
| Vitamin A (IU) | 2 | 0 | 54 | 11 | 0 | 14 | 9 |
| Vitamin B-6 (mg) | 0.591 | 0.21 | Not reported | 0.6 | 0.384 | 0.487 | 0.482 |
| Vitamin C (mg) | 4.2 | 0 | 1.6 | 0.5 | 0 | Not reported | Not reported |
| Vitamin E (mg) | 1.19 | Not reported | 0.5 | 0.8 | 0.05 | 2.44 | 0.08 |
| Vitamin K (µg) | Not reported | Not reported | Not reported | Not reported | 0.9 | 1.1 | 1.9 |
| Water (g) | 11.29 | 9.75 | 5.8 | 4.96 | 8.67 | 13.28 | 8.82 |
| Zinc (mg) | 2.87 | 2.4 | 4.58 | 9.9 | 1.68 | 3.1 | 3.63 |

## 10.3  ANTINUTRITIONAL FACTORS

Super grains are usually correlated with high nutritional value and many health benefits. However, they may contain certain compounds that have negative effects on the absorption of the essential nutrients and are known as antinutritional factors. These compounds interfere with the bioavailability of the nutrients and contribute to the impaired digestion by complexing with nutrients. For instance, phytic acid and saponins are generally correlated with the reduced availability of the iron. Similarly, phytic acid and tannins show resistance in the digestion of the minerals and such effects can be seen at low concentrations of these factors. In the presence of high concentration of fibers, the negative effects of phytic acid and tannins increased by certain folds which can be attributed to the gel-forming ability of the fiber leading to the slow release of nutrient from cellular structure. Also, the gel formed by the fiber interferes with the enzymatic activities, which results in the lower digestibility values [121]. Other antinutritional factors include oxalates, nitrates, and protease inhibitors. In contrast, certain studies show the anti-oxidant potential of the phytic acid thereby contributing to the prevention of cancer and cardiovascular disease [127].

**TABLE 10.2**  Phytic Acid Content in Super Grains

| Grain | Phytic acid content | Ref. |
|---|---|---|
| Amaranth | 0.3%–0.6% | [138, 148] |
| Buckwheat | 10 mg/g | [12] |
| Chia | 7 mg/g | [17] |
| Hemp seed (defatted) | 61.2–74.1 g/kg | [70, 91] |
| Millets | 7–10 mg/g | [162] |
| Quinoa | 10.5–13.1 mg/g | [64] |
| Teff | 1129–1552 mg/100 g (dry matter basis) | [166] |

## 10.3.1  PHYTIC ACID

In many plant tissues, a saturated cyclic acid known as phytic acid is the main storage form of phosphorus. Like other antinutritional factors, phytic acid also binds to certain nutrients which results in the reduced metabolism of such nutrients. Phytic acid has strong affinity for divalent ions attributed to the negative charge present on the structure, which allow it to make stable chelate complex with iron, copper, calcium, zinc, and magnesium. In plant food matrix, it is considered as the prime storage form for phosphorus. It also has the ability to make complexes with certain biomolecules including protein and starch as well as with enzymes in order to reduce their bioavailability. In legumes and cereals, it is mainly found in the hull part with the overall percentage of 1%–3% of the total dry matter [76, 64].

### 10.3.2   PROTEASE INHIBITORS

Proteolytic enzymes play an important in the human body as they are responsible for the metabolism of the proteins. Antinutritional factors like protease inhibitors form undesirable complexes with such enzymes which hinder their activity. In gastrointestinal tract, the complexation of protease inhibitors with trypsin reduces the metabolic activity of the enzyme, thus the pancreases produce more enzymes leading to pancreatic hypertrophy and consequently growth reduction (Tables 10.2 and 10.3). However, these antinutritional factors can be easily destroyed through domestic cooking which is attributed to their thermolabile nature [97, 107]. Super grains like quinoa contain very low levels of protease inhibitors, that is, 1.36–5.04 unit trypsin inhibitor (TIU) per mg, which makes them highly digestible [187] as compared to the lentils (17.8 TIU per mg), soybean (24.5–41.5 TIU per mg) and beans (12.9–42.8 TIU per mg) [87].

**TABLE 10.3**   Trypsin Inhibitor Units (TIU) in Super Grains

| Grain | Trypsin inhibitor content | Ref. |
|---|---|---|
| Amaranth | 1550 TIU/g | [40] |
| Hemp seed (defatted) | 10.8–28.4 TIU/mg | [70] |
| Quinoa | 1.36–5.04 TIU/mg | [64] |
| Teff | 5584 TIU/g | [94] |

### 10.3.3   SAPONINS

Saponins are the water or methanol soluble antinutritional factors with major presence in the plants of Leguminosae family. They are secondary metabolites, produced as defense mechanism for the tolerance of abiotic stresses

[146]. The molecular structure of the saponins include the triterpenoid agly-cone or steroidal; especially, oleanolic acid, hederagenin, serjanic acid, and phytolaccagenic acid, with the presence of specific number of sugar moieties (xylose, glucose, glucuronic acid, galactose, and arabinose) [197]. They are well known for soapy nature in the aqueous solution and this property is well used for the qualitative analysis in various grains. The undesirable affects imposed by the saponins include the haematolysis of red blood cells, which interferes with the normal functioning of the organism. Saponins have the ability to make complexes with the lipids, proteins as well as with certain minerals (zinc, iron) thus lower bioavailability of such nutrients [138, 172]. Also, saponins impart bitter taste to the final product, which results in the reduced consumer acceptability [64]. However, these compounds can be eliminated through the processing techniques technique such as washing. Apart from the undesirable affects, saponins do have certain beneficial prop-erties such as neuroprotective, antimicrobial, anti-inflammatory, analgesic, antithrombotic, immunostimulatory, antioxidant, diuretic, antiviral, hypo-glycemic, and hypocholesterolemic [74]. The saponin content is sometimes used to classify the super grains such as bitter quinoa with more than 0.11% saponins and sweet quinoa with <0.11% saponins (Table 10.4).

**TABLE 10.4**   Saponin Content in Super Grains

| Grain | Saponin Content | Ref. |
|---|---|---|
| Amaranth | 0.09%–0.1% | [138] |
| Hemp seed (defatted) | 69 mg/kg | [70, 91] |
| Quinoa | 0.2–0.4 g/kg (Sweet quinoa) | [64] |
|  | 4.7–11.3 g/kg (Bitter quinoa) |  |

## 10.3.4  TANNINS

Polyphenols are an indigenous part of our food matrix with some beneficial as well as negative effects on the human body. Tannins are classified under the umbrella of polyphenols. They are widely distributed in the nature and well known for their undesirable effects on the human body. Tannins possess the ability to bind with macromolecules including proteins and starch resulting in the reduced bioavailability of such nutrients. However, such complexes are reversible and dependent on the factors like pH. Similarly, it forms chelate complexes with minerals (calcium and iron) and vitamin B12, which leads to lower absorption and reduced nutritional values (Table 10.5). Furthermore, tannins are considered to be responsible for undesirable sensorial properties of the some food products due to their involvement in the enzymatic browning reactions as well as ability to provide astringency flavor [17, 159].

**TABLE 10.5**    Tannin Content in Super Grains

| Grain | Tannin Content | Ref. |
|---|---|---|
| Amaranth | 0.52–0.61% | [44, 138] |
| Buckwheat | 1.6% | [181] |
| Chia | 5 mg/g | [17] |
| Hemp seed (defatted) | 1.36–2.14 g/kg | [70, 91] |
| Millets | 1–4 mg/100 g | [162] |
| Quinoa | 0.53% | [64] |
| Teff | 65–302 mg/100 g (dry matter basis) | [166] |

## 10.3.5  OXALATES AND NITRATES

Nitrates are the essential components of the plants as they are the important nitrogen source for the optimum growth. But their presence in the diet interferes with the functionality of thyroid gland and interferes with the metabolism of the vitamin A. The reduced form (nitrites) of such compounds, through the synthesis of metmyoglobin, lead to cyanosis or in some cases the nitrites interact with amines (secondary or tertiary) resulting in the production of carcinogenic N-nitrous compound [107]. According to WHO, 0.06 and 3.7 mg/kg of body weight are the acceptable daily intake (ADI) levels for nitrite and nitrate ions, respectively [21].

Oxalates are harmful substances and potential risk for the human body. It is not metabolized in human body and excrete through urine. The higher consumption of the oxalates results in the reduced availability of the certain elements, which can lead to hyperoxaluria. This can cause a risk of calcium oxalate stone formation in the kidneys since oxalate and divalent ions are capable of forming insoluble complex in the gut [87, 107, 159]. Moreover, the presence of the oxalic acid in the human diet leads to various harmful effects such as gastrointestinal irritation, reduced minerals availability, impaired blood clotting, and contraction of muscles mainly attributed to the higher amounts of crystalline calcium contents deposits in the cells (Table 10.6). The recommended levels of oxalates in the human diet are estimated to be 50–200 mg per day [107].

**TABLE 10.6**   Nitrate and Oxalate Contents in Super Grains

| Grain | Nitrate Content (mg/100 g) | Oxalate Content (mg/100 g) |
|---|---|---|
| Amaranth | 410–920 [143] | 268 (soluble–33) [72] |
| Finger millet | | 11.3 [8] |
| Pearl millet | | 20 [8] |
| Quinoa | 63.26 [64] | 380 [64] |

### 10.3.6   MISCELLANEOUS

Certain other antinutritional factors like haemagglutinins and cyanogenic glycosides are also present in certain grains. Raw amaranth exhibits an agglutination activity of 1/16 [40]. Defatted hemp seeds contain cyanogenic glycosides at levels of 0.09–0.23 g/kg [70, 91]. Buckwheat causes an allergy which is an IgE-mediated hypersensitive reaction due to binding with IgE. It is uncommon but highly potent especially in children [181].

## 10.4   FUNCTIONAL PROPERTIES

The properties which are responsible for the characteristics of the food system during its preparation, processing, storage, and consumption are known as functional properties. These depend on the macro- and micromolecular composition especially proteins and starch. Functional properties are a reflection of the complex associations among structure, conformation, surrounding food components, and the environment [196]. These are essential while designing of various novel food systems since these can affect the nutritional, organoleptic, and textural properties. Generally, the protein conformation and consequently the solubility, hydration, and gelation characteristics are affected by the apolar amino acid composition. The electrostatic interactions with water are stabilized due to the charged amino acids. Hydrophilic amino acid residues and disulfide linkages affect the water retention and gel formation characteristics [199]. These consequently affect the oil absorption capacity, emulsifying capacity (EC), and emulsion stability (ES) due to the adsorption capacity around oil particles to reduce the oil–water interfacial tension thus inhibiting the separation due to flocculation, coalescing, or creaming. Similarly, the adsorption and rearrangement of the protein molecules at the interface of air and water affects the foaming capacity (FC) and formation of cohesive films around air molecules determines the foam stability [196]. The flavor retention and mouthfeel of the food product depend on the water absorption capacity (WAI) and oil absorption capacity (OAI) since these affect the viscosity of products like dough, soups, and baked products. Gelation, swelling, emulsion properties—EC and ES—and foaming properties—FC and foaming stability (FS)—are responsible for the behavior of the food systems especially during the processing and storage stages [61, 164].

Super grains exhibit better functional properties due to the exceptional macromolecular composition (Table 10.7). For instance, WAI of quinoa flour (147%) and amaranth (209%) is higher than soy flour (130%), pigeon pea flour (138%), and fluted pumpkin seeds (85%). Even the EC of quinoa flour (104%) is higher than pigeon pea (49.9%), soy flour (18%), and benniseed (63%) due to superior protein content and composition [61]. Chia flour also exhibits high WAI since the mucilage (fiber) itself exhibits the capacity to absorb 27× water [124]. The emulsifying properties of whole chia flour (42%) are low but its insoluble fiber-rich fraction exhibits superior ES (53.26%) and EC (94.84%) due to the presence of 28.14% protein in it [50]. Similarly, the least gelation concentration of chia flour is very low (4%) due to the creation of a gel film due to high fiber content [45].

## 10.4   PROCESSING INTERVENTIONS

The nutritive and functional superiority of food can be hindered due to certain compositional and environmental factors. The antinutritional factors highly affect the bioavailability of proteins and minerals along with exhibiting toxicity to the human body. Certain functional properties required for specific products need to be achieved for optimum quality characteristics. This can be achieved by processing the super grains using different treatments at different stages. The evaluation of the effectiveness of the treatment singly or in combination is necessary to determine the best processing methods for achieving a superior product.

**TABLE 10.7**  Functional Properties of the Super Grains

| Grain | WAI g/g | OAI g/g | EC/ES % | FC/FS % | Swelling Capacity (mL/g) | Least Gelation Concentration (%) [Ref.] |
|---|---|---|---|---|---|---|
| Quinoa | 1.44–1.80 [139] | 0.89–1.04 [139] | EC—104% ES—45% [1] | FC—9% FS—4% [1] | 8.55–9.57 [139] | 16% [1] |
| Chia | 5.2 [78] | 1.8 [78] | EC—42% [78] | FC—70% (chia protein isolate) [134] | 8.5 [78] | 4% [45] |
| Teff | 1.36 [46] | 1.35 [46] | | FC—5% FS—60% [46] | | 6% [201] |
| Amaranth | 2.09–2.43 [164] | 1.88–1.95 [164] | EC—2.01% ES—1.2% [3] | FC—15%–30% FS—17%–50% [164] | 2.96 [156] | 7.1% [69] |
| Buckwheat | 1.33 [16] | 1.81 [16] | EC—0.44% [16] | FC—15.47% FS—93.91% [16] | 8.34 [167] | 32% [16] |
| Hemp seed | 1.5–2 [145] | 1.62–1.79 (hemp seed meal protein isolate) | 40–100% [145] | FC—40% FS—5% [145] | | >20% [145] |
| Foxtail Millet | 2.1 [4] | 1.35 [4] | EC—48.2% ES—66.5% [163] | FC—8.8% FS—78.8% [163] | 5.2 [163] | 11% [53] |
| Pearl millet | 1.2 [110] | 1.22 [110] | EC—11.79% ES—7.67% [110] | FC—24% FS—16.69% [110] | 4.06 [132] | 6% [110] |

### 10.4.1  PRETREATMENTS

Quinoa washing or polishing (abrasive peeling) is necessary to remove the saponins especially on the bitter varieties since they are present on the pericarp, but it also reduces the vitamin content of the grain [64]. Moreover, phytic acid content is as high as 8 mg/g after washing, which thus reduces the content of certain minerals like potassium by 46%, iron by 28%, manganese by 27%, and magnesium by 8% [154]. But, saponin removal also improves the protein digestibility by 7% [155]. Generally, washing is employed at domestic levels, but it is inconvenient at industrial level both economically and ecologically. On the other hand, polishing of grains removes the bran completely making the grain devoid of essential nutrients like proteins, minerals, and vitamins. Thus, a combination of washing and polishing is effective for saponin reduction with nutrient loss minimization [25, 64].

Chia seed protein may decrease during soaking due to lixiviation with a decrease in digestibility due to formation of gel, which affect the enzymatic activity adversely. Milling increases the digestibility from 34.18% to 79.8% due to improved exposure and consequently the action of enzymes on all the seed fractions [121]. In case of amaranth, refining is not suggested due to its unique morphology since a high extraction degree (40%) reduces the protein content to 4% [37]. Dehulling of hemp seed reduces or eliminates the cannabinoids which might be present due to contamination from the leaves [70].

### 10.4.2  HEAT TREATMENTS

Heat treatments especially autoclaving increase the protein digestibility due to reduction in protease inhibitors [155]. Washing and drying of quinoa at high temperatures (80 °C) reduces the protein, fat, fiber, and mineral content by 10%, 12%, 27%, and 27%, respectively, which is attributed to protein denaturation, complexation of released amino acids with melanoidins in Maillard reaction, lipid oxidation, enzymatic hydrolysis during initial drying period, and leaching of minerals along with saponins [117]. Tannins in quinoa can be removed effectively by adequate washing and soaking (18–22 h), followed by common domestic process treatments that involve heat treatments like microwaving, autoclaving, boiling, and roasting [25]. Similarly, amaranth exhibits 80% retention of magnesium during steaming and boiling whereas in quinoa, copper is lost up to 17% during boiling. 100 g of cooked amaranth contributes more to the Recommended Nutrient Intake of minerals especially manganese, magnesium, and phosphorus [122].

Starch digestibility increases by roasting and popping of amaranth thereby increasing the GI to 105.81 and 101.26, respectively [35]. Although, popping reduces the content of essential amino acids especially tyrosine and thereby the PER by 14.3%–19.3%, it improves the IVPD by 6%–8% which is attributed to the partial denaturation [68]. Nonenzymatic browning during popping results in significant reduction of aromatic amino acids—phenylalanine, tyrosine, and tryptophan—in amaranth [113].

Roasting significantly improves the protein and fiber content of chia seeds by 20.9% and 17.61%. Micronutrient composition changes also occur in chia seeds during roasting. Vitamin C, iron, and calcium increase by 15.12%, 10.76%, and 1.96%, whereas phosphorus content decreases by 15.46% [78]. Heat treatment of hemp seed reduces the protein digestibility due to partial denaturation of protein [52]. Amino acid content of hemp seed reduces during steaming, whereas the essential fatty acids like LA and ALA increase during roasting [88]. Microwave cooking of millets reduces the oxalate contents significantly but not phytate and tannins. An increase in TDF and insoluble dietary fiber during cooking is attributed to the increased resistant starch [8].

Water and oil absorption capacities of quinoa and amaranth increase significantly during roasting and cooking. Starch gelatinization and protein denaturation during thermal processing improves these functional properties [168]. Roasted chia exhibits significantly low WAI, OAI, swelling power, and EC by values of 48%, 33%, 25.88%, and 7.61% compared to untreated chia [78]. Popped amaranth seeds exhibit superior WAI (5.82) but reduced foaming capacity (12.67%) [95].

### 10.4.3  EXTRUSION

During extrusion, high shear stress and temperature disrupt the chemical bonding, which leads to formation of small particles with improved solubility. Thus, there is a reduction in the content of total and insoluble dietary fibers wherein some fraction of the latter is also transformed into soluble fiber [149]. The in vitro protein and starch digestibility of quinoa increases the extrusion processing [155]. Extruded amaranth exhibits a high PER of 2.5–3.3 [188]. Saponin contents also decrease during extrusion due to destruction of the saponin structure leading to fragment formation [100].

Water absorption and solubility indices increase during extrusion up to 3.05 g/g and 15.87%, respectively, in quinoa [100]. Similarly, water solubility increases by 22.7 and 50% in teff and amaranth [152]. Extrusion of millets at high moisture increases WAI but reduces water solubility, whereas high temperature leads to opposite effects. This is because of reduction in starch granule degradation at high moisture but its depolymerization at high temperature [96].

## 10.4.4  GERMINATION/MALTING

The protein content of chia seed increases during germination mainly due to degradation of carbohydrates (during respiration) and lipid (which act as primary energy source). Moreover, the components of cell wall like hemicellulose, cellulose, and pectic polysaccharides are synthesized during germination, which leads to 65% increase in TDF content [73, 13]. The levels of essential amino acids also increase during germination of chia and amaranth by 6.7–57.9% with no limiting amino acid. The IVPD and PER increase by 4.8%–11.7% and 49%–57%, respectively, in germinated chia and amaranth due to reduction of antinutritional factors like phytic acid, tannins and protease inhibitors [13]. γ-Aminobutyric acid (GABA) in chia seeds increases 11.4-fold due to action of glutamate decarboxylase during germination [73]. The mineral constitution of chia, especially sodium, calcium, iron, manganese, copper and zinc, improve during the germination process [138].

The protein digestibility of amaranth increases to 83.58% at 28 °C for 48 h with significant reduction in phytic acid (30%) and oxalate (38%) but increase in tannin content (47%) [79]. The sugar content of germinated amaranth also increases due to starch and oligosaccharide hydrolysis with the dominance of glucose and galactose [69]. Germination of buckwheat increases the content of linoleic and linolenic acids to 51 and 19%, respectively. The vitamins B1, B6, and C are increased during germination, wherein vitamin C increases to levels of 25 mg/100 g [12].

The endogenous phytase enzyme is activated during the germination process, which leads to hydrolysis of the complexes formed between phytic acid and minerals. Saponins and tannins are solubilized and consequently leached, which causes reduction in their content [85]. The content of saponins, tannins, and phytates of quinoa can be reduced to 0.93 g/100 g, 1.01 mg/100 g and 0.11 mg/100 g, respectively, during germination [85].

WAI, OAI, and foaming properties improve during germination to 3.88 g/g, 3.07 g/g and 11%, respectively, for quinoa [86]. Similar improvement occurs for WAI and water solubility index in amaranth [39]. Malting of millets increases the OAI but reduces the WAI due to exposure of hydrophobic residues of the peptide chains [4].

## 10.4.5  FERMENTATION

The protein (20.62%), vitamin (B1—56.76%, B2—50%) and essential amino acid (lysine—6.46% and threonine—13.98%) contents increase significantly during fermentation with *Lactobacillus casei* with a concomitant decrease in fat (52.05%), fiber (45.87%), and bound phenolic content (40.97%) [106]. The folate content of teff flour increases during fermentation with *Saccharomyces cerevisiae* and *Lb. plantarum* [179]. The IVPD of fermented amaranth improves by 4.8%–7.5% due to phytic acid and tannin hydrolysis [9]. Copper and magnesium are increased in fermented amaranth but no zinc and calcium do not change significantly [113]. Biogenic amines like putrescine and spermidine, which are precursors of carcinogenic nitrosamines, are formed occurs during hemp seed fermentation at safer levels in solid-state fermentation with *Pediococcus acidilactici* and *Pediococcus pentosaceous* than submerged state fermentation. Also, it affects the total PUFA in hemp seed without significantly affecting any single fatty acid [18].

The phytate degradation during fermentation is due to the production of phytase enzyme endogenously and exogenously by the microorganisms. Fermentation with *Lactobacillus plantarum* exhibits a phytate degradation of 83%–85% in quinoa and 64%–80% in amaranth thus improving the mineral bioavailability [38]. Similarly, *Rhizopus oligosporus* reduces the phytate of cooked quinoa grains by 72% after 40 h [59]. Iron, zinc, and copper bioavailability thus increases 3.5–4× and 1.7–2.5× in quinoa and amaranth, respectively, during fermentation [38]. Similarly, 49%–66% and 15% reduction in phytic acid and bound phenolic content occurs in teff leading to improved availability of iron and zinc [165].

Free amino acid content (especially methionine) and soluble protein increase 7–8× with a significant decrease in tannins and TIU activity by 52 and 68.9%, respectively [183]. Thus, it also helps to improve the IVPD in quinoa, amaranth, and finger millets [166]. *Lb. plantarum* and *P. acidilactici* reduce phytic acid and condensed tannins in hemp seed flour by 70%–80% and increase the IVPD to 90% [128]. The phytic acid and bound phenolics are reduced due to enzymes such as phytase, phenolic acid decarboxylase, phenolic acid reductase, and glucosidase produced by LAB like *Lb. casei, Lb. reuteri, Lb. fermentum,* and *Lb. plantarum*, which improves the iron and zinc bioaccessibility [67].

## 10.4.6  MISCELLANEOUS

Ultrasound treatment time improves the hydrophobicity, emulsification properties in vitro starch digestibility but reduces the swelling power and gelation ability due to damage of starch granules by the shearing forces and free radicals created during cavitation. Moreover, these can also cause lipid oxidation and polysaccharide degradation [200]. Combination of mano-thermosonication and ultrasonication improves the functional properties of hemp seed proteins. On the other hand, hydrolysis of hemp seed protein leads to aggregation thereby reducing the interfacial properties like emulsi-fication and foaming. Enzymatic hydrolysis of the hemp seed oil improves the tocopherol content consequently elevating the oxidative stability [103].

## 10.5  DEVELOPMENT OF SPECIALTY FOODS

Due to the superior nutritional composition, consumption of super grains can improve the lifestyle by preventing the risk of certain diseases such as cancer, cardiovascular diseases, and irritable bowel syndrome. These can be used in palatable form as ingredients, partially or completely, in common food products like bread, noodles, cookies, beverages, and pasta to provide functionality, both technologically and nutritionally. The speciality foods from these grains should be consumed by people of all age groups especially those suffering from micronutrient deficiency and celiac diseases.

## 10.5.1  BAKERY PRODUCTS

Artificial improvers in bread can be successfully substituted by amaranth flour which reduces the fermentation time and improves the dough volume [27]. Bread with 25% incorporation of amaranth is highly acceptable with delayed retrogradation and efficient physiological action due to optimum ratio of soluble and insoluble fiber (1:2). It improves the iron, zinc and dietary fiber content which is close to daily requirements of an individual

[118]. Chia flour is approved at levels of <5% by European Commission in bread products. It improves the protein, lipid and mineral profile of the bread. Chia seed incorporated in corn tortillas reduces the starch hydrolysis and thereby the GI due to increased fiber content [186]. Gluten-free cookies from popped amaranth (20% popped flour and 13% popped whole grain) and bread with a ratio of 60:40 for popped and raw amaranth without the use of hydrocolloids are highly promising products for celiac patients [51]. Gluten-free cookies from a combination of chia, millet and buckwheat flour (7.5:40:52.5) can successfully replace the wheat flour cookies [30]. Pound cakes with whole chia flour (15%) can be produced with improved ω-3 fatty acid content [142]. Gluten-free bread from hemp seed and gluten-free crackers from hemp seed meal and decaffeinated green tea leaves are superior functional products due to high amounts of protein, fiber and ω-3 fatty acids [99, 144]. Moreover, hemp seed proteins exhibit a denaturation pattern similar to egg proteins, thus can be used in muffins and cakes without eggs and milk [34, 91]. Incorporation of quinoa flour in gluten-free cakes up to 50% significantly enhances the chemical, physical, and organoleptic qualities with elevated technological and nutritional properties [28].

Breads prepared from quinoa flour (20%) contain significantly high protein, lysine, histidine, and methionine with superior antioxidant activity and aroma profiles compared to 100% wheat flour bread [191]. Teff flour incorporation in bread up to 30%–40% improves the protein, dietary fiber and mineral especially iron concentration with increased in vitro digestibility and antioxidant activity [201]. Teff can be used to prepare gluten-free cookies and muffins with improved nutritional density especially protein, fiber, and mineral [58]. Multi grain cookies with millet and chia flour can be consumed regularly by school going children due to richness of protein and minerals [89]. Cakes and cookies from pearl and foxtail millets can be incorporated in government food programs globally to enhance food security [161]. Gluten-free bread with rice flour and buckwheat (70:30) can be prepared to improve content of protein, calcium, iron, vitamin E, and fiber. Utilization of propylene glycol alginate as a hydrocolloid makes it possible to increase the level of buckwheat to 40% [5, 140].

### 10.5.2  EXTRUDED PRODUCTS

Amaranth can be incorporated in pasta with durum semolina to improve the fiber, protein, and ash with decreased cooking time but increased cooking loss since the amaranth starch and protein (gluten-free) disrupt the gluten-starch matrix of semolina [36]. A 30% substitution with amaranth flour provides optimum nutritional and functional characteristics to pasta [114]. Supplementation with popped amaranth flour provides acceptable organoleptic characteristic with increased protein, calcium, magnesium, and zinc contents [23]. Gluten-free noodles can be prepared from rice flour and corn starch with incorporation of chia seed flour (20%) by using diacetyl tartaric esters of mono (and di) glycerides to improve the zinc, iron, magnesium, potassium, phosphorus, and calcium contents [104]. Chia-corn meal puffs can also be prepared to improve the lipid content of the product [31].

Chia can be used as a thickening agent for gluten-free pasta with rice flour with reduced GI of the product [116]. Pasta formulation with quinoa individually or in combination with wheat flour improves the nutritional quality and the functionality can be enhanced by using structuring agents [191]. Gluten-free pasta prepared from teff and oat composites contains better mineral and dietary fiber content than wheat pasta with reduced GI of 45 [77]. Ready to cook millet flakes improve the functionality of the conventional flakes and thus are highly acceptable [174]. Extruded corn snacks incorporated with 30% buckwheat are potential appetizers with improved nutritional attributes [194].

### 10.5.3   BREAKFAST CEREALS AND NUTRITION BARS

Amaranth grains are usually popped or rolled to be utilized in granola bars or muesli [22]. Chia as a mid-morning snack with yogurt provides short-term satiety [14]. Nutrition bars can be prepared with chia-date-sesame blends with high protein, fiber, and PUFA contents [169]. Energy bars prepared from rice and 20% whole hemp seed powders possess high acceptable organoleptic and nutritional characteristics [131]. Gluten-free bar prepared from quinoa with brown rice and flaxseed is a value-added product with superior protein and bioactive constitution and can be consumed by celiac patients [93].

### 10.5.4   BEVERAGES

Beer may be produced from germinated amaranth (*chichi* in Peru) and *ogi* from its lactic fermentation [119]. Chia and amaranth flours produced after germination and extrusion provide high nutritional and nutraceutical value to beverages thus improving their functionality for utilization by patients of chronic degenerative diseases and obesity [13]. Gluten-free beverages, both fermented and nonfermented, can be also prepared with whole teff grains [201]. Beverages from malted quinoa exhibit high protein content and anti-oxidant activity, thus have antihypertensive and antidiabetic potential [92]. Health drink from barnyard, little, kodo, and finger millets is an economically viable value-added product to provide essential minerals to the human body [129].

### 10.5.5   MEAT PRODUCTS

Incorporation of amaranth protein concentrate in emulsion-type meat product can improve the emulsion and gel properties [44]. Freshwater fish burgers incorporated with whole chia flour (5.92%) exhibit improved ⍵-3 fatty acid content, which is adequate to meet the daily recommendations from 100 g of the product [150]. Low-fat meat products such as restructured ham-like product using chia seeds (1%) and carrageenan (0.5%) are highly acceptable [56]. Common carp restructured meat incorporated with 4–8% chia seed flour contains high fat (LA and ALA) and fiber contents to produce restructured protein network without interfering its thermal transitions [158].

### 10.5.6   FERMENTED PRODUCTS

*Injera* from teff flour is the staple food of Ethopia prepared by natural fermentation generally. Fermentation with lactic acid bacteria like *Lb. buchneri* and *P. pentosaceus* reduces the phytic acid (60%–70%) to a greater extent than natural fermentation with improved bioaccessibility of iron and zinc [65]. Gluten- and dairy-free spoonable products prepared from quinoa by fermentation with the probiotic *Lb. planatrum* exhibit superior nutritional composition with high protein, fiber and mineral profiles and low-fat content [185].

Hemp seed drinks exhibit high amounts of butyrate, propionate, and acetate, which improve the growth of probiotics such as *Bifidobacterium bifidum*, *Lb. planatarum,* and *Lb. fermentum*. Also, the bacterial pathogens are inhibited due to the hydrocarbons such as terpenes [130]. Sourdough fermentation can be employed to improve the organoleptic quality of bread from pearl millet flour to achieve a highly nutritional product in more palatable form [125]. Millets exhibit high prebiotic properties and thus, can be used to prepare symbiotic products. Fermentation with lactic acid bacteria to produce *lassi* from pearl millet is a viable and economically feasible product [180].

## 10.5.7 MISCELLANEOUS APPLICATIONS

Weaning foods can be prepared from teff with pearl millet and legumes with improved content of protein without affecting the content of nonstarch polysaccharide [75]. Nano-composite films formed from the blend from maize starch granules and amaranth proteins, which interact by disulfide linkage and hydrogen bonding, exhibit superior water uptake, water vapor permeability, mechanical behavior, delayed weight loss, and surface hydrophobicity. Folic acid can be successfully photoprotected by encapsulating in amaranth protein isolate-pullulan fibers formed by electrospinning [170]. Amaranth films exhibit antifungal activities against *Aspergillus niger* and *Penicillium digitatum* [44].

Edible films with superior physicochemical, mechanical (UV-radiation shielding and water vapor barrier) and nutritional properties can be prepared using chia flour and maize starch [55]. Gelatin films incorporated with sage oil and hemp oil (1:1) can highly inhibit microbial growth especially *Staphylococcus aureus, Penicillium expansum, Eschericia coli, Saccharomyces cerevisiae,* and *Listeria innocua* [47]. Edible films from quinoa protein and starch exhibit good mechanical properties like low water vapour and oxygen permeability [191]. Pickering emulsions can be formed from hydrophobically modified quinoa starch which shows good interfacial properties and thus can be used for encapsulation of carmine dye [115].

## 10.6   SUMMARY

The super grains can provide special benefits not achieved from the common grains like wheat, maize, and rice. Certain antinutrients may reduce the bioavailability of protein and minerals making it necessary to suitably process these grains to target improved nutrition among patients of celiac disease and micronutrient deficiency. The utilization of these grains as functional foods after optimal processing enhances the organoleptic characteristics thus making them effective delivery vehicles of essential nutrients.

## KEYWORDS

- ancient grains
- antinutritional factors
- functional properties
- processing
- specialty foods
- super grains

## REFERENCES

1. Abugoch, J. L. E. Quinoa (*Chenopodium quinoa* Willd.): composition, chemistry, nutritional, and functional properties. *Advances in Food and Nutritional Research*, **2009**, *58*, 1–31.
2. Acanski, M. M.; Vujic, D. N. Comparing Sugar Components of Cereal and Pseudocereal Flour by GC-MS Analysis. *Food Chemistry,* **2014**, *145*, 743–748.
3. Adeniyi, P. O.; Obatolu, V. A. Effect of Germination Temperature on the Functional Properties of Grain *Amaranthus*. *American Journal of Food Science and Technology*, **2014**, *2*, 76–79.
4. Agrawal, D.; Upadhyay, A.; Nayak, P. S. Functional Characteristics of Malted Flour of Foxtail, Barnyard and Little Millets. *Annals Food Science and Technology*, **2013**, *14*, 44–49.
5. Alvarez-Jubete, L.; Arendt, E. K.; Gallagher, E. Polyphenol Composition and *in vitro* Antioxidant Activity of Amaranth, Quinoa Buckwheat and Wheat As Affected By Sprouting and Baking. *Food Chemistry*, **2010**, *119*, 770–778.
6. Alvarez-Jubete, L.; Arendt, E. K.; Gallagher, E. Nutritive Value of Pseudocereals and Their Increasing Use as Functional Gluten-Free Ingredients. *Trends in Food Science and Technology*, **2010**, *21*, 106–113.
7. Amadou, I.; Gounga, M. E.; Le, G. W. Millets: Nutritional Composition, Some Health Benefits and Processing-A Review. *Emirates Journal of Food and Agriculture*, 2013, 501–508.
8. Amalraj, A.; Pius, A. Influence of Oxalate, Phytate, Tannin, Dietary Fiber, and Cooking On Calcium Bioavailability of Commonly Consumed Cereals and Millets in India. *Cereal Chemistry*, **2015**, *92*, 389–394.
9. Amare, E.; Mouquet-Rivier, C.; Servent, A.; Morel, G.; Adish, A.; Haki, G. D. Protein Quality of Amaranth Grains Cultivated in Ethiopia as Affected by Popping and Fermentation. *Food and Nutrition Sciences*, **2015**, *6*, 38.
10. Ando, H.; Chen, Y-C.; Tang, H.; Shimizu, M.; Watanabe, K.; Mitsunaga, Y. Food Components in Fractions of Quinoa Seed. *Food Science and Technology Research*, **2002**, *8*, 80–84.

11. Arendt, E. K.; Zannini, E. Teff. In: *Cereal Grains for the Food and Beverage Industries*; Cambridge, UK: Woodhead Publishing Limited; **2013**; pp. 351–368.
12. Arendt, E.K.; Zannini, E. Buckwheat. In: *Cereal Grains for the Food and Beverage Industries*; Cambridge, UK: Woodhead Publishing Limited; **2013**; pp. 369–408.
13. Argüelles-López, O. D.; Reyes-Moreno, C.; Gutiérrez-Dorado, R. R.; Sánchez-Osuna, M. F.; López-Cervantes, J. Functional Beverages Elaborated from Amaranth and Chia Flours Processed by Germination and Extrusion. *Biotecnia*, **2018**, *20*, 135–145.
14. Ayaz, A.; Akyol, A.; Inan-Eroglu, E. Chia Seed (*Salvia hispanica* L.) Added Yogurt Reduces Short-Term Food Intake and Increases Satiety: Randomized Controlled Trial. *Nutrition Research and Practice*, **2017**, *11*, 412–418.
15. Ayerza, R.; Coates, W. Protein Content, Oil Content and Fatty Acid Profiles as Potential Criteria to Determine the Origin of Commercially Grown Chia (*Salvia hispanica* L .). *Journal of Industrial Crops and Products*, **2011**, *34*, 1366–1371.
16. Baljeet, S. Y.; Ritika, B. Y.; Roshan, L. Y. Studies on Functional Properties and Incorporation of Buckwheat Flour for Biscuit Making. *International Food Research Journal*, **2010**, *17*, 1067–1076.
17. Barreto, A. D.; Gutierrez, É. M.; Silva, M. R. Characterization and Bioaccessibility of Minerals in Seeds of *Salvia hispanica* L. *American Journal of Plant Sciences*, **2016**, *7*, 2323–2337.
18. Bartkiene, E.; Schleining, G.; Krungleviciute, V. Development and Quality Evaluation of Lacto-Fermented Product Based on Hulled and Not Hulled Hempseed (*Cannabis sativa* L.). *LWT-Food Science and Technology*, **2016**, *72*, 544–551.
19. Baye, K. Teff: Nutrient Composition and Health Benefits. ESSP Working Paper 67. Washington, D.C. and Addis Ababa, Ethiopia: International Food Policy Research Institute (IFPRI) and Ethiopian Development Research Institute (EDRI), **2014**, *67*.
20. Beltrán-Orozco, M. C.; Romero, M. R. Chia: Millenium Food. *Departamento de Graduados e Investigación en Alimentos, E. N. C. B.; I. P. N.;* Mexico, 2003; pp. 22–25.
21. Benevides, C. M. D. J.; Souza, M. V.; Souza, R. D. B.; Lopes, M. V. Anti-nutritional Factors in Foods. *Segurança Alimentar e Nutricional*, **2011**, *18*, 67–79.
22. Bhattarai, G. Amaranth: A Golden Crop for Future. *Himalayan Journal of Science and Technology*, **2018**, *2*, 108–116.
23. Bodroža-Solarov, M. A. R. I. J. A. Quality of Bread Supplemented with Popped *Amaranthus cruentus* grain. *Journal of Food Process Engineering*, **2008**, *31*, 602–618.
24. Borderías, A. J.; Sánchez-Alonso, I.; Pérez-Mateos, M. P. New Applications of Fibers in Foods: Addition to Fishery Products. *Trends in Food Science and Technology*, **2005**, *16*, 458–465.
25. Borges, J. T. S.; Bonomo, R. C.; Paula, C. D. Physicochemical and Nutritional Characteristics and Uses of Quinoa (*Chenopodium quinoa* Willd.). *Temas Agrários*, **2010**, *15*, 9–23.
26. Borneo, R.; Aguirre, A.; León, A. E. Chia (*Salvia hispanica* L) gel can be used as egg or oil replacer in cake formulations. *Journal of the American Dietetic Association.* **2010**, 110, 946–949.
27. Borowy, T.; Kubiak, M. S. Amarantus w piekarstwie. *Przegl Zbożowo-Młyn*, **2012**, *56*, 22–23.
28. Bozdogan, N.; Kumcuoglu, S.; Tavman, S. Investigation of the Effects of Using Quinoa Flour on Gluten-free Cake Batters and Cake Properties. *Journal of Food Science and Technology*, **2019**, *56*, 683–694.

29. Brenneisen, R. Chemistry and Analysis of Phytocannabinoids and Other Cannabis Constituents. In: *Marijuana and the Cannabinoids*; ElSohly, M. A. (Eds.); New York: Humana Press; **2007**; pp. 17–49.
30. Brites, L. T. G. F.; Ortolan, F. Gluten-free Cookies Elaborated with Buckwheat Flour, Millet Flour and Chia Seeds. *Food Science and Technology*, **2019**, *39*, 458–466.
31. Byars, J. A.; Singh, M. Properties of Extruded Chia–corn meal Puffs. *LWT-Food Science and Technology*, **2015**, *62*, 506–510.
32. Cai, Y. Z.; Corke, H.; Wang, D.; Li, W. D. Buckwheat: Overview. In: *Encyclopedia of Food Grains*; Wrigley, C.; Corke, H.; Seetharaman, K. and Faubion, J. (Eds.); Oxford: Elsevier; **2016**; *Volume* 1; pp. 307–315.
33. Callaway, J. C. Hemp as Food at High Latitudes. *Journal of Industrial Hemp*, **2002**, *7*, 105–117.
34. Callaway, J. C.; Pate, D. W. Hempseed oil. In: Gourmet and Health-Promoting Specialty Oils; Moreau, R. and Kamal-Eldin, Afaf. (Eds.); Urbana, Illinois: AOCS Press; **2009**; pp. 185–213.
35. Capriles, V. D.; Coelho, K. D.; Guerra-Matias, A. C.; Areas, J. A. Effects of Processing Methods on Amaranth Starch Digestibility and Predicted Glycemic Index. *Journal of Food Science*, **2008**, *73*, H160–H164.
36. Cárdenas-Hernández, A.; Beta, T. Improved Functional Properties of Pasta: Enrichment with Amaranth Seed Flour and Dried Amaranth Leaves. *Journal of Cereal Science*, **2016**, *72*, 84–90.
37. Caselato-Sousa, V. M.; Amaya-Farfán, J. State of Knowledge on Amaranth Grain: A Comprehensive Review. *Journal of Food Science*, **2012**, *77*, R93–R104.
38. Castro-Alba, V.; Lazarte, C. E. Fermentation of Pseudocereals Quinoa, Canihua, and Amaranth to Improve Mineral Accessibility Through Degradation of Phytate. *Journal of the Science of Food and Agriculture*, **2019**, *99*, 5239–5248.
39. Chauhan, A.; Singh, S. Influence of Germination on Physicochemical Properties of Amaranth (*Amaranthus* spp.) Flour. *International Journal of Agriculture Food Science and Technology*, **2013**, *4*, 215–220.
40. Chávez-Jáuregui, R. N.; Silva, M. E. M. P.; Arěas, J. A. G. Extrusion Cooking Process for Amaranth (*Amaranthus caudatus* L.). *Journal of Food Science*, 2000. *65*, 1009–1015.
41. Cheng, A. Shaping a Sustainable Food Future by Rediscovering Long-forgotten Ancient Grains. *Plant Science*, **2018**, *269*, 136–142.
42. Chinedum, E.; Sanni, S.; Theressa, N.; Ebere, A. Effect of Domestic Cooking on the Starch Digestibility, Predicted Glycemic Indices, Polyphenol Contents and Alpha Amylase Inhibitory Properties of Beans (*Phaseolis vulgaris*) and Breadfruit (*Treculia africana*). *International Journal of Biological Macromolecules*, **2018**, *106*, 200–206.
43. Ciftci, O. N.; Przybylski, R.; Rudzinska, M. Lipid Components of Flax, Perilla, and Chia Seeds. *European Journal of Lipid Science and Technology*, **2012**, *114*, 794–800.
44. Coelho, L. M.; Silva, P. M.; Martins, J. T. Emerging Opportunities in Exploring the Nutritional/Functional Value of Amaranth. *Food and Function*, **2018**, *9*, 5499–5512.
45. Coelho, M. S.; de las Mercedes Salas-Mellado, M. How Extraction Method Affects the Physicochemical and Functional Properties of Chia Proteins. *LWT-Food Science and Technology*, **2018**, *96*, 26–33.
46. Collar, C.; Angioloni, A. Pseudocereals and Teff in Complex Breadmaking Matrices: Impact on Lipid Dynamics. *Journal of Cereal Science*, **2014**, *59*, 145–154.

47. Cozmuta, A. M.; Turila, A.; Apjok, R. Preparation and Characterization of Improved Gelatin Films Incorporating Hemp and Sage Oils. *Food Hydrocolloids*, **2015**, *49*, 144–155.

48. Cozzolino, S. M. F. *Biodisponibilidade de Nutrientes*. 3ª Ed. Brazil: Editora Manole; **2005**; p. 1172.

49. Crescente, G.; Piccolella, S.; Esposito, A. Chemical Composition and Nutraceutical Properties of Hempseed: An Ancient Food with Actual Functional Value. *Phytochemistry Reviews*, **2018**, *17*, 733–749.

50. de Falco, B.; Amato, M.; Lanzotti, V. Chia Seeds Products: An Overview. *Phytochemistry Reviews*, **2017**, *16*, 745–760.

51. de la Barca, A. M.C.; Rojas-Martínez, M. E. Gluten-free Breads and Cookies of Raw and Popped Amaranth Flours with Attractive Technological and Nutritional Qualities. *Plant Foods for Human Nutrition*, **2010**, *65*, 241–246.

52. Deferne, J. L.; Pate, D. W. Hemp Seed Oil: A Source of Valuable Essential Fatty Acids. *Journal of the International Hemp Association*, **1996**, *3*, 4–7.

53. Devisetti, R.; Yadahally, S. N.; Bhattacharya, S. Nutrients and Antinutrients in Foxtail and Proso Millet Milled Fractions: Evaluation of their Flour Functionality. *LWT-Food Science and Technology*, **2014**, *59*, 889–895.

54. Dhingra, D.; Michael, M.; Rajput, H.; Patil, R. Dietary Fiber in Foods: A Review. *Journal of Food Science and Technology*, **2012**, *49*, 255–266.

55. Dick, M.; Henrique Pagno, C.; Haas Costa, T. M. Edible Films Based on Chia Flour: Development and Characterization. *Journal of Applied Polymer Science*, **2016**, *133* (1–9)., 42455

56. Ding, Y.; Lin, H. W.; Lin, Y. L.; Yang, D. J. Nutritional Composition in the Chia Seed and its Processing Properties on Restructured Ham-like Products. *Journal of Food and Drug Analysis*, **2018**, *26*, 124–134.

57. Dini, I.; Tenore, G. D.; Dini, A. Nutritional and Antinutritional Composition of Kancolla Seeds: An Interesting and Underexploited Andine Food Plant. *Food Chemistry*, **2005**, *92*, 125–132.

58. do Nascimento, K. D. O.; Paes, S. D. N. D. Teff: Suitability for Different Food Applications and as a Raw Material of Gluten-Free: A Literature Review. *Journal of Food and Nutrition Research*, **2018**, *6*, 74–81.

59. Duliński, R.; Starzyńska-Janiszewska, A.; Byczyński, Ł.; Błaszczyk, U. Myo-Inositol Phosphates Profile of Buckwheat and Quinoa Seeds: Effects of Hydrothermal Processing and Solid-State Fermentation with *Rhizopus oligosporus*. *International Journal of Food Properties*, **2017**, *20*, 2088–2095.

60. Duodu, K. G.; Taylor, J. R. N.; Belton, P. S.; Hamaker, B. R. Factors Affecting Sorghum Protein Digestibility. *Journal of Cereal Science*, **2003**, *38*, 117–131.

61. El Sohaimy, S. A.; Mohamed, S. E.; Shehata, M. G.; Mehany, T.; Zaitoun, M. A. Compositional Analysis and Functional Characteristics of Quinoa Flour. *Annual Research and Review in Biology*, **2018**, 1–11.

62. El-Alfy, T. S.; Ezzat, S. M.; Sleem, A. A. Chemical and Biological Study of the Seeds of *Eragrostis tef* (Zucc.) Trotter. *Natural Product Research*, **2011**, *26*, 619–629.

63. Fardet, A.; Leenhardt, F.; Lioger, D.; Scalbert, A.; Rémésy, C. Parameters Controlling the Glycaemic Response to Breads. *Nutrition Research Reviews*, **2006**, *19*, 18–25.

64. Filho, A. M. M.; Pirozi, M. R.; Borges, J. T. D. S.; Pinheiro Sant'Ana, H. M.; Chaves, J. B. P.; Coimbra, J. S. D. R. Quinoa: Nutritional, Functional, and Antinutritional Aspects. *Critical Reviews in Food Science and Nutrition*, **2017**, *57*, 1618–1630

65. Fischer, M. M.; Egli, I. M.; Aeberli, I.; Hurrell, R. F.; Meile, L. Phytic Acid Degrading Lactic Acid Bacteria in Tef-Injera Fermentation. *International Journal of Food Microbiology*, **2014**, *190*, 54–60.

66. Flachs, P.; Rossmeis, M.; Bryhn, M.; Kopecky, J. Cellular and Molecular Effects of n−3 Polyunsaturated Fatty Acids on Adipose Tissue Biology and Metabolism. *Clinical Science*, **2009**, *116*, 1–16.

67. Gabaza, M.; Shumoy, H.; Muchuweti, M.; Vandamme, P.; Raes, K. Iron and Zinc Bioaccessibility of Fermented Maize, Sorghum and Millets from Five Locations in Zimbabwe. *Food Research International*, **2018**, *103*, 361–370.

68. Gamel, T. H.; Linssen, J. P.; Alink, G. M.; Mosallem, A. S.; Shekib, L. A. Nutritional Study of Raw and Popped Seed Proteins of *Amaranthus caudatus* L. and *Amaranthus cruentus* L. *Journal of the Science of Food and Agriculture*, **2004**, *84*, 1153–1158.

69. Gamel, T. H.; Linssen, J. P.; Mesallam, A. S.; Damir, A. A.; Shekib, L. A. Effect of Seed Treatments on the Chemical Composition of Two Amaranth Species: Oil, Sugars, Fibers, Minerals and Vitamins. *Journal of the Science of Food and Agriculture*, **2006**, *86*, 82–89.

70. Garcia, A. G. M. *Hemp: Composition Review Plus*. Senior project for Bachelor of Science; California Polytechnic State University, San Luis Obispo, CA; **2017**; p. 83.

71. Gebremariam, M. M.; Zarnkow, M.; Becker, T. Teff (*Eragrostis Tef*) As a Raw Material for Malting, Brewing and Manufacturing of Gluten-Free Foods and Beverages: A Review. *Journal of Food Science and Technology*, **2014**, *51*, 2881–2895.

72. Gelinas, B.; Seguin, P. Oxalate in Grain Amaranth. *Journal of Agricultural and Food Chemistry*, **2007**, *55*, 4789–4794.

73. Gómez-Favela, M. A.; Gutiérrez-Dorado, R. Improvement of Chia Seeds with Antioxidant Activity, GABA, Essential Amino Acids, and Dietary Fiber by Controlled Germination Bioprocess. *Plant Foods for Human Nutrition*, **2017**, *72*, 345–352.

74. Graf, B. L.; Rojas-Silva, P.; Rojo, L. E. Innovations in Health Value and Functional Food Development of Quinoa (*Chenopodium Quinoa* Willd.). *Comprehensive Review in Food Science and Food Safety*, **2015**, *14*, 431–445.

75. Griffith, L. D.; Castell-Perez, M. E.; Griffith, M. E. Effects of Blend and Processing Method on the Nutritional Quality of Weaning Foods Made from Select Cereals and Legumes. *Cereal Chemistry*, **1998**, *75*, 105–112.

76. Gupta, R. K.; Gangoliya, S. S.; Singh, N. K. Reduction of Phytic Acid and Enhancement of Bioavailable Micronutrients in Food Grains. *Journal of Food Science and Technology*, **2015**, *52*, 676–684.

77. Hager, A. S.; Lauck, F.; Zannini, E.; Arendt, E. K. Development of Gluten-Free Fresh Egg Pasta Based On Oat and Teff Flour. *European Food Research and Technology*, **2012**, *235*, 861–871.

78. Haripriya, A.; Aparna, N. Effect of Roasting on Selected Nutrient Profile and Functional Properties of Chia Seeds (*Salvia hispanica*) and Optimization of Chia Seed Based Instant Soup Mix. *International Journal of Food Science and Nutrition*, **2018**, *3*, 200–206.

79. Hejazi, S. N.; Orsat, V.; Azadi, B.; Kubow, S. Improvement of the *in vitro* Protein Digestibility of Amaranth Grain through Optimization of the Malting Process. *Journal of Cereal Science*, **2016**, *68*, 59–65.

80. Hernández-Ledesma, B. Quinoa (*Chenopodium quinoa* Willd.) as Source of Bioactive Compounds: A Review. *Bioactive Compounds in Health and Disease*, **2019**, *2*, 27–47.

81. Himanshu, K.; Chauhan, M.; Sonawane, S. K.; Arya, S. S. Nutritional and Nutraceutical Properties of Millets: A Review. *Clinical Journal of Nutrition and Dietetics*, **2018**, *1*, 1–10.

82. House, J. D. *Evaluating the Quality of Protein from Hemp Seed and Hemp Seed Products Through the use of the Protein Digestibility- Corrected Amino Acid Score Method.* Report; University of Manitoba, Winnipeg; **2007**; p. 44.

83. House, J. D.; Naufeld, J.; Leson, G. Evaluating the Quality of Protein from Hemp Seed (*Cannabis sativa* L.) Products through the use of the Protein Digestibility-Corrected Amino Acid Score Method. *Journal of Agricultural and Food Chemistry,* **2010,** *58,* 11801–11807.

84. Ikumi, P.; Mburu, M.; Njoroge, D. Chia (*Salvia hispanica* L.): A Potential Crop for Food and Nutrition Security in Africa. *Journal of Food Research,* **2019,** *8,* 104.

85. Jan, R.; Saxena, D. C.; Singh, S. Analyzing the Effect of Optimization Conditions of Germination on the Antioxidant Activity, Total Phenolics, and Antinutritional Factors of Chenopodium (*Chenopodium album*). *Journal of Food Measurement and Characterization,* **2017,** *11,* 256–264.

86. Jan, R.; Saxena, D. C.; Singh, S. Effect of Germination on Nutritional, Functional, Pasting, and Microstructural Properties of Chenopodium (*Chenopodium album*) Flour. *Journal of Food Processing and Preservation,* **2017,** *41,* e12959.

87. Jancurová, M.; Minarovičová, L.; Dandar, A. Quinoa-A Review. *Czech Journal of Food Sciences,* **2009,** *27,* 71–79.

88. Jang, H. L.; Park, S. Y.; Nam, J. S. The Effects of Heat Treatment on the Nutritional Composition and Antioxidant Properties of Hempseed (*Cannabis sativa* L.). *Journal of the Korean Society of Food Science and Nutrition.* **2018,** *47,* 885–894.

89. Kanchana, R.; Fernandes, F.; Barretto, K.; Rodrigues, L.; Pereira, S.; D'silva, K. Value Added Food Products from Under-Utilized Soy Beans and Millets—From Laboratory to Industry. *International Journal for Research in Applied Science & Engineering Technology,* **2018,** *6,* 2183–2188.

90. Karunakaran, C. G.; Urooj, A. Millets the Wonder Nutricereal: As Complimentary Food. *EC Paediatrics,* **2019,** *9,* 1–6.

91. Kataria, A.; Ahluwalia, P.; Sharma, S.; Singh, B. Cannabis infused foods. In: *Trends & Prospects in Food Science & Processing Technology*; Prasad, V. M.; Gupta, A.; Singh, B.; Misra, N.; Mani, A. (Eds.); Delhi: Satish Serial Publishing House; **2019**; pp. 145–172.

92. Kaur, I.; Tanwar, B. Quinoa Beverages: Formulation, Processing and Potential Health Benefits. *Romanian Journal of Diabetes Nutrition and Metabolic Diseases,* 2016, *23,* 215–225.

93. Kaur, R.; Ahluwalia, P.; Sachdev, P. A.; Kaur, A. Development of Gluten-Free Cereal Bar for Gluten Intolerant Population by Using Quinoa as Major Ingredient. *Journal of Food Science and Technology,* **2018,** *55,* 3584–3591.

94. Kelbessa, U.; Alemu, F.; Eskinder, B. Effect of Natural Fermentation on Nutritional and Anti-Nutritional Factors of Tef (*Eragrostis tef*). *The Ethiopian Journal of Health Development,* **1997,** *11,* 61–66.

95. Khan, R.; Dutta, A. Effect of Popping on Physico-Chemical and Nutritional Parameters of Amaranth Grain. *Journal of Pharmacognosy and Phytochemistry,* **2018,** *7,* 954–958.

96. Kharat, S.; Medina-Meza, I. G. Extrusion Processing Characteristics of Whole Grain Flours of Select Major Millets (Foxtail, Finger, and Pearl). *Food and Bioproducts Processing,* **2019,** *114,* 60–71.

97. Khattab, R. Y.; Arntfield, S. D. Nutritional Quality of Legume Seeds as Affected by Some Physical Treatments. 2. Antinutritional factors. *LWT-Food Science and Technology,* **2009,** *42,* 1113–1118.

98. Koletzko, B.; Susan, B.; Geoff, C.; Ulysses, F. N. Global Standard for the Composition of Infant Formula: Recommendations of an ESPGHAN Coordinated International Expert Group. *Journal of Pediatric Gastroenterology and Nutrition,* **2005,** *41,* 584–599.

99. Korus, J.; Witczak, M.; Ziobro, R.; Juszczak, L. Hemp (*Cannabis sativa* Subsp. *sativa*) Flour and Protein Preparation as Natural Nutrients and Structure Forming Agents in Starch Based Gluten-Free Bread. *LWT- Food Science and Technology,* **2017,** *84,* 143–150.

100. Kowalski, R. J.; Medina-Meza, I. G. Extrusion Processing Characteristics of Quinoa (*Chenopodium quinoa* Willd.) var. Cherry Vanilla. *Journal of Cereal Science,* **2016,** *70,* 91–98.

101. Lamonthe, L. M.; Srichuwong, S.; Reuhs, B. L.; Hamaker, B. R. Quinoa (*Chenopodium quinoa* W.) and Amaranth (*Amaranthus caudatus* L.) Provide Dietary Fibers High in Pectic Substances and Xyloglucans. *Food Chemistry,* **2015,** *167,* 490–496.

102. Lemke, S. L.; Vicini, J. L.; Su, H. Dietary Intake of Stearidonic Acid-enriched Soybean Oil Increases the Omega-3 Index: Randomized, Double-Blind Clinical Study of Efficacy and Safety. *The American Journal of Clinical Nutrition,* **2010,** *92,* 766–775.

103. Leonard, W.; Zhang, P.; Ying, D.; Fang, Z. Hempseed in Food Industry: Nutritional Value, Health Benefits, and Industrial Applications. *Comprehensive Reviews in Food Science and Food Safety,* **2020,** *19,* 282–308.

104. Levent, H. Effect of Partial Substitution of Gluten-Free Flour Mixtures with Chia (*Salvia hispanica* L.) Flour on Quality of Gluten-Free Noodles. *Journal of Food Science and Technology,* **2017,** *54,* 1971–1978.

105. Li, H. Buckwheat. In: *Bioactive Factors and Processing Technology for Cereal Foods*; Wang, J.; Sun, B.; Tsao, R. (Eds.); Singapore: Springer; **2019**; pp. 137–149.

106. Li, S.; Chen, C.; Ji, Y.; Lin, J.; Chen, X.; Qi, B. Improvement of Nutritional Value, Bioactivity and Volatile Constituents of Quinoa Seeds by Fermentation with *Lactobacillus Casei. Journal of Cereal Science,* **2018,** *84,* 83–89.

107. Lopes, C. D. O.; Dessimoni, G. V.; Costa da Silva, M.; Vieira, G.; Pinto, N. A. V. D. Aproveitamento, Composição Nutricional e Antinutricional da Farinha de Quinoa (*Chenopodium Quinoa*). *Alimentos E Nutricao,* **2009,** *20,* 669–675.

108. Lozano, R.; Naghavi, M.; Foreman, K. Global and Regional Mortality from 235 Causes of Death for 20 Age Groups in 1990 and 2010: A Systematic Analysis for the Global Burden of Disease Study 2010. *The lancet,* **2012,** *380,* 2095–2128.

109. Lutz, M.; Bascuñán-Godoy, L. The revival of Quinoa: A Crop for Health. In: *Superfood and Functional Food—An Overview of Their Processing and Utilization*; Waisundara V and Shiomi N (Eds.); Croatia: InTech; **2017**; pp. 37–54.

110. Mahaam, A.; El, A. H.; Abd Elmoneim, O, E.; Limya, O. M.; Elfadil, E. B. Effect of Different Supplementation Levels of Soybean Flour on Pearl Millet Functional Properties. *Food and Nutrition Sciences,* **2012,** *3,* 124–145.

111. Malomo, S. *Structure-function properties of hemp seed proteins and protein-derived acetylcholinesterase-inhibitory peptides.* PhD. Thesis; University of Manitoba, Winnipeg; **2015**; p. 263.

112. Marcinek, K.; Krejpcio, Z. Chia Seeds (*Salvia hispanica*): Health Promoting Properties and Therapeutic Applications-A Review. *Roczniki Państwowego Zakładu Higieny,* **2017,** *68,* 123–129.

113. Marquez-Molina, O.; Martínez, L. X. L. Effect of Various Process Conditions on the Nutritional and Bioactive Compounds of Amaranth. In: *Nutritional Value of Amaranth*; IntechOpen; **2019**; doi: 10.5772/intechopen.88536.

114. Martinez, C. S.; Ribotta, P. D.; Añón, M. C.; León, A. E. Effect of Amaranth Flour (*Amaranthus mantegazzianus*) on the Technological and Sensory Quality of Bread Wheat Pasta. *Food Science and Technology International*, **2014**, *20*, 127–135.

115. Matos, M.; Timgren, A.; Sjöö, M.; Dejmek, P.; Rayner, M. Preparation and Encapsulation Properties of Double Pickering Emulsions Stabilized By Quinoa Starch Granules. *Colloids and Surfaces A: Physicochemical and Engineering Aspects*, **2013**, *423*, 147–154.

116. Menga, V.; Amato, M.; Phillips, T. D.; Angelino, D.; Morreale, F.; Fares, C. Gluten-Free Pasta Incorporating Chia (*Salvia hispanica* L.) As Thickening Agent: An Approach to Naturally Improve the Nutritional Profile and the *in vitro* Carbohydrate Digestibility. *Food Chemistry*, **2017**, *221*, 1954–1961.

117. Miranda, M.; Vega-Gálvez, A. Impact of Air-Drying Temperature on Nutritional Properties, Total Phenolic Content and Antioxidant Capacity of Quinoa Seeds (*Chenopodium quinoa* Willd.). *Industrial Crops and Products*, **2010**, *32*, 258–263.

118. Miranda-Ramos, K. C.; Sanz-Ponce, N.; Haros, C. M. Evaluation of Technological and Nutritional Quality of Bread Enriched with Amaranth Flour. *LWT-Food Science and Technology*, **2019**, *114*, 108418.

119. Mlakar, S. G.; Turinek, M.; Jakop, M.; Bavec, M.; Bavec, F. Grain Amaranth as an Alternative and Perspective Crop in Temperate Climate. *Journal for Geography*, **2010**, *5*, 135–145.

120. Mohd, A. N.; Yeap, S. K.; Ho, W.Y.; Beh, K. B.; Tan, S.W.; Tan, S. G. The Promising Future of Chia, *Salvia hispanica* L. *Journal of Biomedicine and Biotechnology*, **2012**, 1–9.

121. Monroy-Torres, R.; Mancilla-Escobar, M. L.; Gallaga-Solórzano, J. C.; Santiago-García, E. J. Protein Digestibility of Chia Seed *Salvia hispanica* L. *Revista Salud Pública y Nutrición*, **2008**, *9*, 1–9.

122. Mota, C.; Nascimento, A. C.; Santos, M. The Effect of Cooking Methods on the Mineral Content of Quinoa (*Chenopodium Quinoa*), Amaranth (*Amaranthus* Sp.) and Buckwheat (*Fagopyrum esculentum*). *Journal of Food Composition and Analysis*, **2016**, *49*, 7–64.

123. Muñoz, L. A.; Cobos, A.; Diaz, O.; Aguilera, J. M. Chia seed (*Salvia hispanica*): An Ancient Grain and a New Functional Food. *Food Reviews International*, **2013**, *29*, 394–408.

124. Muñoz, L. A.; Cobos, A.; Diaz, O.; Aguilera, J. M.; Chia Seeds: Microstructure, Mucilage Extraction and Hydration. *Journal of food Engineering*, **2012**, *108*, 216–224.

125. Nami, Y.; Gharekhani, M.; Aalami, M.; Hejazi, M. A. Lactobacillus-Fermented Sourdoughs Improve the Quality of Gluten-Free Bread Made from Pearl Millet Flour. *Journal of Food Science and Technology*, **2019**, *56*, 4057–4067.

126. Navruz-Varli, S.; Sanlier, N. Nutritional and Health Benefits of Quinoa (*Chenopodium quinoa* Willd.). *Journal of Cereal Science*, **2016**, *69*, 371–376.

127. Nawrocka-Musial, D.; Latocha, M. Phytic Acid-Anticancer Nutriceutic. *Polsky Merkuriusz Lekarski*, **2012**, *33*, 43–47.

128. Nionelli, L.; Montemurro, M.; Pontonio, E. Pro-Technological and Functional Characterization of Lactic Acid Bacteria to be used as Starters for Hemp (*Cannabis*

*sativa* L.) Sourdough Fermentation and Wheat Bread Fortification. *International Journal of Food Microbiology*, **2018**, *279*, 14–25.

129. Nishad, P. K.; Maitra, S.; Nilima, J. Physiochemical, Functional and Sensory Properties of Developed Health Drink from Minor Millets. *International Journal of Home Science*, **2017**, *3*, 503–506.

130. Nissen, L.; di Carlo, E.; Gianotti, A. Prebiotic Potential of Hemp Blended Drinks Fermented by Probiotics. *Food Research International*, **2020**, 109029.

131. Norajit, K.; Gu, B. J.; Ryu, G. H. Effects of the Addition of Hemp Powder on the Physicochemical Properties and Energy Bar Qualities of Extruded Rice. *Food chemistry*, **2011**, *129*, 1919–1925.

132. Ocheme, O. B.; Chinma, C. E. Effects of Soaking and Germination on Some Physicochemical Properties of Millet Flour for Porridge Production. *Journal of Food Technology*, **2008**, *6*, 185–188.

133. Ogungbenle, N. H. Nutritional Evaluation and Functional Properties of Quinoa (*Chenopodium quinoa*) flour. *International Journal of Food Science and Nutrition*, **2003**, *54*, 153–158.

134. Olivos-Lugo, B. L.; Valdivia-López, M. Á.; Tecante, A. Thermal and Physicochemical Properties and Nutritional Value of the Protein Fraction of Mexican Chia Seed (*Salvia hispanica* L.). *Food Science and Technology International*, **2010**, *16*, 89–96.

135. Orona-Tamayo, D.; Valverde, M. E.; Nieto-Rendón, B.; Paredes-López, O. Inhibitory Activity of Chia (*Salvia hispanica* L.) Protein Fractions against Angiotensin I-Converting Enzyme and Antioxidant Capacity. *LWT—Food Science and Technology*, **2015**, *64*, 236–242.

136. Orona-Tamayo, D.; Valverde, M. E.; Paredes-López, O. Chia—The New Golden Seed for the 21st Century: Nutraceutical Properties and Technological Uses. In: *Sustainable Protein Sources*; Nadathur, S. R.; Wanasundara, J. P. D. and Scanlin, L. (Eds.); London, UK: Academic Press; **2017**; pp. 265–281.

137. Pająk, P.; Socha, R.; Broniek, J.; Królikowska, K.; Fortuna, T. Antioxidant Properties, Phenolic and Mineral Composition of Germinated Chia, Golden Flax, Evening Primrose, Phacelia and Fenugreek. *Food Chemistry*, **2019**, *275*, 69–76.

138. Pastor, K.; Ačanski, M. The Chemistry behind Amaranth Grains. *Journal of Nutritional Health & Food Engineering*, **2018**, *8*, 358–360.

139. Pellegrini, M.; Lucas-Gonzales, R.; Ricci, A. Chemical, Fatty Acid, Polyphenolic Profile, Techno-Functional and Antioxidant Properties of Flours Obtained from Quinoa (*Chenopodium quinoa* Willd) Seeds. *Industrial Crops and Products*, **2018**, *111*, 38–46.

140. Peressini, D.; Pin, M.; Sensidoni, A. Rheology and Breadmaking Performance of Rice-Buckwheat Batters Supplemented With Hydrocolloids. *Food Hydrocolloids*, **2011**, *25*, 340–349.

141. Petrović, M.; Debeljak, Ž.; Kezić, N.; Džidara, P. Relationship Between Cannabinoids Content and Composition of Fatty Acids in Hempseed Oils. *Food Chemistry*, **2015**, *170*, 218–225.

142. Pizarro, P. L.; Almeida, E. L.; Sammán, N. C.; Chang, Y. K. Evaluation of Whole Chia (*Salvia hispanica* L.) Flour and Hydrogenated Vegetable Fat in Pound Cake. *LWT-Food Science and Technology*, **2013**, *54*, 73–79.

143. Prakash, D.; Pal, M. Nutritional and Antinutritional Composition of Vegetable and Grain Amaranth Leaves. *Journal of the Science of Food and Agriculture*, **1991**, *57*, 573–583.

144. Radočaj, O.; Dimić, E.; Tsao, R. Effects of Hemp (*Cannabis sativa* L.) Seed Oil Press-Cake and Decaffeinated Green Tea Leaves (*Camellia sinensis*) on Functional Characteristics of Gluten-Free Crackers. *Journal of Food Science*, **2014**, *79*, 318–325.

145. Raikos, V.; Neacsu, M.; Russell, W.; Duthie, G. Comparative Study of the Functional Properties of Lupin, Green Pea, Fava Bean, Hemp, and Buckwheat Flours as Affected by Ph. *Food Science & Nutrition*, **2014**, *2*, 802–810.

146. Ramakrishna, A.; Ravishankar, G. A. Influence of Abiotic Stress Signals on Secondary Metabolites in Plants. *Plant Signaling & Behavior*, **2011**, *6*, 1720–1731.

147. Rana, M. Characterization of Chia Seed Flour and Wellbeing Endorsing Possessions. *International Journal of Food Sciences and Nutrition*, **2019**, *8*, 419–426.

148. Rastogi, A.; Shukla, S. Amaranth: A New Millennium Crop of Nutraceutical Values. *Critical Reviews in Food Science and Nutrition*, **2013**, *53*, 109–125.

149. Repo-Carrasco-Valencia, R. A. M.; Serna, L. A. Quinoa (*Chenopodium quinoa*, Willd.) as a Source of Dietary Fiber and Other Functional Components. *Ci^encia e Tecnologia de Alimentos*, **2011**, *31*, 225–230.

150. Riernersman, C. N.; Marí, R. A. Whole Chia Flour as Yield Enhancer, Potential Antioxidant and Input of N-3 Fatty Acid in a Meat Product. *Food and Nutrition Sciences*, **2016**, *7*, 855–865.

151. Ritchie, H.; Roser, M. *Micronutrient Deficiency*. 2017; https://ourworldindata.org/micronutrient-deficiency Accessed on January 30, **2020**.

152. Robin, F.; Théoduloz, C.; Srichuwong, S. Properties of Extruded Whole Grain Cereals and Pseudocereals Flours. *International Journal of Food Science & Technology*, **2015**, *50*, 2152–2159.

153. Ruales, J.; De Grijalva, Y.; Lopez-Jaramillo, P.; Nair, B. M. The Nutritional Quality of Infant Food from Quinoa and Its Effect on the Plasma Level of Insulin-Like Growth Factor-1 (IGF-1) in Undernourished Children. *International Journal of Food Science and Nutrition*, **2002**, *53*, 143–154.

154. Ruales, J.; Nair, B. M. Content of Fat, Vitamins and Minerals in Quinoa (*Chenopodium quinoa* Willd) seeds. *Food Chemistry*, 1993, *48*, 131–136.

155. Ruales, J.; Nair, B. M. Effect of Processing on *in vitro* Digestibility of Protein and Starch in Quinoa Seeds. *International Journal of Food Science & Technology*, **1994**, *29*, 449–456.

156. Sakhare, S. D.; Inamdar, A. A.; Kumar, K. P.; Dharmaraj, U. Evaluation of Roller Milling Potential of Amaranth Grains. *Journal of Cereal Science*, **2017**, *73*, 55–61.

157. Sandoval-Oliveros, M. R.; Paredes-López, O. Isolation and Characterization of Proteins from Chia Seeds (*Salvia hispanica* L.). *Journal of Agricultural and Food Chemistry*, **2013**, *61*, 193–201.

158. Santillán-Álvarez, Á.; Dublán-García, O. Effect of Chia Seed on Physicochemical and Sensory Characteristics of Common Carp Restructured as Functional Food. *Journal of Food Science and Engineering*, **2017**, *7*, 115–126.

159. Santos, M. A. T. D. Effect of cooking on some anti-nutritional factors in broccoli, cauliflower and kale leaves. *Ciência e Agrotecnologia*, **2006**, *30*, 294–301.

160. Satheesh, N.; Fanta, S. W. Review on Structural, Nutritional and Anti-Nutritional Composition of Teff (*Eragrostis tef*) in Comparison with Quinoa (*Chenopodium quinoa* Willd.). *Cogent Food & Agriculture*, **2018**, *4*, 1546942.

161. Shadang, C.; Jaganathan, D. Development and Standardization of Formulated Baked Products using Millets. *International Journal of Research in Applied, Natural and Social Sciences*, **2014**, *2*, 75–78.
162. Sharma, B.; Gujral, H. S. Influence of Nutritional and Antinutritional Components on Dough Rheology and *in vitro* Protein & Starch Digestibility of Minor Millets. *Food Chemistry*, **2019**, *299*, 115–125.
163. Sharma, N.; Goyal, S. K.; Alam, T.; Fatma, S.; Niranjan, K. Effect of Germination on the Functional and Moisture Sorption Properties of High-Pressure-Processed Foxtail Millet Grain Flour. *Food and Bioprocess Technology*, **2018**, *11*, 209–222.
164. Shevkani, K.; Singh, N.; Kaur, A.; Rana, J. C. Physicochemical, Pasting, and Functional Properties of Amaranth Seed Flours: Effects of Lipids Removal. *Journal of Food Science*, **2014**, *79*, 1271–1277.
165. Shumoy, H.; Lauwens, S.; Gabaza, M.; Vandevelde, J.; Vanhaecke, F.; Raes, K. Traditional Fermentation of Tef Injera: Impact on *in vitro* Iron and Zinc Dialysability. *Food Research International*, **2017**, *102*, 93–100.
166. Shumoy, H.; Pattyn, S.; Raes, K. Tef Protein: Solubility Characterization, *in-vitro* Digestibility and its Suitability as a Gluten Free Ingredient. *LWT*, **2018**, *89*, 697–703.
167. Sindhu, R.; Khatkar, B. S. Composition and Functional Properties of Common Buckwheat (*Fagopyrum esculentum* Moench) Flour and Starch. *International Journal of Innovative Research and Advanced Studies*, **2016**, *3*, 154–159.
168. Sindhu, R.; Beniwal, S. K.; Devi, A. Effect of Grain Processing on Nutritional and Physico-Chemical, Functional and Pasting Properties of Amaranth and Quinoa Flours. *Indian Journal of Traditional Knowledge*, **2019**, *18*, 500–507.
169. Singh, J.; Sharma, B.; Madaan, M.; Sharma, P.; Kaur, T.; Kaur, N.; Bhamra, I. K.; Kaur, S.; Rasane, P. Chia Seed Based Nutri Bar: Optimization, Analysis and Shelf Life. https://www.currentscience.ac.in/php/forthcoming/2020/35806.pdf; accessed on July 31, 2020.
170. Singh, N.; Singh, P.; Shevkani, K.; Virdi, A. S. Amaranth: Potential Source for Flour Enrichment. In: *Flour and Breads and Their Fortification in Health and Disease Prevention*; Preedy, V. R.; Watson, R. R. and Patel, V. B. (Eds.); London, UK: Academic Press; **2017**; pp. 123–135.
171. Skov, A. R.; Toubro, S.; Ronn, B.; Holm, L.; Astrup, A. Randomized Trial on Protein vs Carbohydrate in Ad Libitum Fat Reduced Diet for the Treatment of Obesity. *International Journal of Obesity and Related Metabolic Disorders*, 1999, *23*, 528–536.
172. Stuardo, M.; San Martin, R. Antifungal Properties of Quinoa (*Chenopodium quinoa* Willd) Alkali Treated Saponins against *Botrytis Cinerea*. *Industrial Crops and Products*, **2008**, *27*, 296–302.
173. Suri, S.; Passi, S.; Goyal, J. Chia Seed (*Salvia hispanica* L.) a New Age Functional Food. In: *4th International Conference on Recent Innovations in Science Engineering and Management*; New Delhi: India International Centre; **2016**; pp. 286–299.
174. Takhellambam, R. D.; Chimmad, B. V.; Prkasam, J. N. Ready-to-Cook Millet Flakes Based on Minor Millets for Modern Consumer. *Journal of Food Science and Technology*, **2016**, *53*, 1312–1318.
175. Tang, Y.; Li, X.; Chen, P. X. Characterization of Fatty Acid, Carotenoid, Tocopherol/Tocotrienol Compositions and Antioxidant Activities in Seeds of Three *Chenopodium quinoa* Willd. Genotypes. *Food Chemistry*, **2015**, *174*, 502–508.

176. Taylor, J. R.N.; Kruger, J. Sorghum and Millets: Food and Beverage Nutritional Attributes. In: *Sorghum and Millets: Chemistry, Technology, and Nutritional Attributes*; Taylor, J. R. N. and Duodu, K. G. (Eds.); UK: Woodhead Publishing and AACC International Press; **2019**; pp. 171–224.

177. Taylor, J. R.N. Millets: Their Unique Nutritional and Health-promoting Attributes. In: *Gluten-Free Ancient Grains*; Taylor, J. R. N. and Awika, J. M.; UK: Woodhead Publishing; **2017**; pp. 55–103.

178. Taylor, J. R. N. Environmental, Nutritional, and Social Imperatives for Ancient Grains. In: *Gluten-Free Ancient Grains*; Taylor, J. R. N. and Awika, J. M.; London, UK: Woodhead Publishing; **2017**; pp. 1–12.

179. Tesfaye, G. *Optimizing the Folate Content of Injera Using Highly Folate Producing Lactic Acid Bacteria Lactobacillus plantarum; Saccharomyces cerevisiae and Their Combination.* Doctoral Dissertation; Addis Ababa University; 2019; p. 56.

180. Thakur, M.; Tiwari, P. Millets: The Untapped and Underutilized Nutritious Functional Foods. *Plant Archives*, **2019**, *19*, 875–883.

181. Tömösközi, S.; Langó, B. Buckwheat: Its Unique Nutritional and Health-Promoting Attributes. In: *Gluten-Free Ancient Grains*; Taylor, J. R. N. and Awika, J. M.; UK: Woodhead Publishing; **2017**; pp. 161–177.

182. Ullah, R.; Nadeem, M.; Khalique, A.; Imran, M.; Mehmood, S.; Javid, A.; Hussain, J. Nutritional and Therapeutic Perspectives of Chia (*Salvia hispanica* L.): A Review. *Journal of Food Science and Technology*, **2016**, *53*, 1750–1758.

183. Urga, K.; Fite, A.; Biratu, E. Effect of Natural Fermentation on Nutritional and Antinutritional Factors of Tef (*Eragrostis tef*). *The Ethiopian Journal of Health Development*, **1997**, *11*, 61–66.

184. USDA. *United States Department of Agriculture FoodData Central.* 2019; https://fdc.nal.usda.gov/index.html Accessed on January 9, **2020**.

185. Väkeväinen, K.; Ludena-Urquizo, F. Potential of quinoa in the development of fermented spoonable vegan products. *LWT-Food Science and Technology*, **2020**, *120*, 108912.

186. Valdivia-López, M. Á.; Tecante, A. Chia (*Salvia hispanica*): A Review of Native Mexican Seed and its Nutritional and Functional Properties. In: *Advances in Food and Nutrition Research*; Henry, J. (Ed.); USA: Academic Press; **2015**. *Volume* 75; pp. 53–75.

187. Vega-Galvez, A.; Miranda, M.; Vergara, J.; Uribe, E.; Puente, L.; Martinez, E. A. Nutrition Facts and Functional Potential of Quinoa (*Chenopodium quinoa* Willd.). An Ancient Andean Grain: A Review. *Journal of the Science of Food and Agriculture*, **2010**, *90*, 2541–2547.

188. Velarde-Salcedo, A. J.; Bojórquez-Velázquez, E.; de la Rosa, A. P. B. Amaranth. In: *Whole Grains and their Bioactives: Composition and Health*; Johnson, J. and Wallace, T. C. (Eds.); UK: John Wiley & Sons Ltd.; **2019**; pp. 209–250.

189. Vonapartis, E.; Aubin, M.; Seguin, P.; Mustafa, A. F.; Charron, J. Seed Composition of Ten Industrial Hemp Cultivars Approved for Production in Canada. *Journal of Food Composition and Analysis*, **2015**, *39*, 8–12.

190. Wang, Q.; Xiong, Y. L. Processing, Nutrition, and Functionality of Hempseed Protein: A Review. *Comprehensive Reviews in Food Science and Food Safety*, 2019, *18*, 936–952.

191. Wang, S.; Zhu, F. Formulation and Quality Attributes of Quinoa Food Products. *Food and Bioprocess Technology*, **2016**, *9*, 49–68.

192. Weber, W.; Gentry, S.; Kolhepp, A.; McCrohan, R. The Nutritional and Chemical Evaluation of Chia Seeds. *Journal of Ecology of Food Nutrition*, **1991**, *26*, 119–125.

193. WHO (Eds.) *Protein and amino acid requirements in human nutrition.* Report of a joint FAO/WHO/UNU expert consultation; 2007; *WHO Technical Report Series 935*; p. 265.

194. Wójtowicz, A.; Kolasa, A.; Mościcki, L. Influence of Buckwheat Addition on Physical Properties, Texture and Sensory Characteristics of Extruded Corn Snacks. *Polish Journal of Food and Nutrition Sciences*, **2013**, *63*, 239–244.

195. Wolter, A.; Anna-Sophie, H.; Emanuele, Z.; Elke, K. A. *In vitro* Starch Digestibility and Predicted Glycaemic Indexes of Buckwheat, Oat, Quinoa, Sorghum, Teff and Commercial Gluten-Free Bread. *Journal of Cereal Science*, **2013**, *58*, 431–436.

196. Yalcin, E.; Sakiyan, O.; Sumnu, G.; Celik, S.; Koksel, H. Functional Properties of Microwave-Treated Wheat Gluten. *European Food Research and Technology*, **2008**, *227*, 1411.

197. Yendo, A. C. A.; De Costa, F.; Gosmann, G.; Fett-Neto, A. G. Production of Plant Bioactive Triterpenoid Saponins: Elicitation Strategies and Target Genes to Improve Yields. *Molecular Biotechnology*, **2010**, *46*, 94–104.

198. Yoshimoto, Y.; Egashira, T.; Hanashiro, I. Molecular Structure and some Physicochemical Properties of Buckwheat Starches. *Cereal Chemistry*, **2004**, *81*, 515–520.

199. Zayas, J. F. *Functionality of Proteins in Food.* Berlin, Heidelberg: Springer Verlag, **1997**; p. 373.

200. Zhu, F.; Li, H. Modification of Quinoa Flour Functionality Using Ultrasound. *Ultrasonics Sonochemistry*, **2019**, *52*, 305–310.

201. Zhu, F. Chemical Composition and Food Uses of Teff (*Eragrostis tef*). *Food Chemistry*, **2018**, *239*, 402–415.

# INDEX

For Product Safety Concerns and Information please contact our EU
representative  GPSR@taylorandfrancis.com
Taylor & Francis Verlag GmbH, Kaufingerstraße 24, 80331 München, Germany

www.ingramcontent.com/pod-product-compliance
Lightning Source LLC
Chambersburg PA
CBHW060329220326
41598CB00023B/2651

* 9 7 8 1 7 7 4 6 3 9 4 5 0 *